FUNCTIONAL NEUROSCIENCE

HARPER & ROW, Publishers

New York Hagerstown Philadelphia San Francisco London

MICHAEL S. GAZZANIGA
Cornell University Medical College

DIANA STEEN

BRUCE T. VOLPE
Cornell University Medical College

FUNCTIONAL NEUROSCIENCE

Sponsoring Editor: *George A. Middendorf*
Project Editor: *Lois Lombardo*
Designer: *Frances Torbert Tilley*
Senior Production Manager: *Kewal K. Sharma*
Compositor: *The Clarinda Company*
Printer and Binder: *Halliday Lithograph Corporation*
Art Studio: *J & R Technical Services Inc.*

Library of Congress Cataloging in Publication Data
Gazzaniga, Michael S
Functional neuroscience.

Includes index.
1. Brain. 2. Psychology, Physiological.
3. Neurology. I. Steen, Diana, joint author.
II. Volpe, Bruce T., joint author. III. Title.
[DNLM: 1. Psychophsiology. WL103 G291f]
QP376.G38 152 78-21508
ISBN 0-06-042291-2

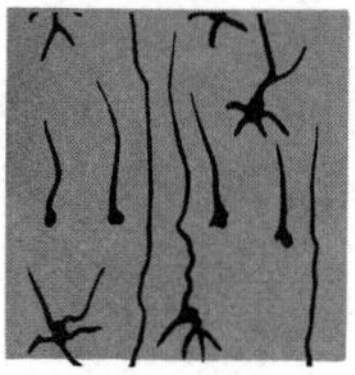

Contents

Preface

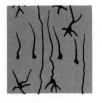

Our purpose in writing this book is to present the foundations of brain and behavioral principles in a tight yet readable format. Often the beginning student in physiological psychology, animal behavior, neuroscience, or whatever this emerging field will eventually be called does not see how basic principle and nervous system action relate to the real, functioning organism. Thus, while learning about the action potential, or rods and cones, or neurotransmitters may be of intellectual interest, the beginning student is frequently at a loss to relate this sometimes difficult information to any realistic framework.

Our solution to this pedological dilemma is to introduce key concepts of brain science by describing real, clinical, neurological, functional disorders—each stemming from an underlying nervous system dysfunction. Each case illustrates a feature of the nervous system and helps in the student's ability to grasp and relate the information. Our purpose is to use clinical case histories to assist in the communication of this information. While we feel all of them are intriguing in their own right, our purpose was not to write a clinical book. We have written, then, a basic science-oriented book which makes use of clinical examples.

It has taken a long time to write this book and there are a lot of people to thank. First is H. Philip Ziegler of the American Museum of Natural History. Philip reviewed the manuscript several times with an editorial acumen we can all only envy. If we have met our goal in bringing together a lively and coordinated book for the neurosciences, it will be largely due to him. We also are grateful to the many students, research fellows, and friends who have given us help, especially Joseph LeDoux and Georg Deutsch. Special thanks are due to Robert Filbey, our illustrator, who continues to provide some of the finest illustrations in the life sciences.

Any thoughts or ideas for improving the text will be welcomed by the authors. We wish the students and the professors good reading.

MICHAEL S. GAZZANIGA
DIANA STEEN
BRUCE T. VOLPE

FUNCTIONAL NEUROSCIENCE

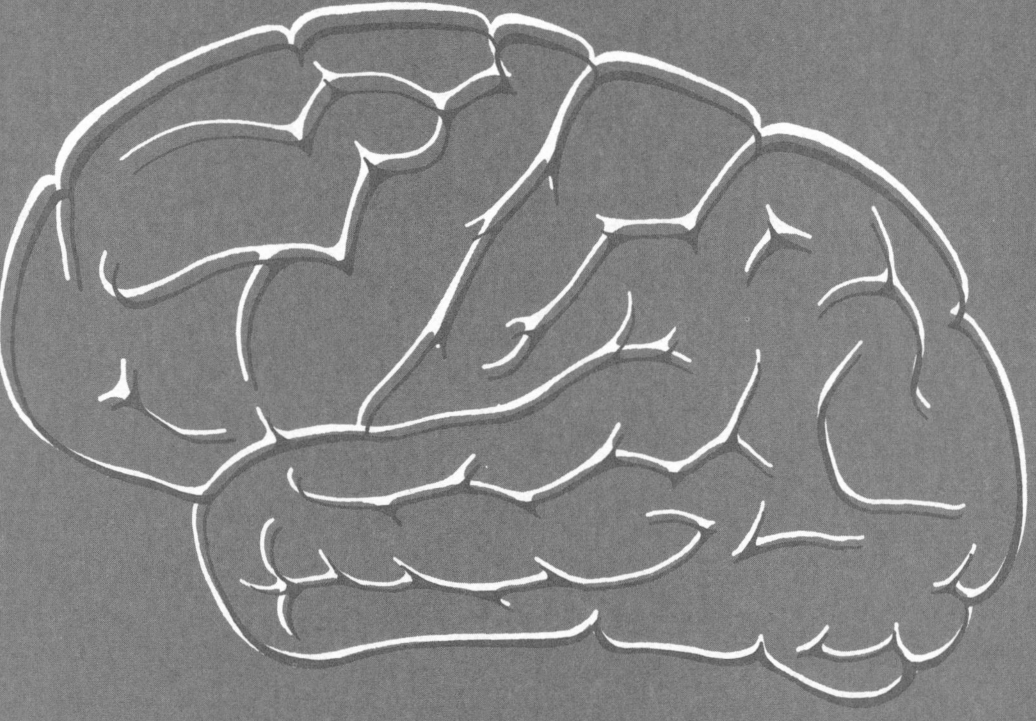

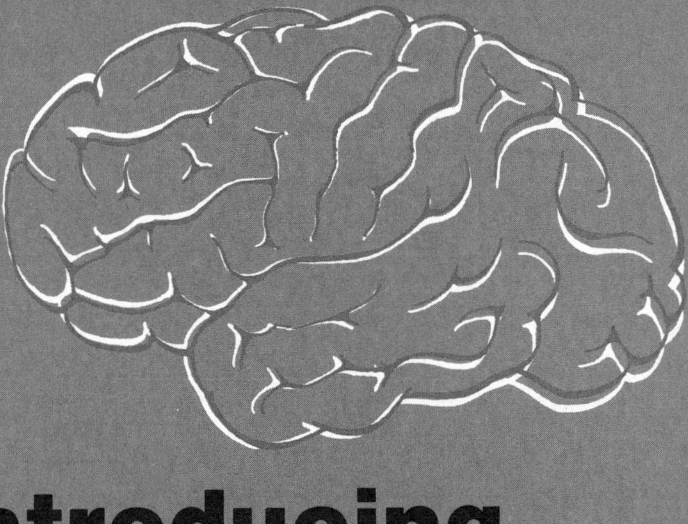

PART I
Introducing Brain Research

CHAPTER 1

Human Models for Neuroscience

Study of the brain and behavior provides the focal point for many modern scientists. Whether in physiology or psychology, neurosurgery or psychiatry, human behavior and its diversity excite a curiosity unparalleled in science. You are about to embark on a journey through that tangled maze of the known and unknown that is called the neurosciences. Our story begins at a separate neuroscience division at a university center.

The university and the medical school provide a productive atmosphere for the research and development of health-oriented questions. Such a multidiscipline division has equal representation from neurophysiology, neurology, psychiatry, and psychology. These new divisions of neuroscience promise breakthroughs for the future.

All of these specialty areas are active in trying to understand the physical basis of behavior. Each week their separate perspectives are brought to bear on a common problem at a meeting called Grand Rounds. This session is held once a week in the afternoon in the amphitheater, a special room constructed so that a patient can be easily examined in front of a large audience of neuroscientists. Grand Rounds, derived from a traditional medical model of case presentation and discussion, serves to stimulate discussion between scientists of different disciplines.

A patient's history is reviewed by a medical resident, and the presentation is usually steeped in medical jargon. Acting like detectives, the neuroscientists carefully listen to the signs, symptoms, and temporal course of the specific dysfunctions caused by the disease. The human nervous system is a fragile network, and disruptions of any kind produce a maze of interrelated problems. It seems that the examining professor always asks the patient the important questions that invariably illuminate the major problem. Proceeding to a brief but pointed physical examination, he demonstrates the key signals of the disease process. Questions about some particular aspect of the patient's problem remain for another faculty member to discuss. And at the end of the round, the professor provides what he thinks are the major points of the case. One can be assured that the major points are almost always questions about the unknowns of neuroscience, and each case provides many unknowns.

In this chapter we shall present both the written transcript of a Grand Rounds and an explanation in simpler terms of what was said in the report. Through this examination of a specific case history, we shall introduce many terms and processes associated with a neurological examination, and thus give you a glimpse of how the information in the following chapters can be integrated and put to use. While we do not expect that all terms in this chapter will be remembered, we do hope that this explanation of a case study will provide a foundation for the chapters and cases to follow.

Quiet comes over the amphitheater as the story of J. A. begins:

The case for discussion at Grand Rounds today is J. A., a 25-year-old man who suffered with herpes simplex encephalitis for which he remained hospitalized for three months. The history of his illness began one week prior to his entry into hospital when he complained of vague fleeting muscle aches and pains, headache, and fever. None of these symptoms responded to aspirin, or bed rest.

Encephalitis, derived from the Greek *enkephalos*, brain, and the suffix *-itis*, inflammation, is an acute inflammation of the brain, the covering of the brain and spinal cord. Added to the meningeal inflammation is the demonstration of deranged function of the whole brain at the four levels of organization: the cerebrum, the cerebellum, the brain stem, and the spinal cord. It is a serious illness that can lead to permanent neurologic deficits or even death. It often begins as a nonspecific, trivial viral illness. By affecting each level of the nervous system, encephalitis may begin with sensory-motor abnormalities and may lead to disorders of speech, memory, and awareness. Each of these functional categories will be studied in greater detail in the chapters that follow. But for now, returning to the case, the isolated causal agents of encephalitis are viruses, and the long list of viruses with potential to damage the nervous system includes the common such as measles or mumps, the less common such as polio, and the rare such as rabies.

By the fifth day of his illness he experienced paresthesias in his right arm. Later, with the fever persisting, he began to behave abnormally. Disoriented to time and place, he paced his apartment ranting unintelligibly.

These symptoms were further clues to a diagnosis of the herpes virus, since viral infections of the nervous system can lead to diverse signs and symptoms. As mentioned, encephalitis may involve dysfunction of any or all levels of the central nervous system, and any of the following combinations of problems reflecting brain dysfunction is possible: convulsions, delirium, or coma; loss of cognitive abilities; paralysis of hemiplegic variety (arm and leg paralysis on the same side of the body); paresthesias (the abnormal spontaneous sensation of tingling) or dysesthesias (disagreeable sensations produced by ordinary stimuli); incoordination, tremor, or rapid involuntary movements. These severe and serious consequences are often preceded by nonspecific, so-called minor illness. The virulence of encephalitis evolves rapidly after this early illness. In fact, herpes simplex encephalitis can be catastrophic: over 50 percent die with the illness. Seizures are common, and clinical signs frequently evolve over the course of the illness that suggest particular involvement of each part of the brain, especially an area called the temporal lobe.

The resident continued:

His wife brought him to a local hospital, where he was noted to be disoriented, delirious, with a fever of 105°F, respirations of 28 per minute, a fast pulse, and a normal blood pressure. His neck was stiff with a positive Kernig's and Brudzinski's sign; his lungs were clear, there were no cardiac murmurs; examination of his abdomen was normal. There were no skin changes.

The general medical physical examination in a patient with encephalitis may present few findings other than fever and stiff neck. Kernig's sign, named after the Russian physician of the nineteenth century, is elicited with the patient lying on his back and flexing knee and hip to 90°. Keeping the hip steady, one attempts to extend the knee. In the presence of meningeal irritation this extension is resisted because the tension exerted on the meninges by the stretching hamstring or thigh muscles causes pain. Brudzinski's sign, named after Kernig's Polish colleague, is elicited by passively flexing the neck of the patient (Figure 1.1). The flexion maneuver, lifting the patient's head off the bed and touching the chin to the chest, also tenses the meninges, and the pain leads to involuntary flexion of the hips.

On neurological examination, other than disorientation and delirium, there was a mild right hemiparesis with right hyperreflexia, increased tone on the right, and a right upgoing toe. Examination of his cranial nerves revealed that he preferred left conjugate gaze, although he could gaze voluntarily in all directions and had full vision. His pupils were equal and reacted normally, his optic disks were flat with normal vessel pulsations, and there was a mild right facial weakness; the remaining cranial nerves were normal.

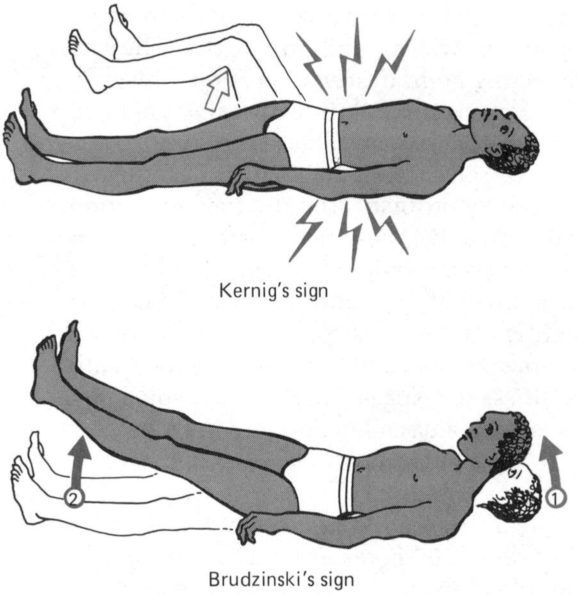

FIGURE 1.1 A positive Kernig's sign is elicited by hip flexion and knee extension that causes pain by stretching the meninges. A positive Brudzinski's sign is elicited by flexing the neck and observing subsequent involuntary hip flexion, again because of pain secondary to stretched meninges.

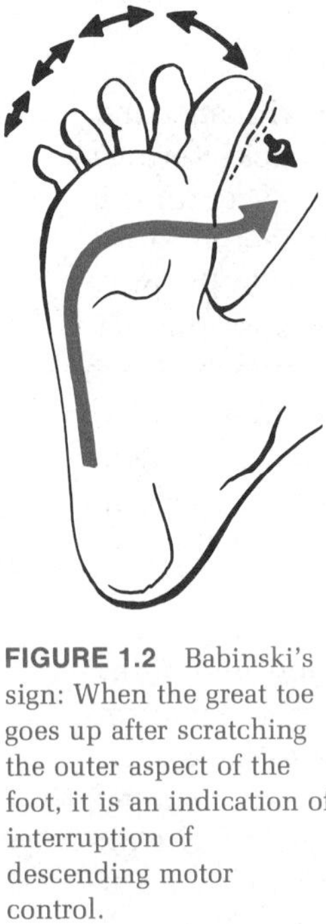

FIGURE 1.2 Babinski's sign: When the great toe goes up after scratching the outer aspect of the foot, it is an indication of interruption of descending motor control.

A right hemiparesis, paralysis of the arm and leg on the right side of the body, suggested motor nerves that originate in the left cerebral hemisphere were disrupted. Tone is the tension maintained in resting muscles, and this quality is usually symmetrical and equal in arms and legs. Increase in tone is often a result of a cerebral lesion and further evidence for disruption of motor neuron paths. Increased resistance to passive flexion, demonstrated by moving the right arm and causing the biceps muscle to flex, consistently focused attention on left cerebral hemisphere dysfunction. The right upgoing toe—called a positive Babinski reflex (Figure 1.2)—particularly reflected left cerebral dysfunction and interruption of the descending motor control tracts. This sign was described by and named after the great Parisian neurologist at the turn of the century. It consists of applying a noxious stimulus, usually a dull object such as a key, to the sole of the foot and stroking the outer aspect. Normally this stimulus produces a downward flexion movement of the great and small toes. In diseases that disrupt the descending motor pathways, this stimulus produces upward movement of the great toe and triple flexion; that is, downward turning of the foot at the ankle and flexion movement of the knee and thigh. This is a positive Babinski response, and although this reflex represents an abnormal sign in adults, the presence of the sign is considered normal in neonates and infants up to about one year of age. The immaturity of the nervous system at this age is marked by the lack of complete, full, specific connections of all the fiber tracts. The movement command originates in the cortex and travels down the spinal cord to synapse on the lower motor neuron still within the spinal cord. In the developing system there is an absence of complete upper motor (hemisphere)-lower motor (spinal cord) connection that leads to a positive Babinski response. The reflex arc, which you will learn more about in Chapter 9, consists of the dorsal sensory root and anterior motor root. This primitive reflex is mature and ready to function immediately at birth. The fine control added by complete connections with the hemispheres develops later in the first year. Neural development is yet another topic that deserves deeper study in a later chapter.

The patient's left gaze preference also suggested focal cerebral disease. In awake, alert patients the eyes are directed straight ahead at rest. Even unconscious patients, with diffuse or bilateral hemisphere disease, have eyes directed straight ahead without involuntary movements. However, when a patient suffers asymmetric damage to a part of the cerebrum called the frontal lobes, the eyes will deviate conjugately and automatically prefer gaze toward the side of the damaged hemisphere. All the signs pointed to left hemisphere dysfunction as J. A. preferred left lateral gaze. The report goes on:

In the first hours of admission, he had a seizure that began with clonic activity in his right arm and quickly generalized to involve his entire body. It stopped spontaneously and by evening he had been transferred to this hospital. Here, he was comatose with eyes deviated to the left and a right hemiparesis. He was treated with anticonvulsants and sent for a CT scan. The scan was normal, except for small ventricles. On return to the floor the staff performed a lumbar puncture which revealed an opening pressure of 300 mm of water; there were 200 red and 50 white blood cells; the protein was elevated to 80 mg% and the glucose was 70 mg% (with a normal simultaneous blood glucose). An EEG was abnormal with bursting periodic sharp activity of the left frontal temporal leads, and a diffusely slow background. The diagnosis entertained was herpes simplex encephalitis, and the appropriate serum and cerebrospinal fluid assays were obtained (and would return later with positive confirmation of the diagnosis).

A lumbar puncture is a painless, low-risk procedure in which a needle enters the spinal cord canal space well below the termination of the spinal cord substance. It allows sampling of the cerebrospinal fluid that flows in the ventricles of the brain, over the convexity of the hemispheres, and down around the spinal cord. There are many by-products of brain metabolism in the spinal fluid, and two components that are frequently assayed are protein and glucose. High values for protein indicate inflammation. Normal values are recorded as high as 50 mg%, and with encephalitis the spinal fluid protein may rise to 200 mg%. Glucose in the spinal fluid represents a complex transport process that reflects the blood glucose level. It is usually considered within normal limits if it is 60 percent of the blood glucose; normal values for blood glucose are 80 to 120 mg%.

The spinal fluid should be clear of all cellular elements. The presence of red blood cells and white blood cells in the spinal fluid is abnormal, and suggests a hemorrhage. Explaining the other laboratory aides: CT is an acronym for computerized tomography. A CT scan is done with a special x-ray machine that produces horizontal cross sections of the brain at any level. The scanner represents a major technological advance, as the procedure is painless and without risk, and the information it gives about the intracranial contents is accurate and specific. The EEG is often less specific. As you will learn later, this procedure measures electrical potential differences between specified areas of the cerebrum through recordings from scalp electrodes. Herpes simplex encephalitis produces focal changes in the electrical pattern over the frontotemporal regions of the brain. The patterns are not specific but may be helpful when they consist of high-voltage sharp waves of a periodic bursting nature. Finally of all these efforts to establish a diagnosis there are assays available that indirectly detect the presence of viruses by locating complex proteins that the human body specifically manufactures to combat virus toxicity. Spinal fluid and blood can be assayed for the presence of herpes simplex virus without actual isolation of the virus itself.

The detailed events of the first three hospital days are particularly important. Although he had no further seizures, he remained lethargic. Early in the morning on the second day his pupils responded sluggishly to light, the left pupil larger than right. His respiration remained normal, ocular movements and ocular reflexes were unimpaired, and his right hemiparesis was unchanged. Within two hours, however, herniation of the temporal lobe and lateral midbrain compression intervened. On ocular reflex testing there was loss of third cranial nerve motor function and an inability to move the left eye. Further, he was no longer moving his left side and he had a left upgoing toe (a positive Babinski response).

This complicated progression of J. A.'s story is based on fundamental neuroanatomy (see Chapter 3). Basically, the skull is a nondistensible structure in an adult. An area of expanding inflammation and hemorrhage can only cause rearrangement of the soft but noncompressible brain tissue. In fact, the only place the brain can move is downward through the large opening at the base of the skull called the foramen magnum (see Figure 1.3). The medulla and spinal cord normally pass

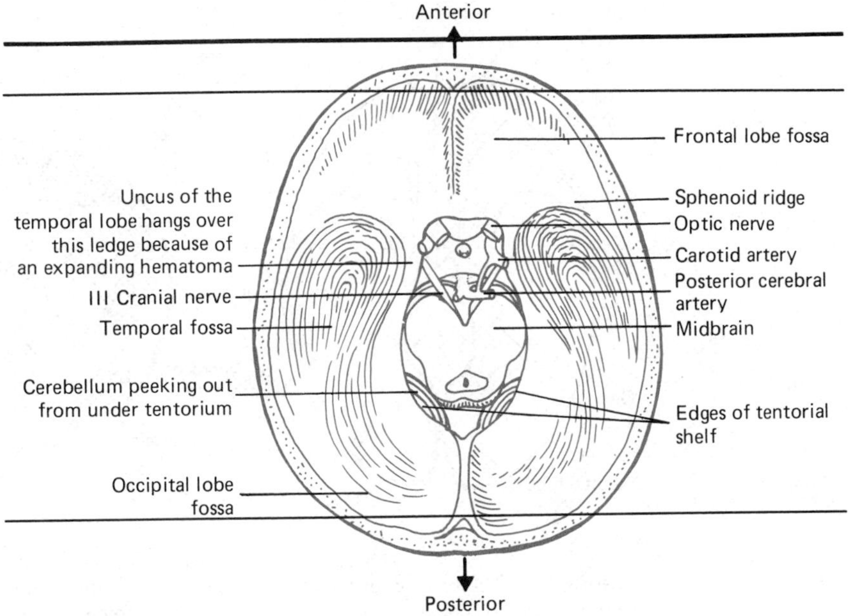

FIGURE 1.3 A depiction of the shelf created by the tentorial sheath. The cerebrum lies on top of the sheath, cerebellum and midbrain are below the sheath. The frontal lobes, temporal lobes, and occipital lobes each have a specific cradle.

through this opening. The cranial vault is partitioned in a horizontal manner by a shelf called the tentorium. This thick, tough sheath forms a platform under which the cerebellum and midbrain lie, and on which the cerebrum lies. Shifting of the intracranial contents results in compression of the brain at several points depending on the location of the initiating expansion. The tentorial shelf, the margins of each part of the skull base, and the foramen magnum may each become incompressible pressure points. Further swelling and shifting caused by the new damage at these pressure points eventually leads to such progressive brain volume increase that the brain squeezes through the only available exit—the foramen magnum.

Given that the uncus is the midventral surface of the temporal lobe (see Figure 1.4), and that the herpes simplex encephalitis involved the left frontotemporal region, and that this area of hemorrhagic inflammation was expanding, the progressive signs of brain compression and herniation are clear (see Figure 1.5). These focal events occurring on the second hospital day were due to swelling of the hemorrhagic area of inflammation. The initial clue was the sudden appearance of pupils of

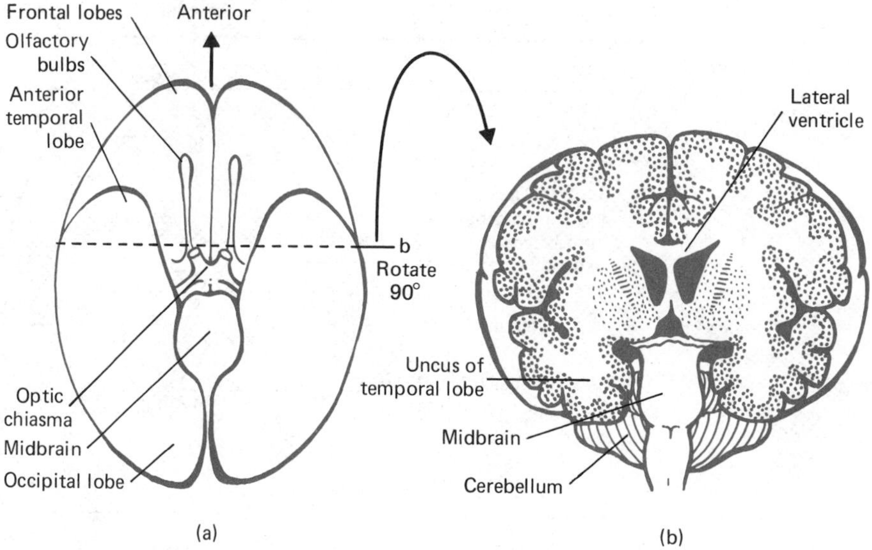

FIGURE 1.4 The relation of the uncus to the temporal lobe. (a) Looking at the brain from the ventral (bottom) side. The perforated line depicts a vertical cut through the brain at that level. (b) The posterior part of the cut brain rotated 90° in order to examine the cut surface.

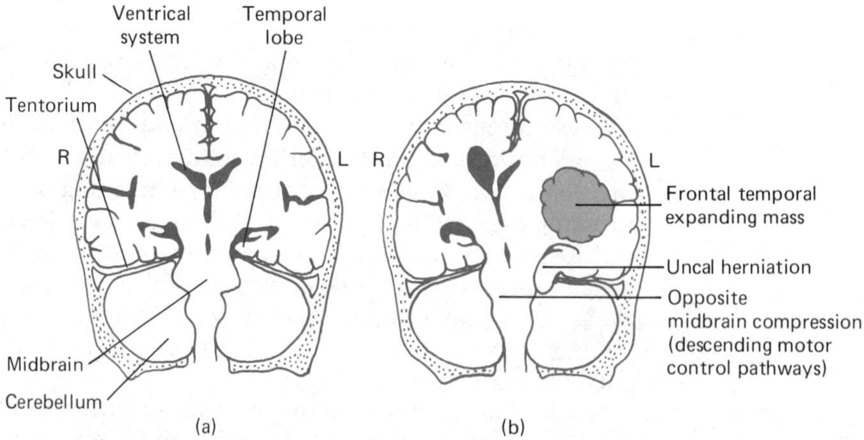

FIGURE 1.5 (a) Vertical cut of a normal brain in relation to the skull and tentorium. (b) Shifting of the uncus over the tentorial sheath and *opposite* compression of the midbrain. Descending motor control pathways at this point in the midbrain are crossing to innervate the opposite body, so disruption of midbrain (R) produces weakness (L).

unequal size, especially as J. A. had not regained consciousness since the seizure. Parasympathetic fibers that dilate the pupils travel on the outside of the third cranial nerve. The left pupil became larger and unresponsive and signaled compression of the third cranial nerve. The expanding temporal mass shifts the inner basal edge of the uncus (basomedial temporal lobe) toward the midline and over the internal edge of the tentorium. The resulting flattening of the midbrain causes it to shift to the opposite side where the descending fibers of the motor control pathways are trapped against the opposite edge. The swollen overhanging uncus then traps the third cranial nerve against the free edge of the tentorium or some other equally resistant skull structure. All this shifting results in an ipsilateral third nerve paralysis (the left pupil in this case) and an ipsilateral hemiplegia (left side again). Remember that the right motor control tracts are trapped as the midbrain shifts away from the expanding lesion left to right. Also remember that the right cerebral peduncle carries fibers from the right cerebral cortex to innervate left-sided motor elements.

He was treated immediately with steroids, mannitol, and with endotracheal entubation. Within one hour the anisocoria disappeared, conjugate eye movements and normal pupillary responses returned; the left hemiparesis receded.

The major clinical lesson is that pressure from shifting mass lesions spreads locally through paths of least resistance in a progressive, contiguous manner. Clinical deterioration continues in an orderly rostral/caudal manner, as if the pressure wave were transecting the brain level by level.

The urgent treatment with mannitol and steroids was aimed at stopping this progression by shrinking all areas of the brain. Its effects were rapid and beneficial. The resolution of the left third nerve paralysis and the left hemiparesis was clear proof that the progressive herniation had been stopped. All efforts could now be focused on rehabilitation and supportive care.

Each day he regained more function and was weaned from the respirator at the end of the first week. The following three months of hospitalization were marked by slow improvement that from day to day was imperceptible. Seizures or brain herniation were never again a clinical problem.

The history continues:

Although he regained complete consciousness late in the third week of admission with improvement of his right hemiparesis, he remained disoriented for time and place. He had dysphasia with difficulty naming objects, but displayed a fluency of propositional speech. In fact, he became quite talkative, in spite of a retrograde amnesia that included all the events of the past three months. He confabulated vividly about recent events and seemed unable to remember any new material, in spite of an adequate remote memory which allowed him to recall many of the details of his life before his illness.

The commanding position of humans in the phylogenetic tree rests on the development of language. Language is that series of symbols that communicate emotions or thoughts through written or spoken words. And a rather tantalizing neurophysiologic structure exists to provide the organization for speech. Most brain mechanisms are organized in either a bilaterally symmetrical representation or a one-sided manner, with each side of the brain responsible for the opposite side of the body. Language and the ability to exercise propositional speech depend, to a great extent, on a single hemisphere, called the dominant hemisphere. Facility with symbolic language occurs after 15 or so years and is subject to influences of social and cultural environment. This is not to say that the opposite hemisphere or nondominant hemisphere is incapable of thinking; some recent experiments indicate the nondominant hemisphere may have latent language ability (more about this in later chapters). In any case, a disorder of language usually reflects dominant hemisphere pathology, and in 90 percent of the population—even the left-handed population—the left hemisphere is dominant.

Naming errors, early in J. A.'s illness, were a function of his delirious and inattentive state early in the course of the illness, but the consistent mistakes he was now making suggested a focal disruption in the left hemisphere. In fact, with the acute early stage of his illness over, all signs pointed to a disorder of the left hemisphere.

The details of the neurobiological basis of human memory remain areas of active research and animated debate. Considering the staggering accomplishments of even ordinary human memory, for example, the ability to carry the meanings of tens of thousands of words, to recognize innumerable faces and visual scenes, to remember the sound of voices or melodies, to perform with grace on center stage or center field, and so on, this immense effort is justified.

In Chapter 10 memory is outlined as a sequence of processes beginning with short-term memory, followed by consolidation of the initial message through unknown mechanisms, and transfer to long-term memory, or permanent memory. The association between elements in the long-term store are woven into a matrix of organization that allows ready access or retrieval at some later time. J. A.'s deficit in this processing schema was profound. His problem with orientation and thinking is also difficult to understand, but we can derive clues that will help in evaluating J. A.'s higher cognitive functions.

J. H. Jackson, a nineteenth century founder of modern neurology, conceived a functional hierarchy of organization in the human brain. In this system those functions last to develop in the ontogeny of the individual human and in the phylogeny of the human species were more fragile. As a result, any perturbation such as a disease, affects more sensitive functions first. The functional capacity of humans deteriorates in the reverse order, with the so-called highest and most complex abilities becoming disordered first. So, although J. A. had recovered almost complete motor function, and even some language ability, certain thinking processes remained severely disordered.

He could care for his own ordinary needs, but this once bright mind was now incapacitated because of his recent memory defect. Clinical evaluation of memory showed superior immediate recall, for he could repeat eight numbers forward and five numbers in reverse. Memories for the events of childhood, college days, and marriage were accurate, but the details of the last five years were patchy and confused. Along this line, he could not recall the names of three familiar objects which he had named just 30 minutes earlier, and if the examiner left the room briefly J. A. could not remember him on his return. Recent memory was impaired, yet remote and immediate capacities were preserved.

Formal psychological testing completed one year after his recovery from encephalitis revealed an overall score of 110 on the Wechsler Adult Intelligence Scale, with a 105 on the verbal scale and a 118 on the performance scale. His memory limitation for recent events had not changed, and he often confused the time sequence of those events subsequent to his hospital discharge. He was aware that several major international events had occurred since he left the hospital, one being the ending of the Vietnam war, but he could not remember the details. He had no difficulty with complicated motor tasks, and once started, easily completed them. In daily functioning he was able to care for himself, and generally found his way around the hospital grounds accurately and appropriately. His wife visited him often, and he certainly displayed a full range of emotions toward her, but would often forget the reason for one feeling or another. Irritated by her on one occasion, he jumped up angry and stormed out of the room and rushed down the hall. Several minutes later, by the time she could catch up with him, he had forgotten not only the entire series of motor responses that led him down the hall, but also the circumstances that so angered him.

With the formal case presentation ended, J. A. was introduced to the assembly. He appeared nervous with all the attention focused on him.

Although this was not his first experience as the focus of discussion at Grand Rounds, he could not recall similar situations—he simply forgot them. As he answered questions it became immediately obvious that his retention lasted only minutes. Pleasant, even somewhat complacent, he displayed little insight into the nature of his difficulty.

The subsequent discussion, after J. A. left the auditorium, consisted of a long series of questions. Many of the first queries dealt with the purely medical aspects surrounding this explosive, rapidly debilitating illness. Why should an otherwise healthy man be so predisposed to an overwhelming viral illness? Once begun, how could the process be stopped or reversed? What caused the areas of inflammation to swell and lead to shifting brain contents within the cranial vault? As for his recovery and permanent deficits, the questions were even more difficult. Why did temporal lobe destruction affect his memory so specifically? Why was his remote, long-term store preserved? How could he have access to his long-term stores and not to short-term stores? What was the relation between his intact immediate memory and his inability to store information? How could he solve the motor problems of self-care with so little verbal access to memory? What were the emotional effects of this illness?

This case presented challenges on many levels for each of the neuroscientists in the audience. It provided a focal point for several disciplines, each with a unique point of view, to examine basic neural mechanisms. Specific motivation varied; for one group it was surgical therapeutics, for another medical therapeutics, and for a third psychiatric therapeutics. For many of the others, therapeutics was not a consideration at all. But certainly each member would agree on one motive, that of seeking to understand the human brain.

That is what this book is about, and we hope to approach the problem in unique ways. Throughout the book we shall illustrate many basic phenomena of brain and behavior by presenting case histories. Through the examination of tangible human problems, we shall approach frontiers of neuroscience.

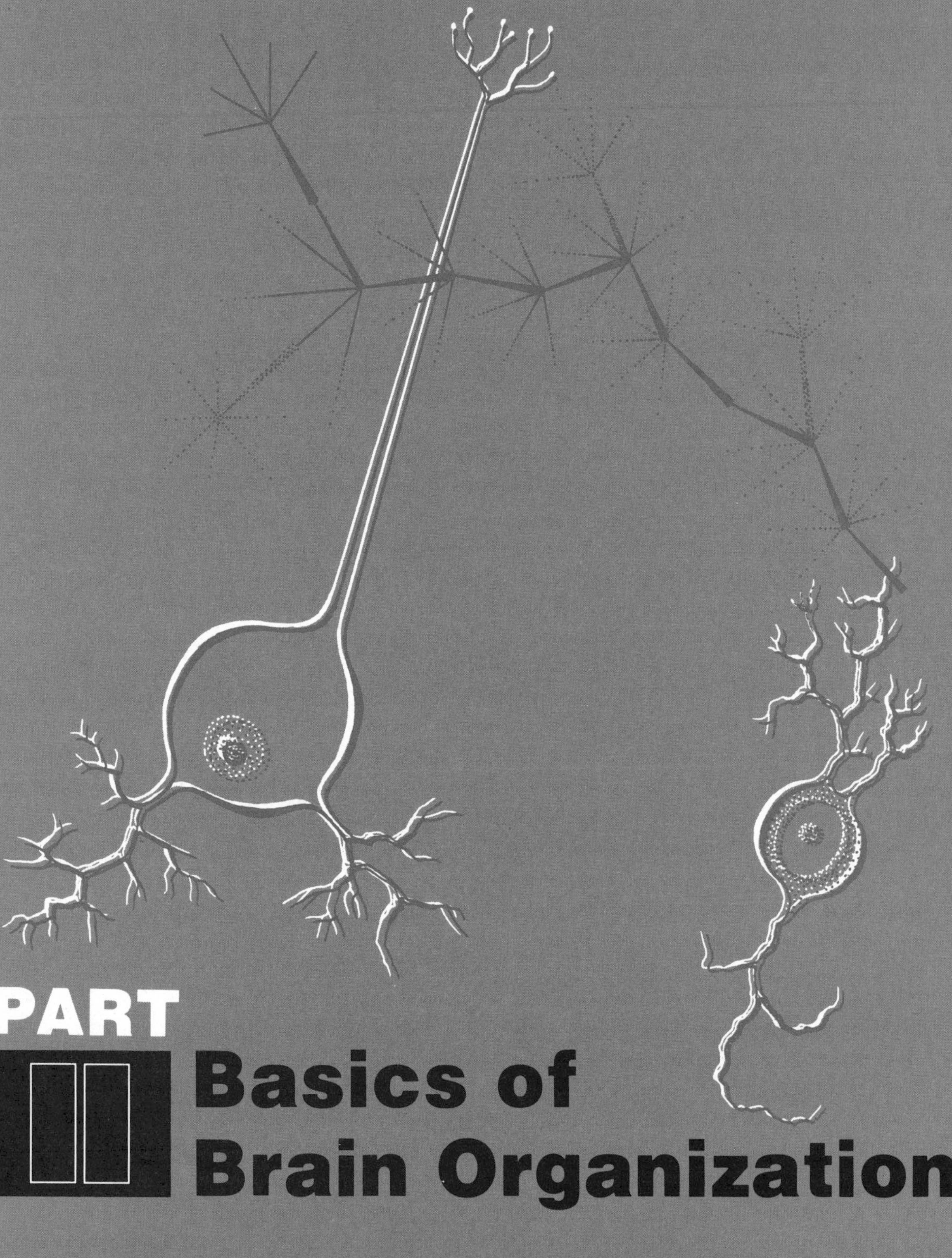

PART II Basics of Brain Organization

CHAPTER 2

Neurons: The Essential Physical Elements for Behavior

Human existence depends on many elements, but without a doubt the most essential element is the neuron, or nerve cell, the basic building block of the entire nervous system. The neuron is an incredible feat of evolutionary engineering. In contrast to other types of cells, a neuron is capable of receiving and sending a "message." Being a cell specialized for communication, a neuron is capable of emitting an electrical impulse. Whereas a nonneural cell, when stimulated, simply accepts the charge passively, a neuron responds dynamically.

A neuron, when stimulated electrically, does not simply pass on a gradually decreasing charge. Rather, the neuron responds actively to electrical stimulation, generating its own fixed-size impulse and transmitting that impulse nondecrementally the entire length of its fiber. Moreover, this neural impulse can be transmitted from one neuron to another. At the neural junction, called a synapse, electrical stimulation can be transferred. However, the neuron receiving the charge fires only when the electrical stimulus is strong enough to exceed a fixed threshold. The receiving neuron is then "turned on" and transmits its fixed-size electrical current. In other words, the neuron has two kinds of response properties, for the propagation of neural impulses is accomplished in both a decremental and a nondecremental fashion.

Like the circuits of a computer, a single neuron is binary; that is, it is either "on" or "off." But transfer of impulses between neurons occurs in a more complicated way. While in the initial phase of receiving stimulation, the neuron is affected directly by input. Every cell has an electrical charge, and the electrical charge inside the neuron changes continuously in response to the amount of stimulation received within a given time period. However, if that stimulation reaches a certain critical point, the neuron responds digitally, or in one way only: by sending an impulse that is always of the same strength. The frequency of impulses transmitted may vary with the amount of stimulation, but the size of the impulse never changes.

Thus, the signal transmitted from neuron to neuron is always the same and carries meaning according to where it comes from and where it goes. For example, if your finger is touching an object, the sensory receptors in your skin stimulate the appropriate neurons. That is, the touch receptors are "turned on," and by transmitting impulses to the appropriate area of the brain, they signify the nature of the object. Similar processes occur in most systems that receive sensory information. Although the thought processes involved in learning and memory call into play more complex neural circuitry, all functions of the brain nevertheless occur through vast networks of neurons being turned on and off. But, before examining complex brain functions, we must consider the basics, so we shall first consider the behavior of a single neuron (of which there are upwards of 10 billion to 12 billion in the human brain), and determine the operating pattern of this cell unit. In later chapters, we shall proceed to higher levels of organization and see how the simple units are integrated and function together to produce not only the elementary neural functions common to all animals, but also the complex thought processes attributed only to humans.

The Anatomy of the Neuron

Surprisingly, a *neuron*, or nerve cell, though unique in its ability to transmit information, is structurally similar to any other cell (Peters et al., 1976). Like all other cells, the neuron has a *soma* (cell body), but in addition, the neuron also has *processes*, or fibers extending from the cell body. The processes are called dendrites and axons, *dendrites* being commonly defined as fibers that receive information and *axons* as fibers that transmit information (Figure 2.1). Both the soma and the processes are surrounded by a *cell membrane*, which, like the membranes of other cells, is semipermeable, allowing some substances to enter and excluding others. All cell membranes are believed to be composed of two layers of lipids (fatty substances), but the unique feature of the nerve cell membrane is the presence of special protein molecules that lie along the inner and outer surface of each layer of lipids. These protein molecules are believed to play a role in controlling the permeability of the membrane by acting as receptors for specific substances, which, if introduced into the cell, will produce the electrophysiological response that is unique to the nerve cell. Thus, the protein receptors are important in controlling the input and output of information transmission.

The soma is filled with a substance called *cytoplasm* (Figure 2.2). Within the cytoplasm of the neuron are various organelles (miniature "organs") that play an important and critical role in the development of

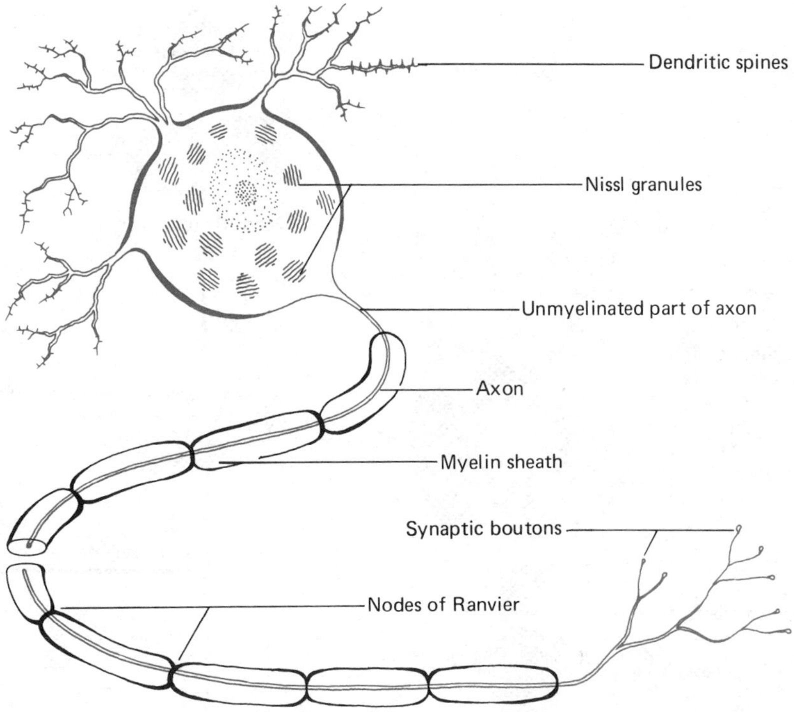

FIGURE 2.1 An example of a "typical" neuron, with the basic dendritic processes, as well as the cell body, axon, and the synaptic boutons indicated.

the cell, impart rigidity to the cell, and synthesize materials necessary for the functioning of the cell. Examples of such organelles are those comprising the *endoplasmic reticulum* (ER), which are bits of membrane (composed of protein, as are all cell membranes) scattered throughout the cytoplasm. These bits of protein may be classified as either smooth or rough, depending on the presence of small, closely adhering particles called ribosomes. The rough ER (with ribosomes) is sometimes folded into structures called *Nissl bodies,* and is believed to be the site of the synthesis of proteins, including those protein receptors involved in information transmission between cells. The smooth ER (without ribosomes), when organized into stacks, is called the *Golgi apparatus,* and plays a role in the "packaging" of the chemical substances involved in the transmission of information between nerve cells. The chemical substances are "packaged" or contained in small but very important structures called *vesicles,* which, when stimulated by a neuronal impulse, release their chemical (Collier and McIntosh, 1969).

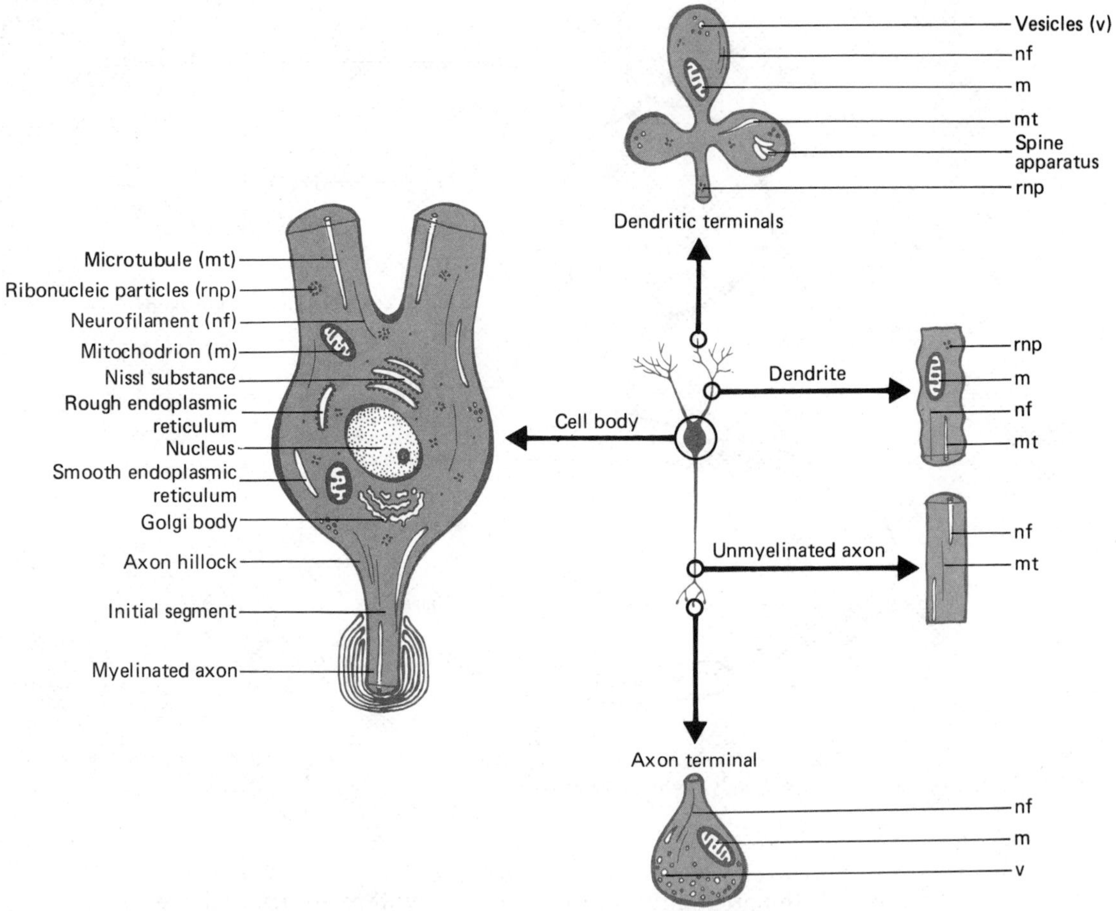

FIGURE 2.2 Various aspects of a neuron. Most of the structures schematically drawn are visible only with electronmicroscopy. (After Shepherd, 1974.)

Neurofilaments and *microtubules* are both elongated structures composed of protein, and also play an important role in development. While neurofilaments have not yet been positively connected with a specific function, microtubules are thought to provide cellular support, and may also play a role in transporting various substances within the cell, since they are found at nerve terminals along the axon, as well as in the cytoplasm. *Mitochondria,* of course, as in all cells, supply energy for metabolism by synthesizing ATP.

Axoplasm, the fluid within the axon, is in some respects similar to the cytoplasm of the cell. Axoplasm and cytoplasm, being more or less continuous with each other, have identical concentrations of chemical substances such as potassium, sodium, and chloride, and thus have the same ionic properties. However, the axon is dependent on the cell body for the manufacture of the chemicals needed at the axonic terminals where intercellular communication takes place (Hodgkin, 1964). The all-important organelles that synthesize the chemical substances (called transmitters) are largely restricted to the cytoplasm of the cell body, so it is thought that the cytoplasm acts as a factory, manufacturing the substances needed at the terminals for transferring information to other cells. The substances that are manufactured in the cytoplasm are then transported down through the axoplasm to the terminal through a process called axoplasmic transport. The microtubules mentioned previously are thought to play a role in this process.

Distinguishing Cellular Features

The processes, those elements branching out from the cell body that receive and transmit signals, are the distinctive features of a neuron. The usual distinction made between the two processes is that a dendrite receives a signal from an adjacent cell, and passively conducts the impulse the short distance to its cell body. An axon transmits a signal for the cell, actively conducting the impulse, sometimes over great distances, to another cell. While this generalization is valid most of the time, there are exceptions to the rule. A dendrite may make contact with a second cell, rather than conducting the impulse to its own cell body, and an axon may sometimes receive an impulse from another axon. In addition, some dendrites have been observed to actively conduct impulses in a manner similar to that of the axon. In general, however, the distinction can be made that dendrites are involved with receiving local signals, and axons are involved with transmitting conducted impulses.

Distinguishing Groups of Cells

Neurons may be categorized according to the number of major processes they have. As the terms suggest, a *unipolar cell* has one process, a *bipolar cell* has two, and a *multipolar cell* has more than two major processes (Cajal, 1955).

In the unipolar cell, one process performs the functions of both receiving and conducting impulses. The process thus serves as a dendrite as well as an axon. For example, sensory receptors in the skin, when stimulated, generate impulses that are both received and actively transmitted towards the spinal cord by the same process. A bipolar cell has one axon and one dendrite. Examples of bipolar nerve cells may be found in the sensory receptor cells of the eye, ear, and nose. All other cells are multipolar. They have many processes for input (the dendrites), and thus have a large receptive field (receive impulses from a wide area).

However, they possess only a single process for output, the axon. Multipolar cells, being the most common kind of nerve cell, are further divided into *Golgi type I* or *type II*, according to the length and branching of the cells' axons. Long-line neurons, or type I neurons (sometimes called macroneurons) (Figure 2.3), have long axons with few branches which carry the neuron impulse for long distances. Local circuit neurons, or type II neurons (sometimes called microneurons), have short axons, which branch repeatedly. These type II neurons are commonly called interneurons, since their main function is to conduct impulses to other neurons in the immediate area.

Obviously the function of the axon is an important one. The sad story of Sal shows what can happen when the axon is damaged or restricted in some way.

Sal sold newspapers from an enclosed corner stand, some said for 30 years. It was probably longer.

Sunday morning is a quiet time for most, but not for a New York

FIGURE 2.3 There are three major types of nerve cells in the brain. Macroneuron: a typical bipolar cell such as the primary efferent neuron in the spinal ganglia; or a common neuron with its typically long distal axon. Microneurons: a small neuron that always has proximal and distal dendrites.

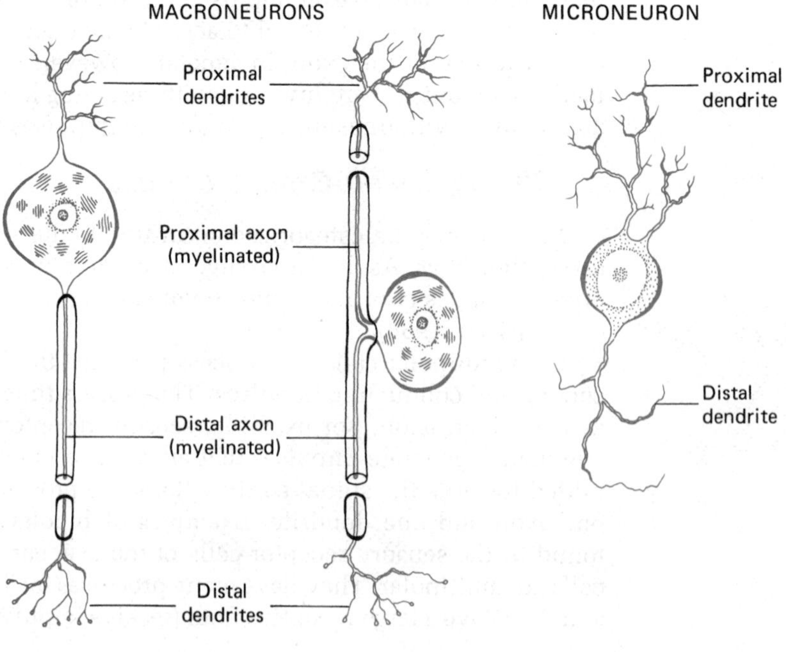

newspaper man. Assembling the encyclopedic Times *is a chore that begins Saturday night. This Sunday, Sal seemed more upset than usual, and the reason was soon apparent. On his way to work he noticed he had difficulty grasping his coffee cup. The failure of his right hand made him useless in the sequential task of folding the Sunday* Times. *In fact, when he moved his right arm 90° from his body his right hand, fingers too, fell limply, unable even to resist gravity. Really, he had no ability to extend his hand or fingers, and although flexion of the hand and opposition of the fingers was possible, the mechanical disadvantage of grasping with the hand flexed was overwhelming. Sal suffered a "wrist drop," so called because the wrist acts as a fulcrum for grasping and finger movement, and without the fulcrum, movement of the fingers is difficult. The muscles of the upper arm and the shoulder were strong, so he could at least carry single sections of the newspaper to the assembly board. Further, he complained of a small area of numbness to touch over the right hand. His ability to sense other modalities such as heat, cold, touch, and painful stimuli was otherwise intact.*

This extension paralysis baffled Sal. He had been eating erratically for some time now, and for sure, he had lost 35 pounds in the last five years. He had been drinking alcohol more frequently, and last night he did drink more than usual. Could there be a connection between these habits and his wrist problem? He remembered falling asleep in the chair near the bar last night. So deep was his sleep that the bartender had left him there all night, and this morning Sal found himself in exactly the same position that he had assumed much earlier with his arm folded over the back of the chair, acting as a pillow for his hand. It was no surprise that the pressure from the chair on an area of his upper arm, where the radial nerve courses superficially, interrupted nerve transmission and resulted in paralysis.

The wrist drop in this case is caused by this area of focal radial nerve destruction and subsequent interruption of action potential transmission. It is commonly called "Saturday night palsy," since an inebriated person will often slump over and pass out in an awkward position, placing extreme pressure on nerves that pass from the spinal cord through the shoulder and forearm to innervate the hand. In other words, Sal's unusual sleeping position the night before had placed pressure on the nerve that innervates the hand as it passes through the arm. Consequently the nerve was unable to transmit impulses down the arm to the hand. The most vulnerable points of the nerve as it leaves the armpit are its bony relations around the middle third of the upper arm and around the elbow. Although Sal retained upper arm power, he suffered a wrist drop and numbness. These symptoms indicated the pressure must have damaged the radial nerve as it traveled around the humerus.

The treatment for a condition such as Sal's is designed to relieve that pressure, allowing the nerve to heal. Use of an upwardly cocked splint that will put the hand in full extension is part of the treatment program. In addition, the paralyzed muscles of extension should be massaged and exercised, and electric stimulation should also be applied. In pressure palsies the prognosis is uncertain. Whether or not the nerve will heal depends on how severely the nerve has been squeezed, and on the duration and extent of compromised circulation to the axons. Weight loss with disappearance of protective fat, the toxic effect of alcohol, and poor nutrition also play some role in the pathogenesis of this injury.

Thus we see that the axon plays an essential role in the chain of neural commands. Without it working properly, the peripheral muscles cannot work normally. From here we shall look more closely at this important neural fiber.

The Physiology of the Neuron

The neuron transmits information through a series of electrochemical phenomena. Just as certain anatomical features of the neuron are similar to those of other cells, so are some physiological properties of the neuron common to all cells. An essential function of any cell is metabolism, that is, utilizing various nutrients to produce energy. All cells have electrical properties, and all cells have selectively permeable membranes. A nerve cell, however, is different in that its membrane has developed special properties that enable it to receive, and more important, to *send* electrical impulses. While nonneural cells are capable of performing various functions, they are not active in the sense that a neuron is active. Only a neuron is capable of sending a message. The uniqueness of the neuron's physiology lies in the fact that the neuron is electrically excitable. Other cells, when stimulated electrically, simply accept the charge passively. A neuron, when stimulated electrically, responds actively, with a programmed series of movements of charged particles called the action potential. This physiological response involves the membrane potential, the action potential, and the synaptic potentials (see Stevens, 1966).

The Resting Membrane Potential

One of the essentials for learning how nerve impulses are transmitted is study of the nerve membrane and how it functions. It is the permeability of the membrane that to a large extent controls the electrochemical phenomena.

To understand the membrane potential, it is necessary to realize some basic bioelectrical properties. First, as in all electrical systems, ions tend to seek a balance in charge: negative ions attract positive ions, and vice versa. Second, ions also follow a concentration gradient, moving from an area of high concentration to one of lower concentration. According to the principle of diffusion, ions of the same element separated by a semipermeable membrane will try to achieve a balance in concentration, moving from a region of high concentration to one of lower concentration in an effort to equalize the distribution.

Three terms important in studying the neuron are *hypopolarization, hyperpolarization,* and *depolarization*. Hypopolarization means that the inside of the cell is more positive with respect to the outside, and hyperpolarization means that the inside of the cell is more negative with respect to the outside. Depolarization means that a positive charge has been applied to the membrane, thus lessening the potential difference measured across the membrane between the normally negative charge inside the cell, and the normally positive charge outside the cell.

Like other cells, nerve cells have a difference in electrical charge between the inside and the outside of the cell. This difference defines a cell that is polarized. In the normal resting state of the neuron, the polarity is maintained by a dynamic balance of certain of the chemical ions on each side of the neuron cell membrane. The outside has a net positive charge and the inside has a net negative charge.

Neuronal cells are not different from other cells of the body, in that there are relatively high concentrations of sodium and chloride outside the nerve cell (the extracellular fluid) and a relatively high concentration of potassium inside (neural cytoplasm or axoplasm) (Curtis and Cole, 1940). The inside of the nerve cell also has large macromolecules of protein that have a negative charge. The sum of charges on the inside of the membrane, and the sum of charges on the outside of the membrane lead to a potential difference across the neuronal membrane. This potential difference is called the resting membrane potential, and is due largely to the distribution of potassium ions.

The ionic flow between the cytoplasm or axoplasm and extracellular fluid is controlled by the semipermeability of the nerve cell membrane. The membrane is much more permeable to potassium ions (50 to 100 times more) than to sodium or chloride. Selective permeability is not unique to the neuron. Many cell membranes are semipermeable, admitting some substances to the interior of the cell and restricting others (and vice versa—the membrane permeability works both ways). This semipermeability, an inherent property of the nerve cell membrane, is believed to operate by means of "gates," or holes in the membrane, which allow some ions through, but refuse others. Hence, because of the nerve cell's permeability, potassium ions, which are normally concentrated inside the cell, easily move to the outside of the cell because of the natural tendency to balance ionic charge. As potassium ions move out, however, the inside of the cell is left with a negative charge because of the large negative protein molecules inside the cell, which cannot pass through the membrane. Eventually, potassium momentarily reaches an equilibrium point. That is, potassium no longer leaks out of the cell because a balance of potassium ions (the potassium equilibrium point) has been reached. At this point, the difference in electrical charge between the inside and outside is measured, and the difference is called the resting membrane potential (see Katz, 1966).

The Sodium-Potassium Pump

One might think that if potassium has reached its equilibrium point, cellular ionic flow might stop. However, as in most living organisms, change is the basis of life. Thus, the cell maintains a *dynamic* state of polarity, and the ionic flow never stops. Even though potassium reaches an equilibrium point, there are other ions affecting the charge across the membrane, and the state of equilibrium for potassium is only momentary. While potassium was leaking out, sodium was leaking in, though at a much slower rate than potassium, because the permeability of the membrane, as already described, is much more (50 to 100 times more) favorable to potassium than to sodium. As a result, when potassium has reached a state of equilibrium, sodium, because of its slower diffusion rate, has not. It continues to leak in. If this process continued, eventually the entire ionic composition of the cell would be reversed. However, nature will not allow that, and has a way of restoring the original concentrations of ions. Sodium is actively transported to the exterior at a rate much faster than it could passively diffuse, and potassium is transported to the interior by a process called the "sodium-potassium pump." This "pumping action" is activated by metabolic energy that is derived from the breakdown of ATP. The passive diffusion of potassium and sodium ions is overcome by the activation of this natural "pump" response, during which the membrane permeability allows sodium to be forced out of the cell, and potassium to be pumped back.

The "pump" is believed to operate as an exchange arrangement, ejecting a sodium ion from the cell while bringing a potassium ion into the cell, though the ratio of sodium to potassium varies from 1:1 to 3:1, depending on the specific biochemical properties of the substance. Once the original concentrations (potassium inside and sodium outside the cell) are reached, the pump action decreases and the process of passive diffusion starts again (see Cooke and Lipkin, 1972).

Experimental Models: Squid Axon Much of what is known about membrane potentials is derived from work done on the giant axon of the squid (Figure 2.4). The axon used for experiments is the large fiber leading from the head to the tail, which is involved in the squid's reflex

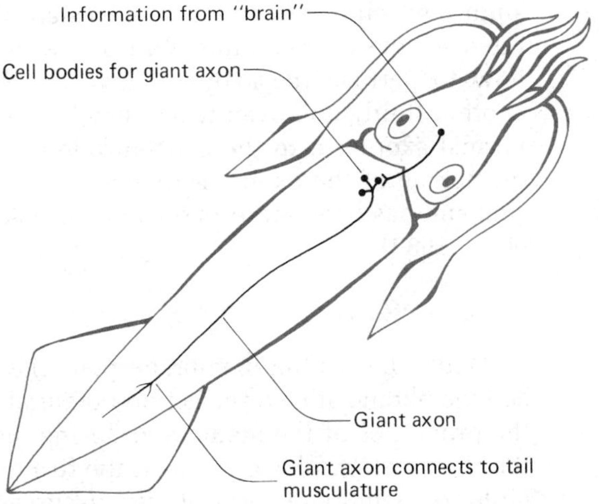

FIGURE 2.4 Simple drawing of the squid, which shows the approximate location of the giant axon. (After Young, 1936.)

action of flicking its tail quickly in order to escape from danger. This axon measures up to 1 mm in diameter, as compared to other axons, which are only 1/100 mm. Because of its relatively large size, the axon is easily studied by inserting a tiny glass tube called a micropipette into the interior, and measuring the electrical charge of the axoplasm inside. By simultaneously recording the charge of the extracellular fluid, the resting membrane potential (the difference between the two charges) can be determined (Figure 2.5). Both the axoplasm and the extracellular fluid of the squid are easily duplicated. Axoplasm can be replaced by a watery solution with the proper ionic concentration of sodium, potas-

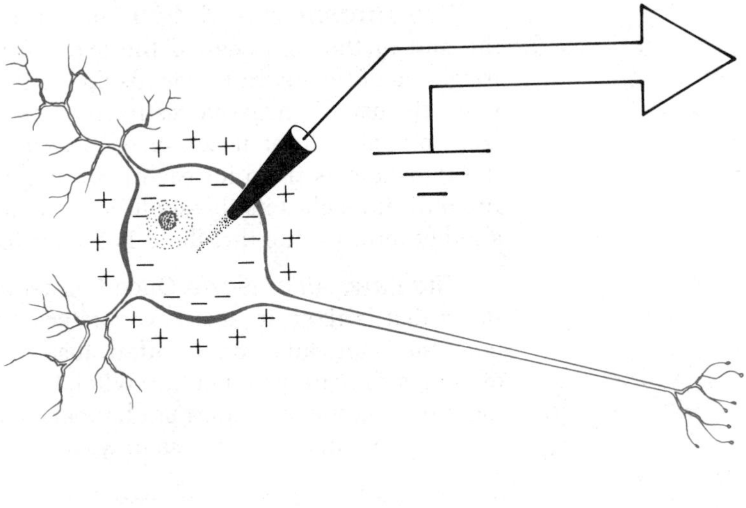

FIGURE 2.5 In order to measure the resting potential of a neuron, a microelectrode must be inserted into the nerve cell. A typical 70-millivolt potential difference always finds the cell negative with respect to the outside.

sium, and chloride, and substances similar to seawater can be substituted for the extracellular fluid of the squid. Researchers have learned how to perfuse the axon (remove the axoplasm and replace it with another fluid), and even when they have used substances differing from normal axoplasm in the concentrations of sodium, potassium, etc., the membrane of the axon has displayed the same impermeability to chloride and has been more permeable to potassium than to sodium (Baker et al., 1962).

The Neuron in Action

While the resting membrane potential reflects the properties of the cell membrane at rest, the action potential, as the term suggests, reflects the properties of the membrane during the active phase of the neuron, the electrical "explosion" that is the firing of the neuron. The same principles of membrane permeability discussed in connection with the resting membrane potential form the basis for the more exciting function of the nerve cell, the transmission of information.

Information transfer occurs through the unique physiological property of the nerve cell membrane, which is its response to a depolarizing current. Whereas other cells respond passively to a depolarizing current accepting the charge, a nerve cell responds actively. A depolarizing current of sufficient strength applied to a neuron triggers an electric impulse during which sodium rushes in and potassium rushes out of the cell (Curtis and Cole, 1940). This impulse is known as the action potential. It is this response, the "firing" of the neuron, which is considered the "on" state of the neuron. The action potential lasts only 0.2 to 0.5 msec; the firing response is then "turned off" automatically, and the nerve cell membrane is restored to its resting potential.

The Threshold of Action The action potential normally arises at the part of the soma called the axon hillock (Cole, 1968). The initial triggering of the neuron depends on the membrane potential, and occurs when the usually negative resting membrane potential becomes depolarized (brought closer to zero). A specific level of depolarization called the *threshold* is fixed for each neuron, and the neuron simply will not fire until it reaches its threshold level of depolarization. For this reason, another term for the threshold is the critical firing level (CFL).

The Law: All or None Once the neuron reaches threshold, an impulse that is fixed in size is generated at the axon hillock. The action potential is an "all or none" affair. Just as an electric light is either on or off, depending on whether the switch has been flipped, the action potential either happens or does not happen. There are no "weak" action potentials generated in response to weak stimuli, and there are no "strong" action potentials generated in response to strong stimuli. The neuron is either "on" or "off," and the strength of the action potential is fixed for each fiber.

The Action Potential

Basically, the action potential is an electrical charge that is propagated down the axon until it gets to a synaptic terminal, where it is converted to a stimulus (synaptic potential) affecting another neuron (Figure 2.6). The initial charge occurs at the first segment of the axonic membrane. It reaches its limit (a fixed size) and subsides, but generates an identical charge that is manifest in the adjacent patch of membrane. This pattern is repeated until the action potential reaches the terminal.

The effect of the charge can be measured on the membrane. If the electrical charge of the membrane is monitored, the path of the action potential can be followed down the axon. In a resting state, the axonic

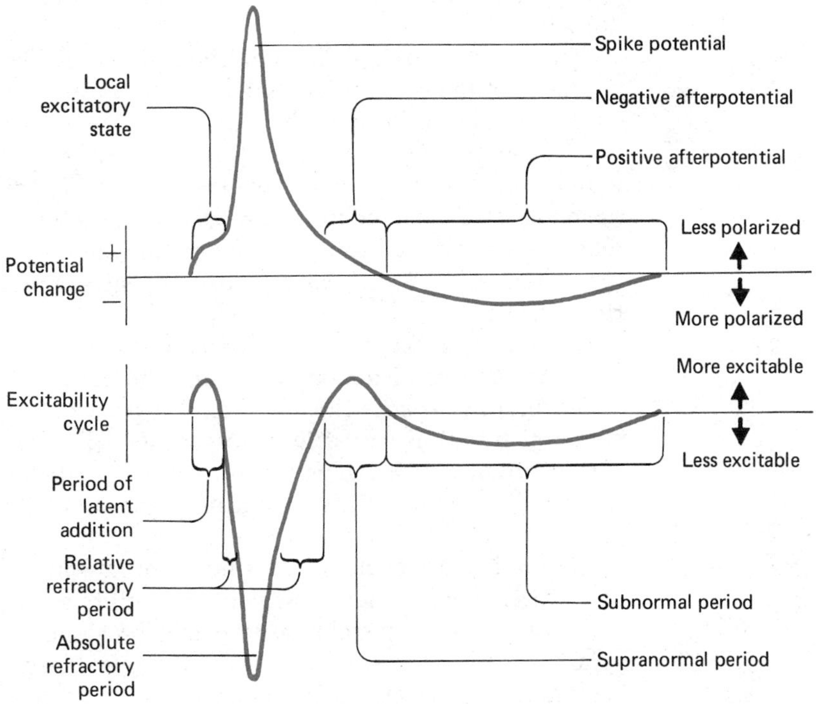

FIGURE 2.6 The change of potential as a spike traverses an axon. In the top portion, the potential differences that mark the ion flux and the current flow are indicated, while on the bottom, possible further response states (the probability of the neuron firing again during these ion flux changes) are shown.

membrane is polarized, with the inside of the axon having a more negative charge than the outside. The resting membrane potential, as you will recall, is the voltage difference across the membrane generated by the negative charges inside the axon and the positive charges outside the axon. The resting membrane is highly permeable to potassium, and slightly permeable to sodium, yet when a stimulus is applied to the membrane, the membrane loses its polarity (becomes depolarized), and consequently the permeability changes, and the action potential is propagated down the nerve. When this depolarization occurs, sodium permeability increases, so the sodium ions outside the axon rush in. Since they carry a positive charge, they cause the membrane potential to be highly positive (more positive inside the axon than outside). However, the increase in permeability to sodium is short-lived (0.2 to 0.5 msec). When the equilibrium for sodium is reached, the charge starts to subside, sodium ions begin to flow back out, and potassium ions flow back in to restore the resting membrane potential. Here again, as in the resting membrane potential, original ionic concentrations are restored by the sodium-potassium pump at a rate faster than could be achieved by passive diffusion.

The sequence of ionic flow outlined above may be described in terms of phases of the action potential, with the various phases caused by the changes in permeability of the membrane. The peak of the action potential, the point at which the membrane is most positively charged, is due to the high concentration of positive sodium ions inside. At this point, the polarity of the membrane is reversed (the cell is more positive inside than out, as opposed to its normal resting state of being more negative inside than out). This peak is called the spike potential (Hodgkin and Huxley, 1952).

The falling phase of the action potential, during which the membrane loses its positive charge and, through the action of the sodium-potassium pump, is restored to its normal negative state (the resting membrane potential), is called the afterpotential (Figure 2.7). Following the afterpotential is a brief period during which the membrane is again slightly depolarized. This period of slight depolarization is called the prepotential.

Naturally, the excitability of the neuron varies with the phases of polarity, excitability being the neuron's ability to respond to a stimulus that will cause the membrane to reach threshold and again reverse its polarity. During the spike potential, the membrane cannot be depolarized, since it has already reversed its polarity. Hence, this period is called the absolute refractory (unresponsive to stimulus) period. During the afterpotential, the original concentrations of ions are being restored by the sodium-potassium pump. A stronger than normal stimulus is needed to get the membrane to threshold, since the difference between

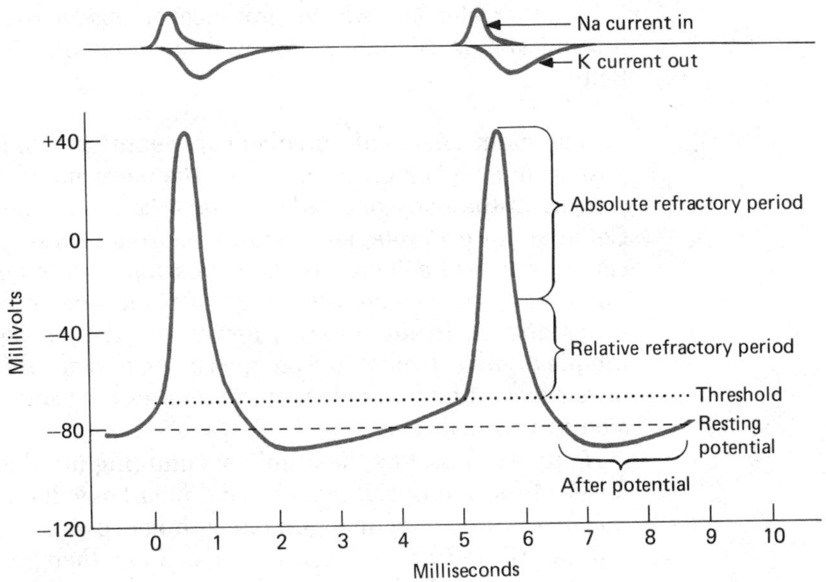

FIGURE 2.7 The sequence of ion flux and current flow that occurs with the generation of action potentials.

the membrane potential and the threshold is greater than the usual difference between the resting membrane potential and the threshold. Hence, this period is called the relative refractory period, meaning it is possible for the membrane to be stimulated, but it is relatively harder than usual since the membrane is somewhat resistant to stimulation. As the membrane potential gets closer to its normal resting state, it is relatively easy to stimulate the neuron because half the task of depolarizing the membrane is already done. Since the membrane is hypopolarized (positive inside), even a small stimulus can push it up to threshold. This period is called the prepotential, or the period of facilitatory hypopolarization. Thus, an intense stimulus may generate more *frequent* impulses, but the size of each individual impulse will not vary. If an impulse does not come during this period of facilitatory hypopolarization, the membrane usually returns to its resting potential. However, some neurons overcompensate and again become, for a short time, more difficult to stimulate, this time because the membrane is more polarized than normal. This period of hyperpolarization is caused by an over-zealous sodium-potassium pump, which pumps out too many sodium ions, leaving a stronger than normal negative charge inside the cell. However, passive diffusion again brings the membrane potential to its resting potential level, and the membrane is receptive to and can process any stimuli.

Another element whose presence or absence is crucial to neural transmission is calcium, as you will see in reading the following case of Betty.

The main chemicals involved in neural transmission are sodium, postassium, and chloride. However, there are many other chemical substances in the body and each of them can affect neural transmission. Calcium, for example, will depress neuronal transmission in high concentrations while increased transmission occurs with low concentrations. Very low concentrations of calcium may cause unstable resting states and an irritable nerve. Because of the particular ionic makeup unique to each element, the charge varies, and accordingly, the presence or absence of any one element, no matter how small, affects transmission in various ways.

Betty was upset by the numbness and tingling she was feeling in her fingers, toes, and lips. It had been a difficult day at the Epilepsy Foundation offices, and after an argument with her co-worker she could not control herself and broke down in tears. Since then she had experienced numbness and tingling (paresthesias) in her extremities for which she had no explanation. Although paresthesias like this were a common occurrence in her life, never had they lasted 12 hours. Sitting in the emergency room, composure regained, she waited to be seen.

This 25-year-old woman had suffered from epilepsy of unknown origin since age 14, but had been seizure free for almost eight years. In fact, this visit to the emergency room was the first time she had seen a physician in years. Treatment with Dilantin over the last five years had allowed her to finish college and then work at the Epilepsy Foundation. Aside from her seizure history she enjoyed good health.

Her examination was striking. When the blood pressure cuff was inflated around her upper arm, her hand flexed at the wrist, and her fingers assumed the shape of a cone. The posture of her hand changed when the blood supply was decreased by inflating the blood pressure cuff. This phenomenon is called a positive Trousseau's sign. The next phase of the examination involved tapping on the jaw muscle to excite the branches of the facial nerve. When the muscle was tapped, Betty began having repetitive twitching movements of the muscles around her nose and mouth. This was a positive Chvostek's sign. Both the hand flexion and the facial twitching were continuous muscle contractions—and the ease with which both were elicited suggested that a decreased threshold of excitability existed in Betty's nervous system. What could have caused this decreased threshold of excitability? Obviously, her body chemistry was off balance: It was likely that Betty had either too much or too little of a certain chemical, thus altering the normal ionic balance.

The fact that muscles contracted easily indicated that the chemical culprit was one involved in muscle contraction. One such chemical is calcium. It plays an important role in regulating the permeability of the neuronal cell membrane to sodium and potassium; it plays an additional role in coupling neuronal excitation with muscular contraction. Indeed, Betty's lab report confirmed the hypothesis of a lowered concentration of calcium. Her blood calcium returned from the lab at 5.3 mg%, while the normal range is 9 – 11 mg%.

She was admitted to the hospital that day, and a complicated evaluation revealed that her chronic seizure disorder was due to persistent hypocalcemia related to an undiscovered endocrine abnormality. Tetany, continuous muscle spasm, is a sign of neuronal and neuromuscular hyperexcitability, and may develop from a number of conditions, including hypocalcemia. In this case hypocalcemia, probably of a long-standing nature, had caused peripheral as well as central signs of increased excitability and decreased threshold.

So we see that the balance of chemicals in the body is extremely important. Something as simple as neglecting to correct a calcium deficiency can result in a serious disorder such as epilepsy; or, in its less severe manifestation, in the numbness and tingling Betty felt earlier, along with the tetanic muscular contractions elicited by pressure. Altering the chemistry of the body in any way, whether by diet, drugs, or disease, is a complicated business, and the results can be far-reaching due to an intricate series of cause-effect relationships. The truth of the matter is that every function of the body depends on the basic action of the nerve cell membrane and its chemical processes. Whether or not its action proceeds normally depends on the delicate balance of many chemical substances. An upset of this balance can result in a higher than normal rate of firing, a lower than normal rate of firing, or in the most severe cases, no firing at all.

In the following sections we shall examine other functions of the neuron that are also electrochemical processes dependent on ionic transfer and balance. First we shall look at how a neural impulse is transmitted from the cell body down the axon.

Propagation of the Action Potential

A unique feature of the neuron is that it is able to conduct its impulses nondecrementally. Once threshold is reached in the cell body and the neuron impulse has originated in the axon hillock, the impulse begins to travel down the axon regeneratively. It does not get weaker along the way, because it is amplified and relayed by each part of the axonal membrane. The initial electrical charge causes a depolarization of the axon, resulting in increased permeability to sodium. The sudden influx of sodium ions causes an electrical current, which, in turn, stimulates the next patch of the axon, depolarizing it, and allowing another sudden influx of sodium ions, which again generates an electrical current.

Once an impulse has been initiated, the cell is incapable of generating another impulse immediately because of the refractory periods discussed earlier. These refractory periods insure that the action potential will travel in the proper direction, "proper" being the direction leading away from the stimulus, toward the outlying terminal. Because the membrane cannot be excited immediately after the action potential, the impulse moves forward to a "fresh," unstimulated patch of membrane. Thus, the process of ionic flow moves all the way down the axon (Hille, 1976).

The speed at which the impulse travels varies with the size of the axon, impulses generally traveling faster in large axons than in small. However, the speed is steady and sometimes slow in all axons, ranging from 2 to 200 mph, depending on the fixed speed for the axon.

The presence or absence of myelin also affects the speed of conduction. Myelinated axons propagate impulses much faster, because every section of the axonal membrane does not have to go through the depolarization process. Instead, impulses are propagated from one unmyelinated, exposed area of the axon (a node of Ranvier) to another, thus proceeding much more rapidly than if the entire length of the axon had to depolarize progressively. Such conduction is called saltatory conduction, from the Latin word meaning to skip or jump. The insulated areas of the axons are not involved at all in transmission; they may be anesthetized with no effect on the propagation, but if anesthetic is applied to the nodes of Ranvier, conduction is virtually stopped.

Recently, certain dendrites have been observed to propagate impulses in a manner similar to axonal propagation. However, it is believed that only certain patches of dendritic membrane are excitable.

The Synapse: Site of Information Transmission

The end tip of the axon (the axonic terminal) is called a button, bouton, knob, or end-foot. A dendritic terminal (which usually receives an impulse from an axon) is called a varicosity, knob, spine, or gemmule. The terminals almost, but do not quite, make contact with a part of another neuron (either a dendrite, an axon, or occasionally the cell body).

These junctions, or to be more accurate, "near junctions," are called synapses, and the space between the terminal and the other neuron is called the *synaptic cleft* (The Synapse, 1976).

Synapses are classified according to their structural components. Axodendritic synapses are formed when an axon meets a dendrite. Axosomatic synapses occur when an axon meets the cell body. Axoaxonic and dendrodendritic synapses follow the same pattern of terminology (axon on axon and dendrite on dendrite). Additionally, there are more complicated synapses involving more than two cells, called serial synapses, or involving feedback, called reciprocal synapses.

Synaptic Anatomy

The usual synaptic pattern is axodendritic, where the axonic terminal forms a synapse with the dendritic terminal. The depolarizing or hyperpolarizing response (depending on whether the synapse potential is excitatory or inhibitory), which occurs at the dendritic terminal, is then passively transmitted by the dendrite to the cell body. There it affects a portion of the membrane, interacting with other synaptic potentials that have arrived at the cell body at the same time, or perhaps earlier at the same place.

Less common, but not unusual, are the axosomatic synapses, where the axon forms a synapse with the cell body itself or with short dendritic stumps coming directly from the cell body.

The separation between cells ranges from a synapse called a tight junction, in which the membranes actually fuse, to a gap junction, in which the membranes are barely separated, to the most standard synapse, in which the membranes are placed in juxtaposition (side by side), separated by a small synaptic cleft (Figure 2.8).

The Physiology of Synaptic Transmission

Although the action potential plays an essential role in the transmission of information throughout the nervous system, it cannot accomplish this feat alone. A second function is necessary to transmit the impulse to another neuron, for the action potential is largely intraneuronal. That is, it travels from the cell body (specifically, the axon hillock) to the axon terminal. The axon terminal is separated from the other cell by a space—admittedly a very small space, but in most cases, sufficiently

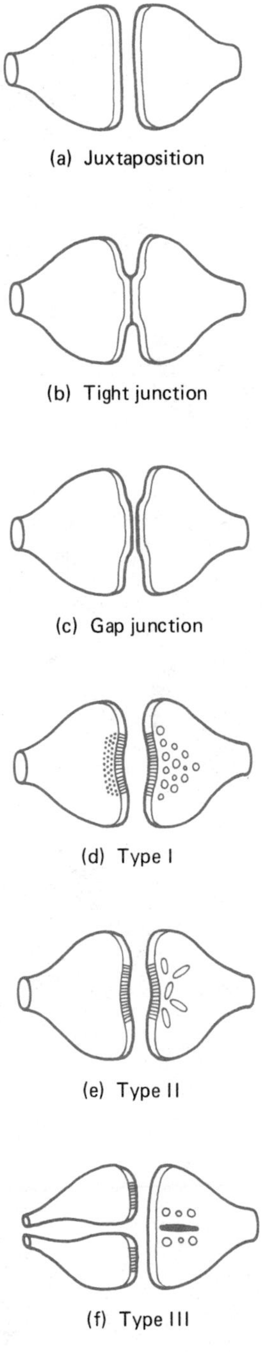

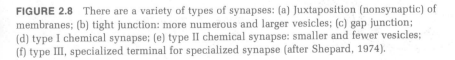

FIGURE 2.8 There are a variety of types of synapses: (a) Juxtaposition (nonsynaptic) of membranes; (b) tight junction: more numerous and larger vesicles; (c) gap junction; (d) type I chemical synapse; (e) type II chemical synapse: smaller and fewer vesicles; (f) type III, specialized terminal for specialized synapse (after Shepard, 1974).

large to require a means other than an electrical impulse for transferring an impulse to another cell. The "near junction" formed by the terminal and the other cell is called a synapse, as we have described, and it is through synaptic transmission that an impulse is sent to the receiving neuron. At the synapse, the cell that is transmitting the impulse is called the presynaptic cell; the cell that is receiving the impulse is called the postsynaptic cell (Eccles, 1964). The response of the postsynaptic cell membrane is called the postsynaptic potential, or more commonly, the *synaptic potential.*

Synaptic Potentials The action potential and the synaptic potential are closely related. The action potential is the stimulus for generating a synaptic potential, and subsequently the synaptic potentials cause the depolarization of the postsynaptic cell, bringing it to threshold, so that it generates an action potential, and thereby continues the neural message along to its destination (Figure 2.9). Thus, the entire sequence of events is that an impulse is transmitted down an axon to a terminal, where a synaptic potential is generated; the synaptic potential travels to the postsynaptic cell body, and there, given sufficient depolarizing stimuli (either a strong synaptic potential or several small ones), an action potential is generated.

However, although the action potential and the synaptic potential are similar in some respects, there are differences between them. The action potential is a conducted response, which is amplified and relayed along its way down the axon. The synaptic potential, on the other hand, is largely a local response, usually originating at the dendritic terminal and passively traveling down the short dendrite to the membrane of the cell body, and sometimes occurring on the cell body itself (in the case of axo-somatic synapses). The action potential is of a fixed size, an all or none affair; the synaptic potential is a graded response: Its size varies, depend-

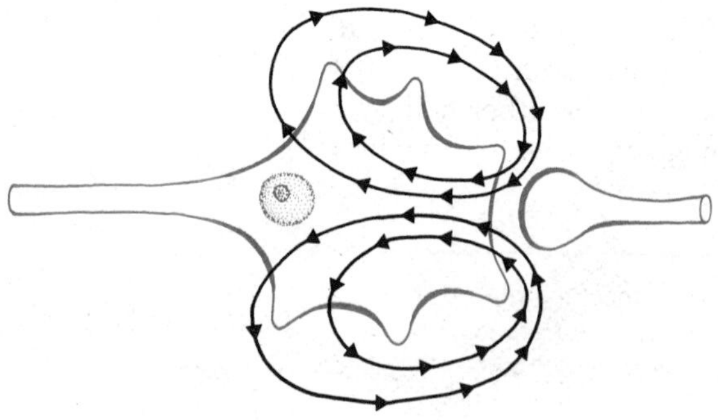

FIGURE 2.9 The decrease of negativity that accompanies cell discharge spreads to areas not directly in the site of synaptic discharge.

ing upon the interaction of other inputs coming into the cell. Rarely does a neuron fire with input from only one source. It is at the synapse that multiple inputs converge, and through their combined effects on a cell, they may or may not cause it to fire. Integration of input occurs at the synapse through a process of summation, and the important "decision" to fire or not to fire is made as a result of the total electrical input affecting a neuron. The synaptic potential also seems to be more complicated than the action potential. For instance, there are two modes of synaptic transmission, electrical and chemical. To further complicate matters, the effect of the chemical synaptic response varies. It may either excite or inhibit the firing response (the action potential) of the postsynaptic cell. An excitatory postsynaptic potential is commonly referred to as an EPSP, and an inhibitory postsynaptic potential is called an IPSP.

Spatial and Temporal Summation A synapse seldom acts alone; each neuron usually has hundreds and sometimes thousands of synapses. Assimilating all the inputs coming in may seem to be a formidable task; however, a system of simple algebra prevails. Both spatial and temporal summation are used. If enough small synaptic potentials arrive at the cell at the same time, even at different places on the cell membrane, the sum of their depolarizing (or hyperpolarizing) effects may be enough to bring the receiving (postsynaptic) cell to threshold, thus triggering the action potential through spatial summation. The synaptic potentials may also add up in time. Each synaptic potential lasts for a short time, ranging from 2 to 20 msec. Thus, if a second EPSP follows the first within 2 to 20 msec, the second EPSP will have a greater than normal effect on the cell membrane because of the depolarization of the cell membrane triggered by the first EPSP. In other words, depolarization of the cell membrane may be facilitated by a temporal summation of excitatory potentials.

The Electrical Synapse

Though not common in the mammalian brain, electrical synapses do exist. Electrical synapses reflect greater speed in transmission, since there is no 0.2 to 0.5-msec delay between the cells as in the chemical synapses. One type of electrical synapse is the gap junction, which has a very small cleft with a low-resistance electrical pathway between the cells (Bennett, 1974).

The Chemical Synapse

The most common and the most complicated synapse is the chemical synapse (Krnjevic, 1974). For many years, the transmission between neurons was thought to be electrical, since the reaction of the postsynaptic cell membrane is an electrical response. However, the 0.2 to 0.5-msec delay between the impulse coming from the presynaptic terminal and the depolarization of the postsynaptic cell membrane could not be explained in terms of electrical transmission. Eventually it was hypothesized that the reaction had to be chemical.

It is now known that chemical synapses work through a combination of chemical and electrical phenomena. The basic pattern is that the electrical impulse (the action potential), when arriving at the nerve terminal, triggers the release of a chemical substance stored in the vesicles that are concentrated in the knob or bouton (terminal). (Figure 2.10) This chemical substance, called a transmitter, travels across the synaptic cleft and interacts with the membrane of the receiving cell, changing the membrane permeability. Depending on the characteristics of the transmitter and of the membrane of the receiving cell, the transmitter causes an electrical reaction in the cell: The membrane either depolarizes or hyperpolarizes, thus bringing the cell either closer to or farther away from threshold.

The last stage of the sequence of events involved in the synaptic potential is the reaccumulation of the transmitter by the cell that released it from the presynaptic membrane. This "recycling process" is common to all but one of the known transmitters. In the exceptional case, the transmitter (a compound) is broken down into its basic components, and one

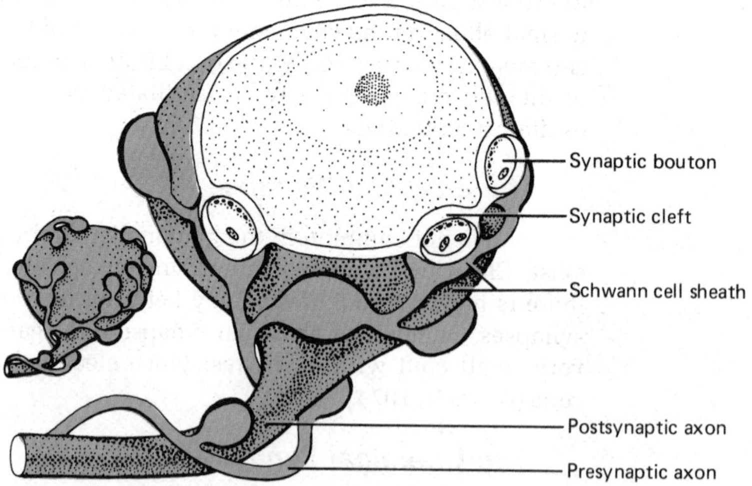

FIGURE 2.10 Structural features of chemical synapses. Shown is an example of synaptic boutons distributed on a ganglion cell in the heart of a frog. (From Kuffler and Nichols, 1976.)

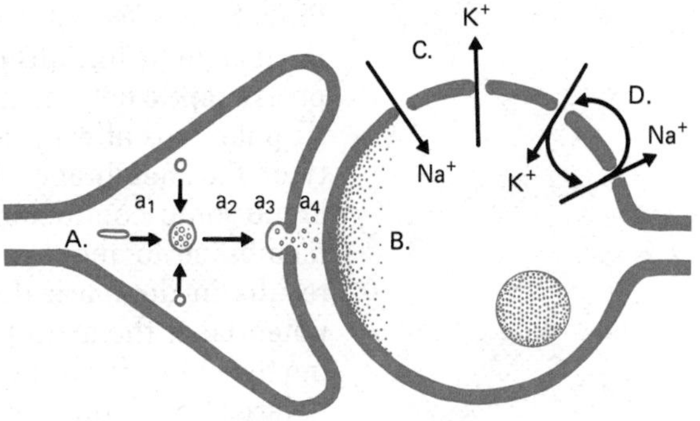

FIGURE 2.11 The many activities involved in the transmission of neural information from one cell to another. A, chemical substances are synthesized (a_1), and packaged (a_2) in the presynaptic cell. This package of transmitters then interacts with the presynaptic membrane (a_3) and releases neurotransmitter into the synaptic cleft (a_4). The transmitter is then cleared from the synaptic space by reuptake and by enzyme hydrolysis in order to control the effect on the postsynaptic membrane. B indicates the postsynaptic membrane. There is some evidence that it is this area that determines whether a given transmitter has a hyperpolarizing or depolarizing effect. In C, membrane changes in depolarization are thought to cause gates to open up in the membrane, by rapid change in the conformation of membranal protein. D marks the repolarization of the membrane, with the active replacement of ions that have been previously described.

of these components is taken up by the presynaptic terminal where it is used to manufacture more transmitter. Although transmitters are synthesized in the nerve terminal, the catalysts for the reaction that produces the transmitter must come from the cell body (Figure 2.11).

Transmitters: Fuel for Synaptic Transmission

Knowledge of transmitters and how they work is still somewhat limited, but there are some hypotheses that appear to be valid. Transmitters will be discussed in detail in Chapter 5, but here we shall explain the basic principles of how transmitters work. First, it seems that they are stored in and released in packets called quanta (one packet = one quantum). Small structures called vesicles contain the transmitter. These vesicles line up along the presynaptic cell membrane (at the terminal), and in response to a depolarization of the presynaptic terminal, fuse with the membrane, thus discharging their contents (the quanta) to the extracellular fluid. The released transmitter flows across the synaptic cleft and interacts with the protein receptor molecules of the postsynaptic cell membrane, causing a synaptic potential. The depolarization of the presynaptic nerve terminal is not the only crucial factor for the liberation of the transmitter, however. A second requirement is that calcium be present in the extracellular fluid. Although it has been conclusively demonstrated that a sufficient concentration of calcium is necessary for release of the transmitter, the exact interaction of calcium with the transmitter release system has not yet been found out (Hubbard, 1973).

Any one neuron is capable of secreting only one transmitter, although the effect of that transmitter may be to depolarize or hyperpolarize (excite or inhibit) depending on the makeup of the receptors in the postsynaptic cell membrane. Both excitatory and inhibitory postsynaptic potentials affect the membrane potential by changing the permeability of the membrane. An *excitatory* potential increases the transmembrane ionic conductances to sodium and potassium, thus forcing the membrane to move toward the sodium equilibrium potential, which results in depolarization and the subsequent generation of the action potential at the axon hillock. An *inhibitory* potential works by increasing the chloride permeability of the membrane, which results in a hyperpolarization of the membrane.

Axoplasmic Transport of Transmitters

The transmitter secreted by each neuron is manufactured in the terminal of the neuron. The blueprint for manufacturing the specific transmitter substance comes from DNA, found in the nucleus of the cell, and a means of sending the necessary "materials and instruction" down to the terminal from the cell body is required. An in-depth description of the transport means has not yet been devised, but the following sequence of events is believed to take place.

DNA produces RNA, which moves out of the nucleus and attaches to the ribosomes on the rough ER. Here amino acids are attached to the RNA and are lined up in the proper sequence by RNA, thus determining the specific enzymes necessary for the production of each transmitter. But, since the actual synthesis of the transmitter takes place in the terminal, the enzymes must be transported from the soma to the terminal. A carrier called the microtubule is believed to play a role in actively transporting these substances to the terminal (passive diffusion must be discounted, for some terminals are so far from the cell body that transport by diffusion might literally take years). The system of active conveyance is called axoplasmic transport, and it is presumed that metabolism provides the energy for transport and regulates the flow.

Summary

The basic building unit of the nervous system, the neuron, is seen to be a varied structure. Its essential function is to propagate an electrical impulse from dendritic processes to the cell body and down the axon to the axon terminals. In most neurons, this impulse leads to release of any number of chemical transmitters that have the effect of either inhibiting or exciting the postsynaptic cell, and so conduct the impulse through the network of nerves.

The semipermeable membrane plays a major role in governing the action of a neuron through maintenance of specific permeability for each charged ion. Generating an action potential, and transferring it from one neuron to another, involves a complex yet basic chain of events. Depolarization of the cell membrane from its resting potential results in the action potential being fired. Changes in the permeability of the membrane to sodium and then potassium lead to charge generation and current flow. The action potential is conducted down the axon, often speeded along its way by the presense of myelin. This protein-containing cell wraps the axon with electrical insulation and causes saltatory conduction as the charge skips from one nonmyelinated area to the next.

The synapse has fast become a hotbed of research interest. A summation of input on the cell membrane at the synaptic junction may result in excitation or inhibition of the subsequent cell depolarization. The neuron discharges a chemical that diffuses across the synaptic cleft to interact with a specific receptor area on the adjacent neuron. This interaction causes changes in the membrane permeability and subsequent transmission of the action potential. The variability and plasticity this system allows is enormous, for the chemical transmission may excite or inhibit the affected neuron.

Research with these biochemicals or transmitters is also revolutionizing neurobiology. Their synthesis from precursors, their storage, release, and binding on the postsynaptic membrane, and their subsequent degradation or reuptake into the presynaptic neuron have provided a handle to manipulate and ultimately to attempt to understand the functions of the nervous system.

Through the case examples, it becomes clear that the system is tenuous and delicate. Disruption caused by direct pressure, or biochemical or hormonal imbalance may upset orderly transmission.

This interruption of orderly transmission in the central nervous system may lead to seizures, general discharges of many neurons without any apparent synchrony. In the peripheral nervous system this disruption may lead to anesthesia, the inability to sense touch, heat, cold, pain, or even the ability to know the limbs' position in space (proprioception). It may also lead to paralysis, for the motor nerve may also be involved.

Besides learning about the intriguing studies that have uncovered many of the physiological mechanisms of the single neuron, one must also grasp the possible philosophical implication of the interrelationship of these all or nothing neuronal complexes. Does the multibillion neuronal system allow us to be free? More about that later.

References

Baker, P. F., A. L. Hodgkin, and T. I. Shaw. 1962. Replacement of the axoplasm of giant nerve fibers with artificial solutions. *J. Physiol.* *164*:330–354.

Bennett, M. V. L. 1974. Flexibility and rigidity in electronically coupled systems. In: M. V. L. Bennett, ed. *Synaptic Transmission and Neuronal Interaction*. New York: Raven Press.

Cajal, Raymon y, S. 1955. *Histologie du Système Nerveux*. Vol. II. Madrid: C. S. I. C.

Cole, K. S. 1968. *Membranes, Ions, and Impulses*. Berkeley: University of California Press.

Collier, B., and F. C. McIntosh. 1969. The source of choline for acetylcholine synthesis in a sympathetic ganglion. *Can. J. Physiol. Pharmacol.* *47*:127–135.

Cooke, I., and M. Lipkin. 1972. *Cellular Neurophysiology*. New York: Holt, Rinehart and Winston.

Curtis, H. J., and K. S. Cole. 1940. Membrane action potentials from the squid giant axon. *J. Cell. Comp. Physiol.* *15*:147–157.

Eccles, J. C. 1964. *The Physiology of Synapses*. Berlin: Springer-Verlag.

Hille, B. 1976. Ionic basis of resting and action potentials. In: E. Kandel, ed. *Handbook of the Nervous System*. Bethesda, Md.: American Physiological Society.

Hodgkin, A. L. 1964. *The Conduction of the Nervous Impulse*. Liverpool University Press.

Hodgkin, A. L., and A. F. Huxley. 1952. Currents carried by sodium and potassium ions through the membrane of the giant axon of *Loligo*. *J. Physiol.* *116*:449–472.

Hodgkin, A. L., and B. Katz. 1949. The effect of sodium ions on the electrical activity of the giant axon of the squid. *J. Physiol.* *108*:37–77.

Hubbard, J. I. 1973. Microphysiology of vertebrate neuromuscular transmission. *Physiol. Rev.* *53*:674–723.

Katz, B. 1966. *Nerve, Muscle, and Synapse*. New York: McGraw-Hill.

Krnjevic, K. 1974. Chemical nature of synaptic transmission in vertebrates. *Physiol. Rev.* 54:418–540.

Kuffler, S. W., and J. G. Nicholls. 1976. *From Neuron to Brain*. Mass.: Sinauer Associates, Inc.

Peters, A., S. L. Palay, and H de F. Webster. 1976. *The Fine Structure of the Nervous System*. Philadelphia: Saunders.

Shepard, G. M. 1974. *The Synaptic Organization of the Brain*. New York: Oxford University Press.

Stevens, C. F. 1966. Molecular basis for postjunctional conductance increases induced by acetylcholine. *Cold Spring Harbor Symp. Quant. Biol.* *40*:169–174.

The Synapse. 1976. *Cold Spring Harbor Symp. Quant. Biol.* *40*.

Young, J. Z. 1936. The giant nerve fibers and epistellar body of cephalopods. *Quart. J. Microsc. Sci.* *78*:367–386.

CHAPTER 3

Fundamentals of Brain Anatomy

Grace was the 18-year-old daughter of Dr. and Mrs. Vincent Row. She was a talented and intelligent young woman who graduated in the top of her school class and who quite successfully finished her freshman year at college. Summer had been a particularly exciting time, full of many new experiences. She spent most of the time managing and working at a greasy spoon restaurant on the beachfront. The hectic pace of working, or partying most of the night and sleeping late in the morning, was de rigueur in this summer community.

One of her summer activities was romance. How could she help noticing him? After all, he was also a manager of the restaurant and, like herself, a one-fifth share owner. The relationship blossomed and grew, and even lasted after the summer's end. All fall one or the other would make the 150-mile car trip to visit each weekend. The horror came on a cold, rainy winter night. It was his turn to make the trip, and while making a particularly sharp turn, his car skidded out of control. He died instantly when the car hit the embankment. Grace was overwhelmed with grief and could not be consoled by anyone. In an impulsive gesture the following evening she took all 25 Seconal tablets that remained in her mother's room. She fell on her bed crying herself to sleep—maybe forever.

Fortunately her father checked on her sometime later and noticed the opened Seconal bottle immediately. Grace was rushed to intensive care in deep coma.

Her examination in the intensive care unit revealed the progressive orderly loss of gross brain function, which you will come to learn about in this chapter. First she was flaccid (limp) and motionless, unresponsive to voice or visual threat. This meant her higher cerebral cortical functions were depressed. She was, however, responsive to pain, withdrawing each limb nonreflexively as various mildly noxious tactile stimuli were applied. There were other signs suggesting reversible de-

pression of cortical function. This was important. If she had responded instead with reflex postures to somatic stimulation it would have suggested she had done irreversible damage to her midbrain.

Vestibular and cerebellar functions were similarly depressed. These systems were tested by employing midbrain reflexes. For example, her pupils were in mid-position (3–5 mm) and were reactive to light. The oculocephalic reflex, commonly called the doll's-head eye movement, was also present. In performing this maneuver the eyelids are held open and the head briskly rotated from side to side. A positive response, indicating a functioning but depressed midbrain, consists of contraversive conjugate eye deviation. In other words, if the head is rotated to the left the eyes deviate to the right much in the manner of a child's old-fashioned doll.

These clinical tests indicated the condition of various parts of Grace's brain. For example, the pupillary reflex gave information about the midbrain, since it is dependent on the anatomic patternings of the pupillary fibers in the high midbrain. The oculocephalic reflex revealed the condition of the vestibular and oculomotor nuclei.

Finally, but most unfortunately, her respirations were slow, uneven, and shallow. This is a common feature of coma caused by barbiturates. Respiration always tends to be depressed, at least as much as somatic-motor function, sometimes more. She needed respiratory assistance and a special tube was placed in her trachea, and attached to an automatic ventilator. Although she might need respiratory assistance for several days, chances were excellent for full recovery. While other life-supporting functions were being maintained or aided by drugs or mechanical means, her body would be ridding itself of the barbiturates. They would be metabolized in her liver and excreted by her kidney.

Her waking-up process would be a progressive and orderly return of function. First, as her brain stem area recovered, respirations would occur spontaneously and maintain adequate ventilation. Then, spontaneous movement would return, followed quickly by return of voluntary gaze. As the forebrain recovered, that is, as consciousness returned, the midbrain reflexes would be overcome by conscious, willful activity. She would lose her so-called doll's eyes and look where she pleased when her head was briskly rotated from side to side. Finally she would speak and understand, although longer time than that would be needed to heal her grief.

For our purposes Grace's accident teaches many lessons about the organization of the central nervous system. The business of this chapter is to outline the main features of brain anatomy. It is knowledge that is crucial not only for what follows in this book, but also for use in emergency situations such as the sudden onset of coma.

General Terms

Studying the organization of the nervous system requires knowledge of some basic directional terms used for determining locations in the brain. The brain, being an object, has three dimensions: top or bottom, front or back, and side or middle. The terms used for studying the brain are those used in any anatomical study: Top and bottom are *dorsal* and *ventral* (one's back being considered the top, as in animals that walk on all fours). Front to back (head to tail) is called either *rostral* to *caudal* or *anterior* to *posterior*. The sides and the middle of the brain are designated *lateral* or *medial*, respectively (Figure 3.1). Although the human brain has a right angle because of the human's upright posture, the same directional terms are used for all organisms. One need only "straighten the right angle out" as if a human crawled on all fours to apply the directions to the human. This is especially important in the lower part of the brain and the spinal cord to get dorsal (back) and ventral (front) regions correct.

In addition to these three sets of directional terms, there are three different planes used for sectioning the brain. Since it is quite difficult to study the anatomy of a whole brain, it is necessary to cut into the brain in order to see particular structures. Normally, one of three planes is used for sectioning. The most common cut used, dorsal to ventral, is

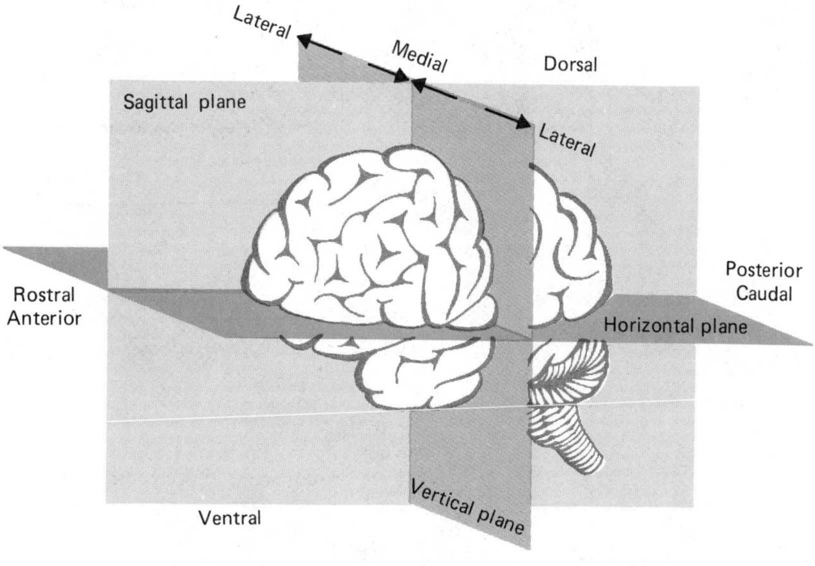

FIGURE 3.1 Directional terms in the nervous system. (Adapted from Isaacson et al., 1971.)

analogous to the plane used for slicing a loaf of bread. This plane is called the *coronal*. A second plane is again a vertical cut, this time at a right angle to the coronal plane. This cut, analogous to the way in which a hot dog bun is split, is in the *sagittal* plane. The last plane, which may be compared to the cut in a hamburger bun, is the *horizontal* plane (parallel to the base of the brain).

The Nervous System Divided

The two main divisions of the nervous system are the *central* and *peripheral* nervous systems (Figure 3.2). Terminology for neural tissue in the central nervous system differs from terminology used for the pe-

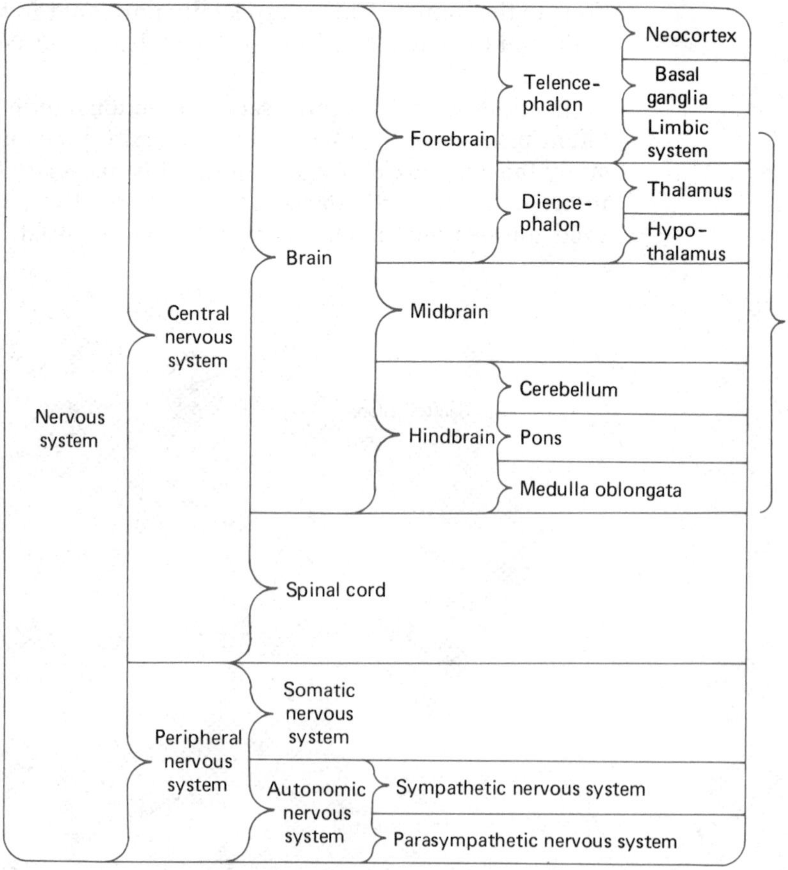

FIGURE 3.2 Organization of the nervous system. (Adapted from Isaacson et al., 1971.)

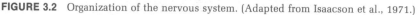

ripheral nervous system. Neural fibers (axonic processes) are called *tracts* within the central nervous system, and are called *nerves* in the peripheral nervous system. Masses of cell bodies are called *nuclei* when they lie within the central nervous system, and *ganglia* when found in the peripheral nervous system.

Peripheral Nervous System (PNS)

The PNS serves as a communication network, its main job being to transport impulses to and from the CNS. Virtually all neural fibers outside the CNS are part of the peripheral nervous system. The peripheral system has two main divisions: the *somatic division* and the *visceral division*. The nerves in each division can be further grouped into afferents and efferents. While *afferents* carry incoming or approaching impulses to the CNS, *efferents* carry outgoing or effective messages from the CNS. Thus, the peripheral nerves fall into one of four categories: *somatic afferents, somatic efferents, visceral afferents,* and *visceral efferents.*

The somatic division runs our interactions with the external world. Its afferents are the fibers headed for the brain from the receptors in the eyes, nose, skin, and the other sensory organs. In contrast, the somatic efferents carry commands for movement from the brain to the muscles of the body.

We are generally aware of excitation of the somatic afferents and efferents, for they are the basis of perception and movement. However, the activity of the visceral nerves generally goes unnoticed. As their name implies, these nerves carry messages concerning the viscera, or internal organs and glands. The heart, liver, kidneys, salivary glands, and so on, are all connected to the CNS by way of the visceral afferents and efferents. Thus, the visceral nerves mediate interactions with the internal environment, just as the somatic nerves mediate interactions with the external environment.

The visceral efferent system is also referred to as the *autonomic nervous system*. The autonomic nervous system has two divisions. One division, the *parasympathetic*, may be compared to the routine maintenance crew of a town. This system insures that the daily, routine aspects of bodily functioning are carried out, for example, breathing, digestion, and sleep. A second system, however, is called into play for what might be termed "emergency" action, just as a town might call in extra maintenance crews to prepare for and cope with emergency situations. This second division of the autonomic nervous system, the *sympathetic* division, innervates organs when more than routine functions are needed, as in stressful situations calling for more energy. Thus, if a person who is frightened of dogs sees a large German shepherd approaching, the sight of the dog will likely elicit a fear reaction. That is, the person's heart will beat faster, perspiration may begin, arm hairs may become erect. While this fear reaction is going on, normal bodily functions cease. Digestion stops, and normal rates of breathing, pulse rates, and blood pressure are changed. However, after the person has safely passed the dog or overcome the fear, the parasympathetic nervous system takes over, resuming its regulation of normal bodily functions.

The cell bodies of the different divisions of the PNS are located in different regions of the nervous system. The cell bodies of the somatic afferents are located in the *dorsal root ganglia*, a collection of cell bodies just outside the dorsal (sensory) part of the spinal cord (Figure 3.3). The afferent fibers from the ganglia form a nerve bundle (the *dorsal root*) that feeds into the spinal cord. The cell bodies of the visceral afferents, in contrast, are actually in the dorsal part of the spinal cord (Figure 3.4). Thus, the visceral afferent system does not involve the dorsal root ganglia.

The cell bodies of the efferent fibers of both the somatic and visceral systems are in the ventral (motor) part of the spinal cord. The somatic efferents leave the cord in the *ventral root* and terminate on the muscles of the body. The visceral efferents are localized depending on whether

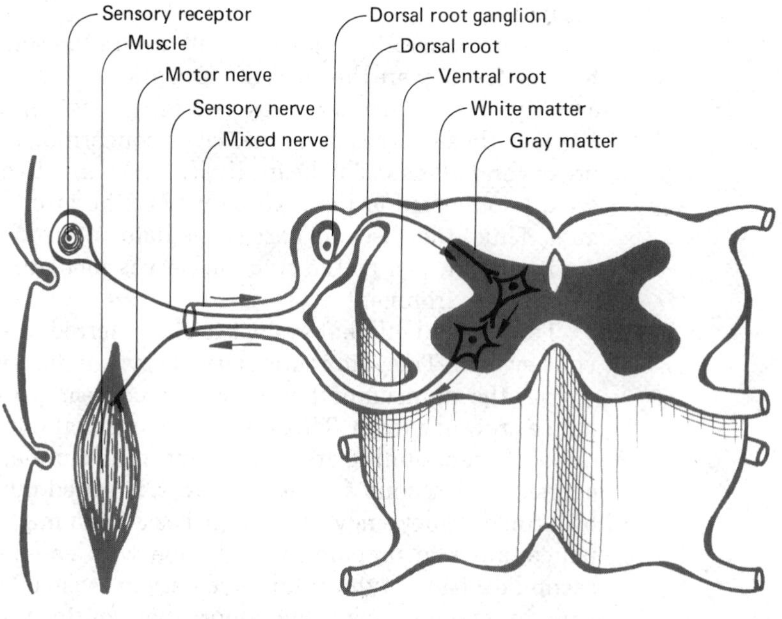

FIGURE 3.3 Somatic afferents bring information into the central nervous system. The somatic efferents are the motor neurons that innervate muscles.

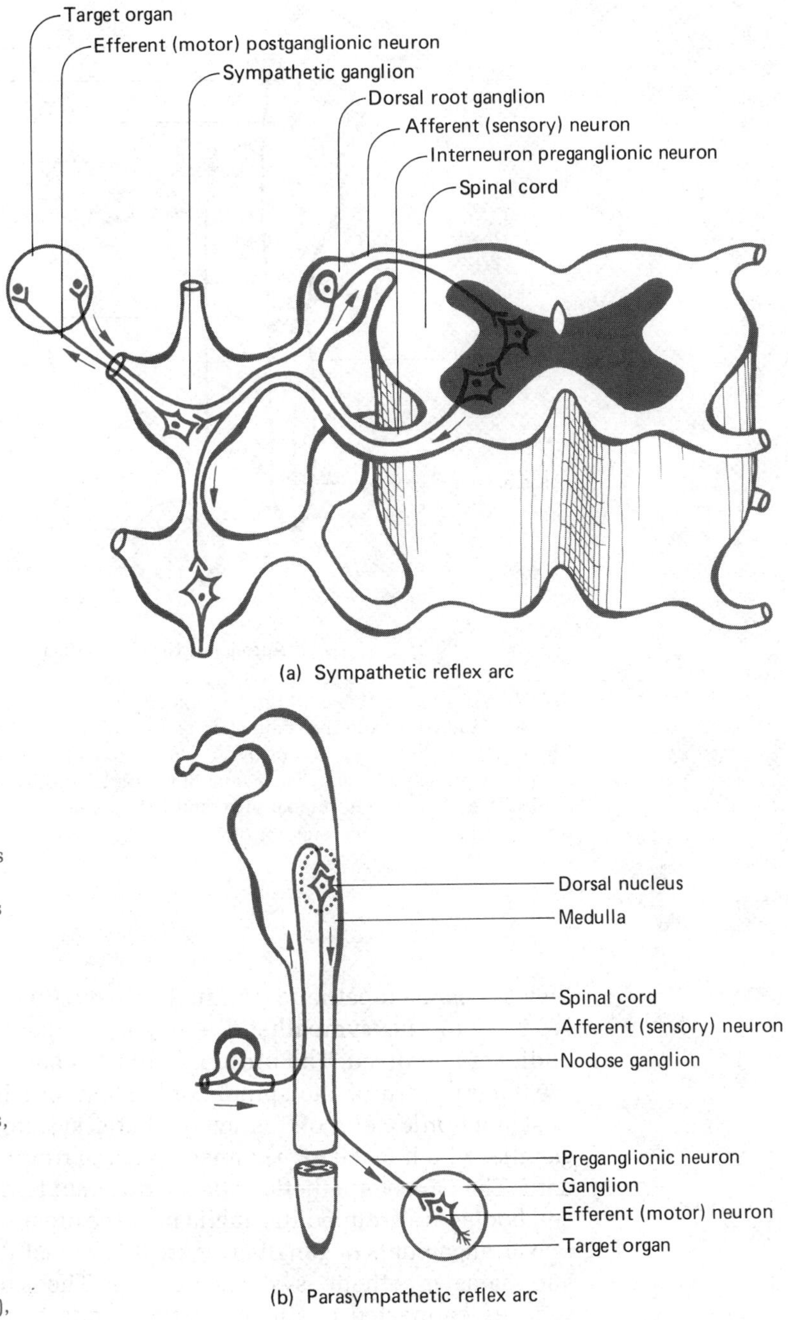

FIGURE 3.4 Autonomic reflex arcs. Visceral afferents and efferents. Part (a) depicts the visceral afferents for the sympathetic autonomic nervous system. Visceral afferents do not differ substantially from somatic afferents. The visceral efferents of the sympathetic reflex arc (a) differ from somatic efferents, with synapse in the sympathetic ganglion adjacent to the spinal cord, before projecting to distant target organs. In the parasympathetic organization, depicted in (b), the efferent fiber projects to a ganglion, adjacent to the target organ.

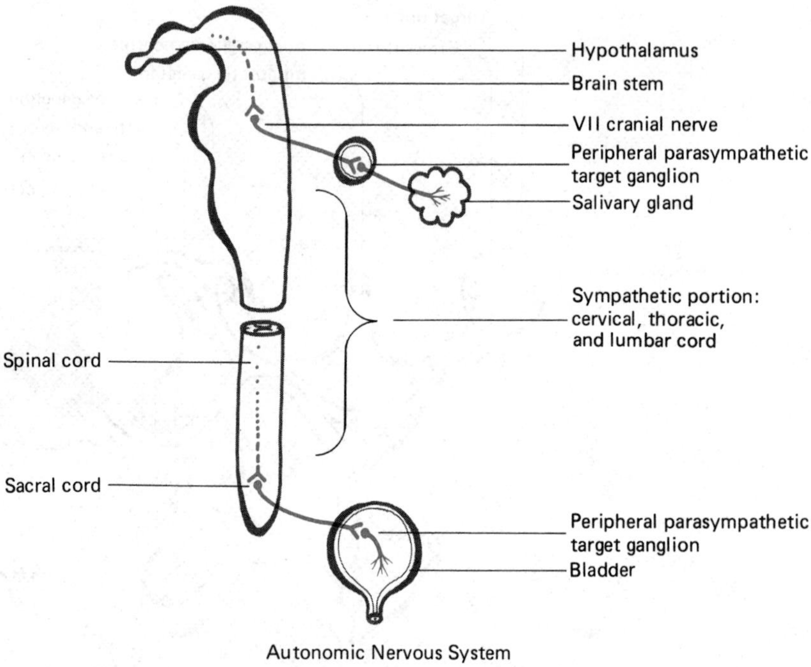

FIGURE 3.5 Sympathetic and parasympathetic organization. The parasympathetic division originates from the brain stem and from the sacral division of the spinal cord (the most caudal part). It is thus often referred to as the craniosacral division of the autonomic nervous system. The sympathetic division arises from segments of the spinal cord in the thoracic and lumbar area, and is thus referred to as the thoracolumbar division of the autonomic nervous system.

they are parasympathetic (routine) or sympathetic (nonroutine). Actually, in both the sympathetic and parasympathetic systems, two cell bodies are involved. The *preganglionic cell bodies* of both systems are in the ventral horn of the spinal cord. Then, outside the spinal cord, the *postganglionic cells* of the sympathetic system form the sympathetic ganglia, which make up a connected chain running parallel to the spinal cord. The parasympathetic cells are different in that their postganglionic cell bodies are grouped in ganglia near the organ being innervated. These two arrangements of ganglia (Figure 3.5) reflect the way the sympathetic and parasympathetic systems operate: The sympathetic (emergency) with its connected chain of ganglia, tends to excite all the organs to which it is connected at once, whereas the parasympathetic (routine), which has its ganglia located in various places near each organ that is being innervated, acts in a more specific manner, stimulating particular organs rather than indiscriminately stimulating all at once.

PNS: The Spinal and Cranial Nerves

The PNS can also be classified into spinal and cranial nerves. The cranial nerves contain the afferents and efferents (both somatic and visceral) of the head and neck region, and the spinal nerves contain the afferents and efferents of the body and visceral regions below the neck.

There are 12 pairs of *cranial nerves* in all, numbered in the order of their entrance to the brain stem in a rostral to caudal direction, and named according to the cranial area to which they are connected (Figure 3.6). A silly mnemonic device has been used for years by students of the brain to remember the cranial nerves: "On old Olympus's towering top, a Finn and German vend some hops" (see Table 3.1). The cranial nerves are "mixed," containing both afferent and efferent fibers. The spinal nerves are also mixed, but unlike the cranial nerves, which remain mixed, the *spinal nerves* separate into afferent and efferent components near the spinal cord and form the dorsal and ventral roots of the cord. The 31 pairs of spinal nerves each arise from a particular segment of the spinal cord and are named according to that segment (Figure 3.7).

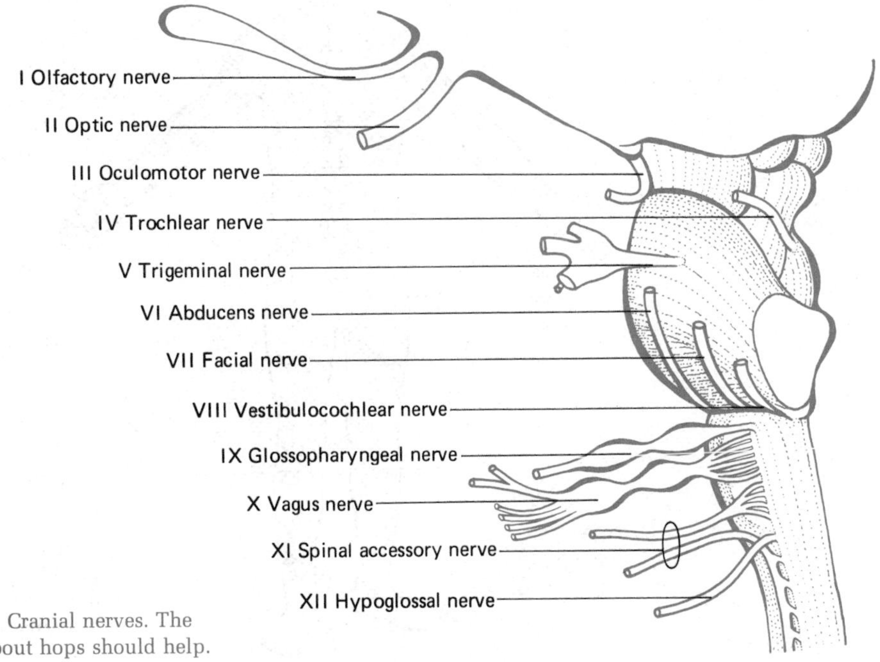

FIGURE 3.6 Cranial nerves. The mnemonic about hops should help.

TABLE 3.1 The Cranial Nerves

Number	Name	Functions
I	Olfactory	Smell
II	Optic	Vision
III	Oculomotor	Eye movement
IV	Trochlear	Eye movement
V	Trigeminal	Masticatory movements Sensitivity of face and tongue
VI	Abducens	Eye movements
VII	Facial	Facial movements
VIII	Auditory vestibular	Hearing Balance
IX	Glossopharyngeal	Tongue and pharynx, swallowing,
X	Vagus	Heart, blood vessels, viscera
XI	Spinal accessory	Neck muscles and viscera
XII	Hypoglossal	Tongue muscles

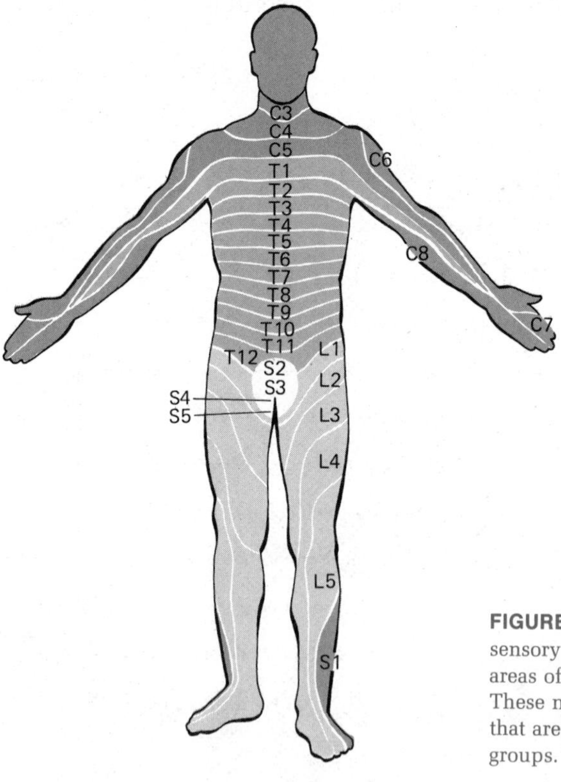

FIGURE 3.7 Spinal nerves receive sensory information from specific areas of the body called dermatomes. These nerves also innervate muscles that are organized in myotomal groups.

Central Nervous System (CNS)

The peripheral nervous system does not process the afferent information it collects; nor does it issue the efferent commands it carries to the muscles and viscera. It functions only as a receiver and sender for the CNS. The central nervous system is the control center of the organism, for it is in the CNS that the input from the PNS is processed and the output to the PNS is programmed. Before considering the two main divisions of the CNS, the brain and the spinal cord, we shall examine the protective tissue that insulates these vital organs from the rest of the body.

Protection for the CNS

Nature has provided the CNS with special protective mechanisms. Both parts of the CNS, the brain and the spinal cord, are covered with three insulating layers called the meninges (Figure 3.8). These layers are named descriptively: The outer layer (the *dura mater*) translates from the Latin to "tough mother." Indeed, the dura mater is a very tough layer of tissue. The second layer is the *arachnoid layer*, meaning spiderweb, and as its name suggests, it is a thick fibrous mass. The name for the innermost layer, *pia mater*, means literally "tender mother." This is a soft layer that actually comes in contact with the neural tissue of the brain and spinal cord.

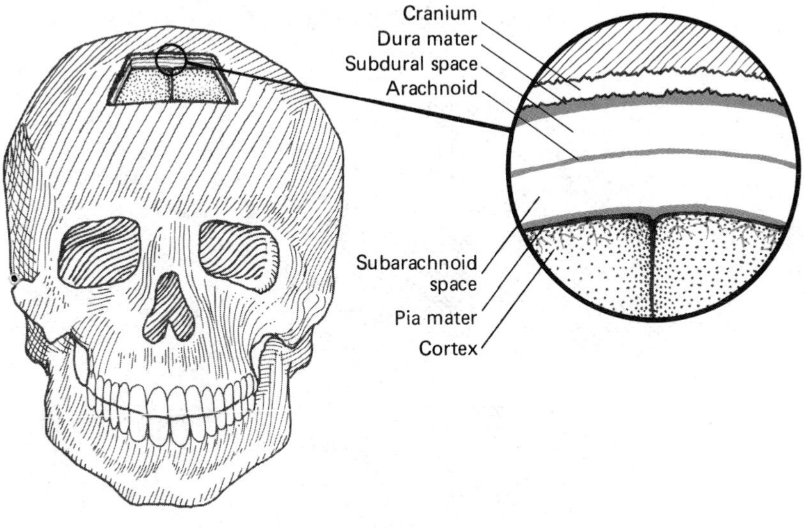

FIGURE 3.8 Meningeal layers of the brain. These layers include the pia mater, which is directly on the surface of the cortex, followed by the arachnoid system. Enveloping the whole brain is the very thick dura mater.

In between these layers flows the *cerebrospinal fluid*, which circulates through the brain, mainly in four cavities called *ventricles* (Figure 3.9), and also runs through the center of the spinal cord. The cerebrospinal fluid carries nutrition to the central nervous system (as does blood to the rest of the body), and also serves as a cushioning agent for the tender tissues of the central nervous system.

A final protective mechanism is the *blood-brain barrier*. This is a molecular mechanism that filters nutrients out of the blood and into the cerebrospinal fluid, and also selectively prevents or delays the entrance of other chemical substances that might be harmful to the delicate and crucial chemical balance of the brain.

The Spinal Cord

The spinal cord, as part of the central nervous system, is responsible mainly for receiving sensory information transmitted by the peripheral nervous system and sending it to the brain, and for transferring the motor commands from the brain to the muscles by way of the peripheral nerves. The spinal cord is also responsible for reflex processing (see Chapter 9). All incoming (afferent) and outgoing (efferent) fibers of the nervous system, with the exception of the cranial nerves, run through the spinal cord. Not surprisingly, the spinal fibers going up to the brain are called *ascending fiber tracts*, and the fibers coming down from the brain are called *descending fiber tracts* (Figure 3.10).

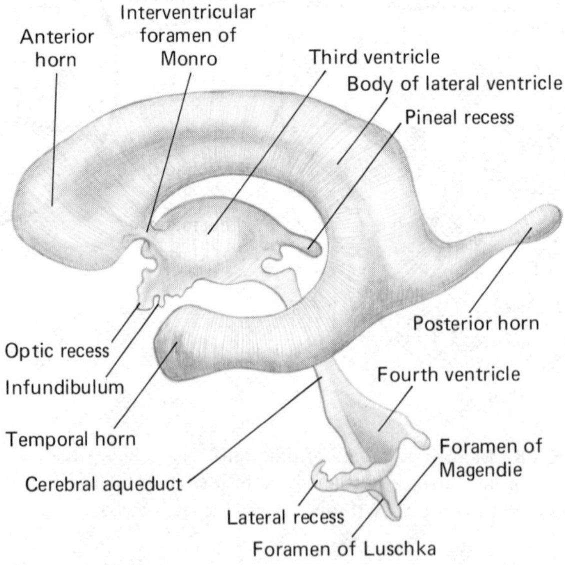

FIGURE 3.9
The ventricular system of the brain seen from a direct lateral view.

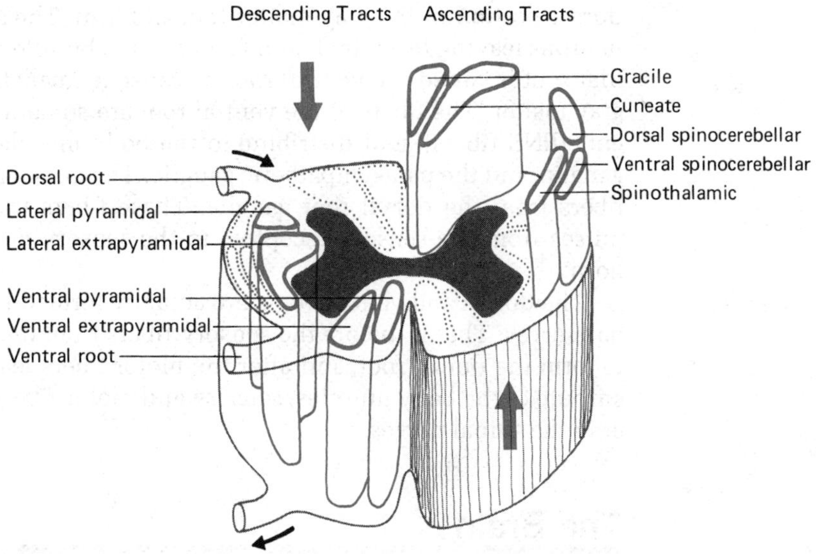

FIGURE 3.10 Ascending and descending tracts of the spinal cord. These tracts make up the white matter of the cord. Tracts in the dorsal part of the white matter are generally sensory tracts carrying information to the brain. The ventral white matter mainly contains descending motor fibers.

Anatomy of the Spinal Cord

The spinal cord begins at the base of the brain, just below the skull. The cord, which is made up of the ascending and descending fiber tracts (*white matter*) and cell bodies of neurons (*gray matter*), is protected by the bony structure of the vertebral column, and like the brain, is immediately surrounded by the three layers of *meninges*. In the center of the cord is the *central canal*, which is filled with cerebrospinal fluid. The cord, as is most of the body, is bilaterally symmetrical; that is, if it were cut through the central canal, the two halves would be identical. The fiber tracts and the cell bodies form a butterfly-shaped design in the cord; cell bodies and unmyelinated axons being the gray butterfly (see Figure 3.10).

The cell bodies making up the gray matter of the cord are of three classes: Two classes are neurons whose axons make up the descending and ascending fiber tracts, including *motoneurons (motor neurons)* and *sensory neurons*. The third class is composed of interneurons, the function of which, as their name suggests, is to interconnect spinal neurons near one another.

The motoneurons are concentrated in the ventral portion of the gray matter (ventral horn) and the sensory neurons are concentrated in the dorsal portion of the gray matter (dorsal horn). The axons of the motorneurons leaving the spinal cord form a nerve bundle or root. This particular root is called the *ventral root*, because it emanates from the ventral gray matter. The fibers of the ventral root are somatic and visceral efferents (PNS fibers), and distribute to the body muscles, the sympathetic ganglia, and the parasympathetic ganglia. The *dorsal root* is composed of fibers from the dorsal root ganglia. These fibers transmit sensory impulses from the sensory receptors to the sensory neurons of the dorsal horn.

The dorsal and ventral roots are actually formed from the mixed spinal nerves. That is, before the sensory fibers from the receptors separate to form the dorsal root, and after the motor fibers leave the ventral root enroute to the body muscles, sensory and motor fibers are mixed together in the spinal nerves.

The Brain

Fortunately, the 12 billion neurons of the brain are well organized, so the process of studying the brain is not without an inherent pattern. The brain may be divided into three fundamental areas: the *hindbrain*, the *midbrain*, and the *forebrain*. As one would logically expect, these areas are the back part, the middle, and the front part of the brain. Each of these areas may be further subdivided into different structural components, either groups of nuclei or fiber tracts.

The Hindbrain

The hindbrain controls basic functions essential to life itself. As you will remember, Grace would first regain the ability to breathe on her own as her hindbrain was the first brain area to recover from the effects of the drug overdose. The brain and spinal cord come together in the hindbrain, much of which retains the tubular formation of the spinal cord (Figure 3.11). There is no distinct dividing line between the two. Two structures of the hindbrain included in what is called the *brain stem* are the *medulla* and the *pons*. A third hindbrain structure, the *cerebellum*, is the largest of the three, and is technically not considered part of the brain stem.

FIGURE 3.11 Schematic cross-sectional view of the medulla (a) and pons (b). The level of the section is shown by the line through the brain stem in the midsagittal views of the brain. (Adapted from Thompson, 1967).

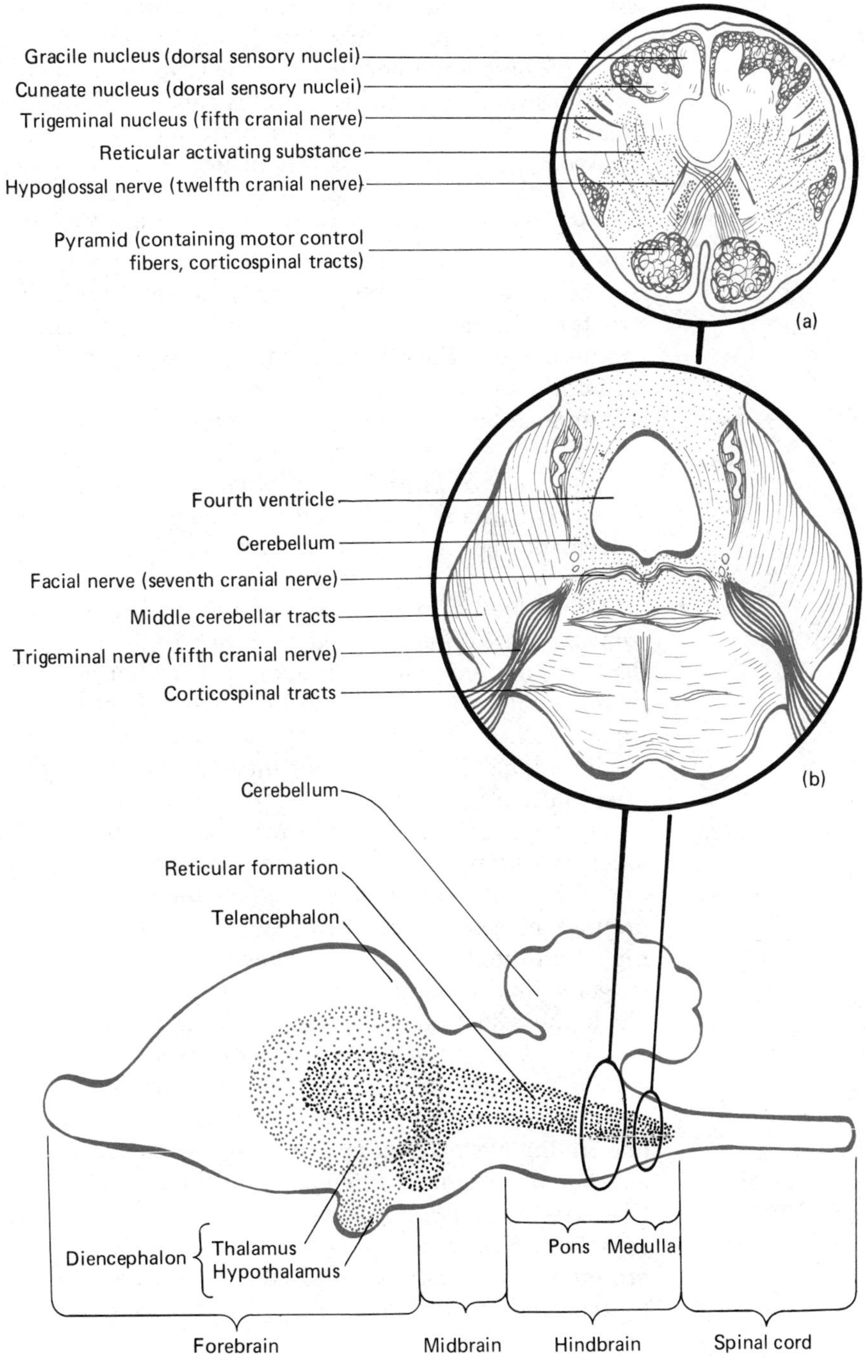
Gracile nucleus (dorsal sensory nuclei)
Cuneate nucleus (dorsal sensory nuclei)
Trigeminal nucleus (fifth cranial nerve)
Reticular activating substance
Hypoglossal nerve (twelfth cranial nerve)
Pyramid (containing motor control fibers, corticospinal tracts)
(a)
Fourth ventricle
Cerebellum
Facial nerve (seventh cranial nerve)
Middle cerebellar tracts
Trigeminal nerve (fifth cranial nerve)
Corticospinal tracts
(b)
Cerebellum
Reticular formation
Telencephalon
Diencephalon
Thalamus
Hypothalamus
Pons
Medulla
Forebrain
Midbrain
Hindbrain
Spinal cord

The Medulla The medulla is often described as an extension and enlargement of the spinal cord (see Figure 3.11). All of the descending and ascending fiber tracts pass through the medulla, and in addition, many of the cranial nerves enter the CNS in the medulla. However, unlike the spinal cord, the medulla is capable of higher-order processing. Many of the vital reflexes of the body such as heart rate, breathing, and digestion are controlled wholly or in part by nuclei in the medulla.

The Pons A second brain stem structure of the hindbrain is the pons, literally "the bridge." As its name suggests, the pons serves as a connecting structure, linking the brain stem with the first major brain structure, the cerebellum. Like the medulla, the pons contains ascending and descending fiber tracts and the nuclei of some of the cranial nerves. An additional function of the pons is to link the two halves of the cerebellum together through a large bundle of transverse fibers.

The Cerebellum This bulblike posterior extension serves to coordinate both afferent and efferent systems. Without the cerebellum each movement may be very difficult. Ed's saga is a prime illustration.

Ed tended bar at McGlade's on the weekends now that he had retired from the post office. He had not come to the job at McGlade's by accident. A longtime patron, so long in fact that he had his own stool, Ed merely switched his place to the other side of the bar. But he held his liquor well, as they say, and for him the signs of inebriation were less the lurching gait, and more the intricate spinning of one incredible story after another.

No one made much of his complaint one weekday morning of a left-sided posterior headache. He had had headache problems in the past, and now, with the added insult of alcohol, this posterior headache aroused no special concern. But the pain continued throughout the night and into the next day. On the morning of the third day Ed could no longer walk a straight line. It was true that he had been drinking excessively these last three days, for alcohol numbed the pain, but his gait could not entirely be explained by drunkenness.

The main features of this gait were wide separation of the legs, as if to broaden his base of operation. Unsteadiness and irregularity of length and timing of step, that is, some steps were short and quickly executed, others longer than he intended, caused him to lurch from side to side. Changes in direction or position were becoming impossible to manage smoothly. Rising from a chair, stopping suddenly, or simply turning around caused such irregular swaying of the trunk that he almost fell. By the fifth day his equilibrium was so disordered he could not stand without assistance. But gait disorder was not a defect in antigravity muscle support, or ability to step, or propulsion. Ed's problem with movement represented incoordination of sensory information, balance information, and visual information so that motor activity, particularly that required to make rapid adjustments in postural changes, could not be carried out effectively. Furthermore, his headaches never stopped. Another clue to Ed's condition was that he displayed rapid jerking of his eye movements (nystagmus) when gazing in horizontal directions. All this suggested definite cerebellar pathology.

The examination confirmed each aspect of the history, for his gait and movements were completely ataxic. Lack of coordinating ability, called ataxia, was more prominent on his left leg and arm than on the right. Radiologic evaluation revealed a mass in the left posterior lobe or neocerebellum, and subsequent surgery led to removal of an abscess. A month more of hospitalization was required for rehabilitation, and although Ed could not toss darts with his former winning ways, he could get the glass of ale to his mouth without spilling a drop. His gait improved and the stories again filled the hours spent at McGlade's.

In some sense, the cerebellum, the site of Ed's problem, can be thought of as a primitive brain. It is specialized for sensory-motor control, and through the peduncles it is connected to sensory and motor cell groups in the cerebral cortex, brain stem, and spinal cord. The cerebellum is thus particularly well developed in animals capable of graceful and intricate movements, such as cats and porpoises.

The cerebellum can be divided into two hemispheres. Each cerebellar hemisphere has a cortex, which covers the underlying fiber masses (white matter) and the deep cerebellar nuclei. The cortex has three lobes. The *flocculonodular lobe* is phylogenetically the oldest part, and is called the *archicerebellum*. The *anterior lobe* is called the *paleocerebellum*. The *posterior lobe* is the newest part, and is called the *neocerebellum*. Thus, while all vertebrates have the archicerebellar and paleocerebellar lobes, the neocerebellum is more typical of mammals (Figure 3.12).

Damage to the cerebellum or its fiber tracts produces a variety of disturbances in sensory-motor control, as we have seen. Cerebellar ataxia, as Ed had, is a disturbance where voluntary movement is clumsy and disorganized. Another cerebellar disturbance is hypotonia, where muscle tone is reduced. Tremor of the muscles during movement and asthenia (muscle weakness) are also common. Finally, affected patients often find it difficult to carry out rapid movements. These and other aspects of cerebellar functioning will be explored when we examine sensory-motor integration in Chapter 10.

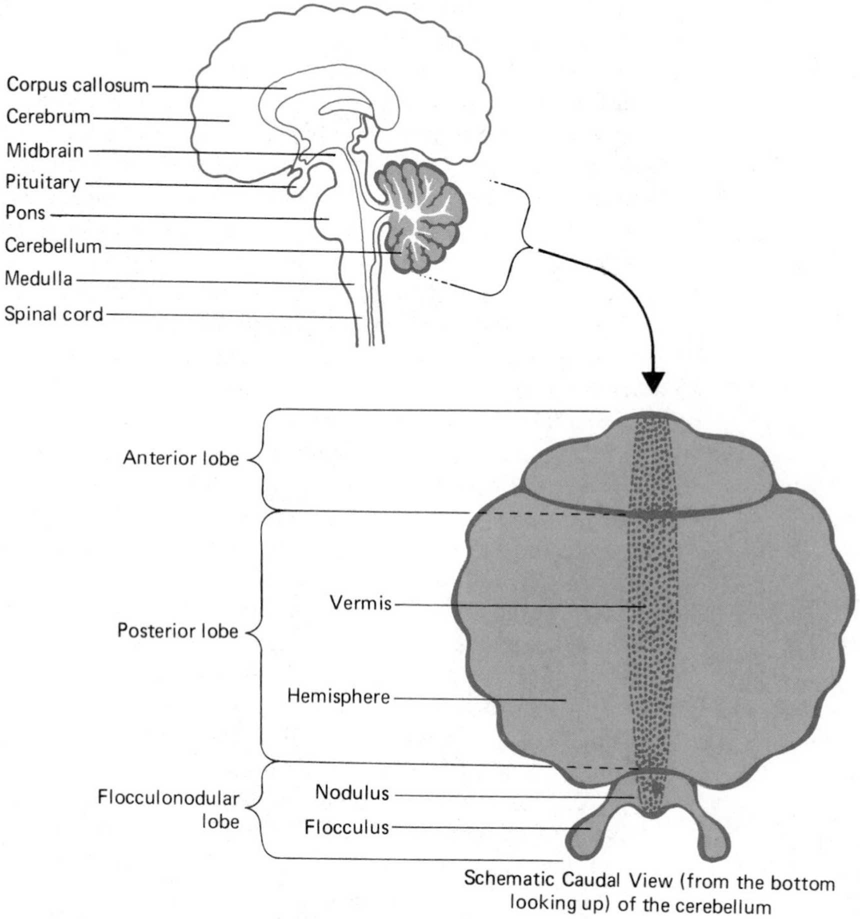

FIGURE 3.12 The cerebellum. This structure is critically involved in sensory-motor integration.

The Midbrain

Like the medulla and pons of the hindbrain, the *midbrain* is considered part of the brain stem, being largely a connecting structure, linking the hindbrain with the forebrain. The midbrain continues the tubular arrangement of the medulla and pons below it, consisting of a central canal filled with cerebrospinal fluid surrounded by gray matter, which in turn is covered with white matter. The dorsal portion of the midbrain is called the tectum; the ventral part is called the tegmentum.

The Tectum The *tectum*, sometimes called the roof of the midbrain, is important mainly because of two pairs of pea-shaped groupings of nuclei on the dorsal side. These enlarged areas are called the superior and inferior colliculi (Figure 3.13). The *superior colliculi* are involved with the processing of visual information, and in animals without well-developed cerebral (not cerebellar) cortices, the superior colliculi serve as the primary area of visual processing. In animals with a well-developed cerebral cortex, the superior colliculi seem to be involved primarily in visual reflexes, but may also mediate higher-order processing. The *inferior colliculi* are involved with the processing of auditory stimuli. In Chapters 6 and 7 the visual and auditory functions of the colliculi will be considered in detail.

The Tegmentum Through the ventral portion of the midbrain, the *tegmentum*, pass all the ascending and descending fiber tracts between the hindbrain and the forebrain. The tegmentum also contains some important nuclei, those of the third and fourth cranial nerves, which innervate the muscles of the eye. In addition, the tegmentum contains part of the reticular formation, a complex network of cell bodies and fibers that extends through the middle of the brain stem from the hindbrain to the forebrain.

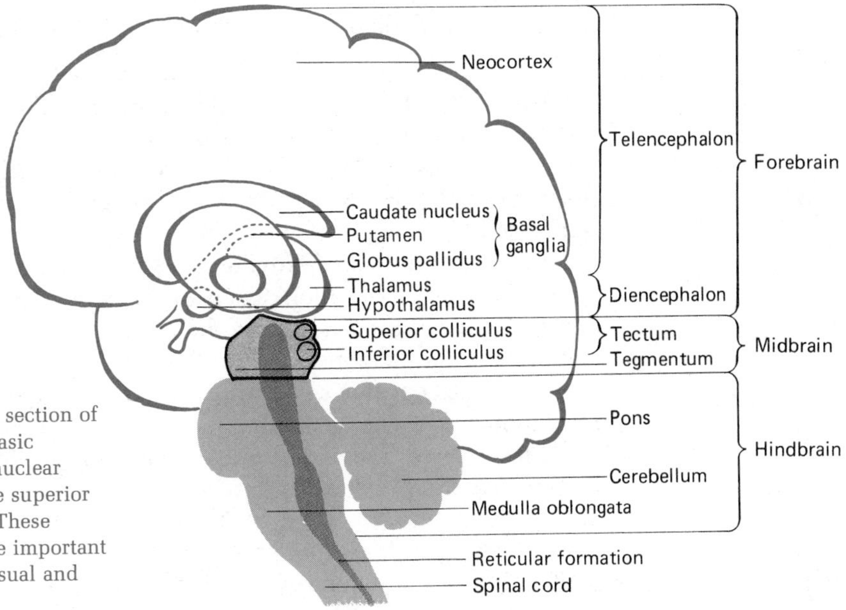

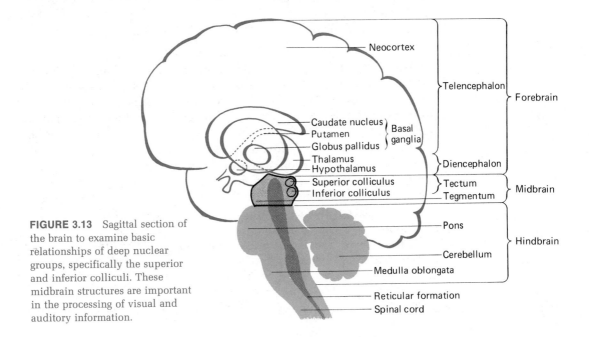

FIGURE 3.13 Sagittal section of the brain to examine basic relationships of deep nuclear groups, specifically the superior and inferior colliculi. These midbrain structures are important in the processing of visual and auditory information.

The Reticular Formation

The *reticular formation* is a somewhat different part of the brain. Rather than being a discrete structure, such as the tectum or cerebellum, the reticular formation is more like a system, composed of a network (reticulum) of small nerve cells and fibers extending through the central part of the brain stem from the medulla and pons through the tectum and tegmentum and on to the thalamus. This network of cells functions as an activating center for the organism, "arousing" the cortex so that incoming sensory information can be deciphered. Though all sensory signals go to the cortex, along the way they send short fibers (collaterals) to the reticular formation, so that the cortex is first stimulated in a general sense by the reticular formation and then is ready to receive specific sensory information.

As we shall see in Chapter 13, when we examine states of awareness, important functions of the reticular formation are the regulation of the organism's level of arousal (sleep-wakefulness) and the maintenance of attention mechanisms. Each of these functions can be selectively disrupted by reticular formation lesions.

The Forebrain

Grace was not fully conscious until her forebrain recovered from the effects of the drug, for it is the forebrain that controls the highest functions of the brain, such as abstract thinking. The forebrain is the most highly developed section of the brain. The main structures of the forebrain are the thalamus, the hypothalamus, the basal ganglia, and the cortex.

The Thalamus The *thalamus*, an oval-shaped structure located just anterior and dorsal to the midbrain, is a complex collection of nuclei that serves, among other functions, as an integrating center for the senses (Figure 3.14). One way of grouping the many thalamic nuclei is on the basis of where the nuclei project: (1) extrinsic projection, (2) extrinsic association, and (3) intrinsic.

The extrinsic projection or sensory relay nuclei receive sensory input and transfer the information to the cortex. "Relay nuclei," however, is somewhat of a misnomer, since it has been shown that the nuclei are in some cases capable of altering (or even acting upon) the sensory information.

The extrinsic association nuclei receive input from other areas within the thalamus and project to nonspecific areas of the cortex (those areas that are not directly identified with any sensory or motor function, but that are known simply as association areas).

The intrinsic nuclei differ from sensory relay and association nuclei

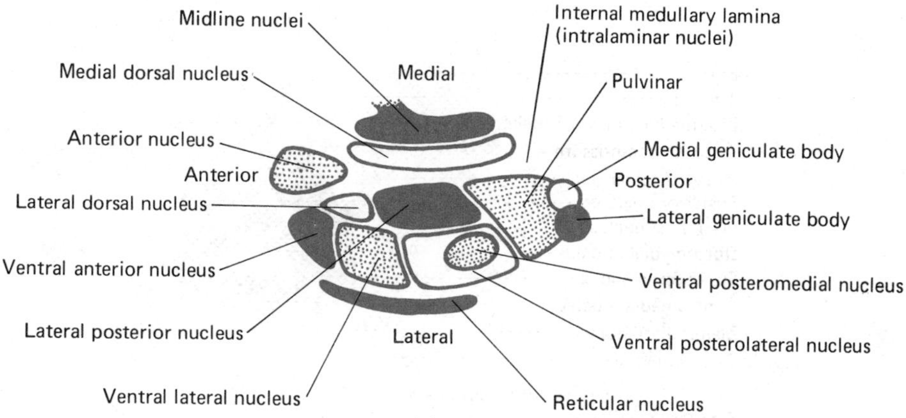

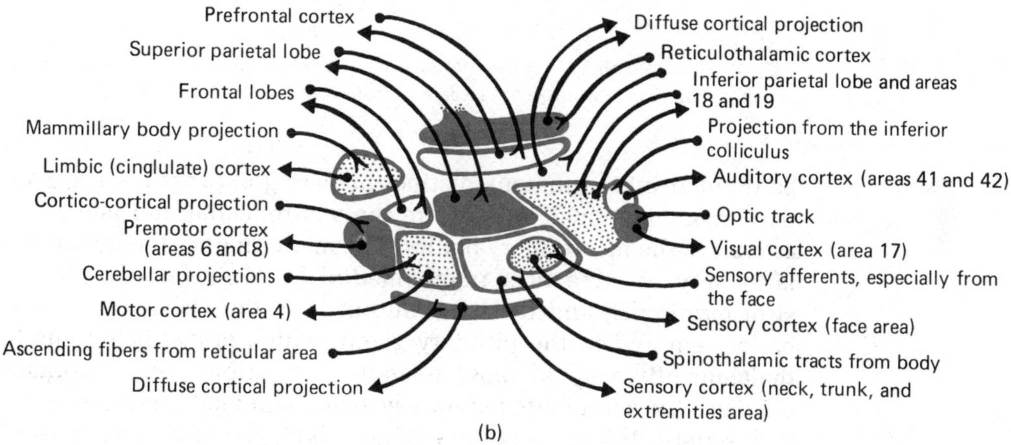

FIGURE 3.14 (a) Three-dimensional representation of the various thalamic nuclei and their afferent connections and efferent projections. This section is a horizontal cut through the left thalamus. Part (b) shows the functional relationships of the nuclei from the same horizontal cut. (Adapted from Isaacson et al., 1971.)

in that they do not project to the cortex. Instead, they provide intrathalamic communication and link the thalamus with the reticular formation and the limbic system.

The Hypothalamus The *hypothalamus* is about the size of a peanut. This tiny collection of cell bodies is located, as its name suggests, below the thalamus. In spite of its size, the hypothalamus can

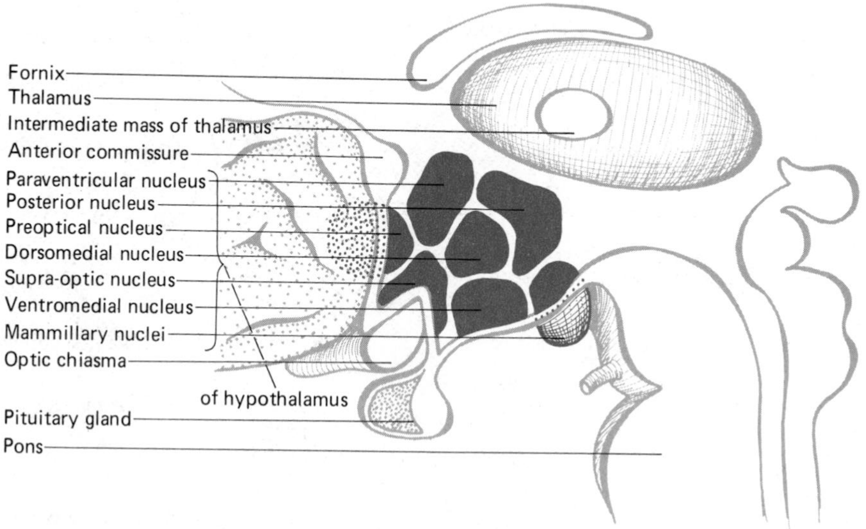

FIGURE 3.15 Schematic representation of the hypothalamus, and its relation with the adjacent thalamus and pituitary. (Adapted from Netter, 1974.)

be divided into numerous distinct nuclear groupings (Figure 3.15). Of particular functional interest are the ventromedial and lateral nuclei, as well as the mammillary bodies. The main input to the hypothalamus is by way of three fiber tracts (*medial forebrain bundle, fornix,* and *stria terminalis*) and the main output is to the visceral nuclei of the brain stem and to the pituitary gland, which is just below the hypothalamus. By way of these efferent connections, the hypothalamus regulates the autonomic nervous system. Such vital functions as hunger and satiety, thirst, osmotic pressure, body temperature, respiration, circulation, and hormonal regulation are all believed to be critically dependent upon the hypothalamus, and these will be considered, along with the role of the hypothalamus in emotion, in Chapter 11, which treats motivational and emotional mechanisms.

The Basal Ganglia The basal ganglia are not actually ganglia at all, given the fact that they are a collection of cell bodies within (not outside) the central nervous system and thus should properly be called nuclei rather than ganglia. However, accepting this discrepancy in terminology, one should know that the basal ganglia are located in the central part of each cerebral hemisphere, just under the cortex (Figure 3.16).

There are three main cell groupings in the basal ganglia: the *caudate nucleus*, the *globus pallidus*, and the *putamen*.

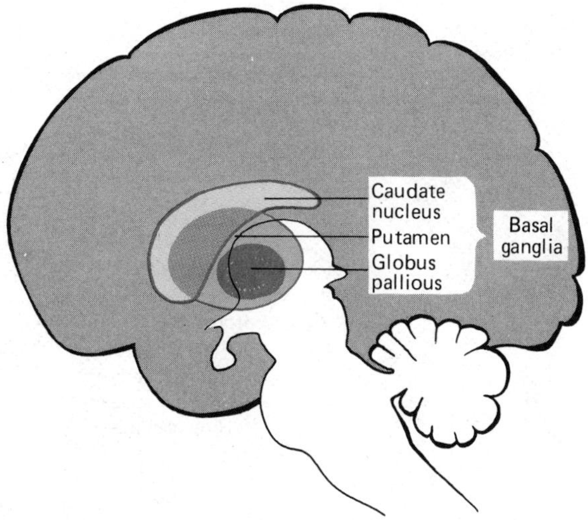

FIGURE 3.16
The basal ganglia, as viewed from the lateral aspect.

These cell populations and their fiber connections are believed to play an important role in sensory-motor control, as suggested by observations of patients with basal ganglia lesions. For example, in Parkinson's disease, there is severe degeneration of the basal ganglia. Such patients have muscular rigidity. Interestingly, however, there is a difference in how well the muscles function, depending on whether the patient is trying to intitiate a slow movement or a fast movement. The patient has almost no difficulty with high-speed movements, but finds it quite difficult to initiate slow movements. As you will recall from an earlier discussion, this is in direct contrast to what happens when a person's cerebellum is damaged. Cerebellar patients suffer a muscle tremor when they are moving rather than when they are at rest, and they have trouble initiating rapid movements.

The Limbic System

The *limbic system* is, in a sense, like the reticular formation. It is not a localized collection of neurons, but instead is spread throughout parts of the brain stem and forebrain. Included in the limbic system are the *mammilary bodies of the hypothalamus*, the *anterior nucleus of the thalamus*, the *cingulate cortex*, the *entorhinal cortex*, the *hippocampus*, the *septal nucleus*, the *amygdala*, and the various *olfactory nuclei*. Many of these structures are interrelated by the *fornix*, the *stria terminalis*, the *median forebrain bundle*, the *anterior commissure*, and other tracts shown in Figure 3.17. These fiber connections link some of the limbic structures in a circular pathway called *Papez circuit*. This cir-

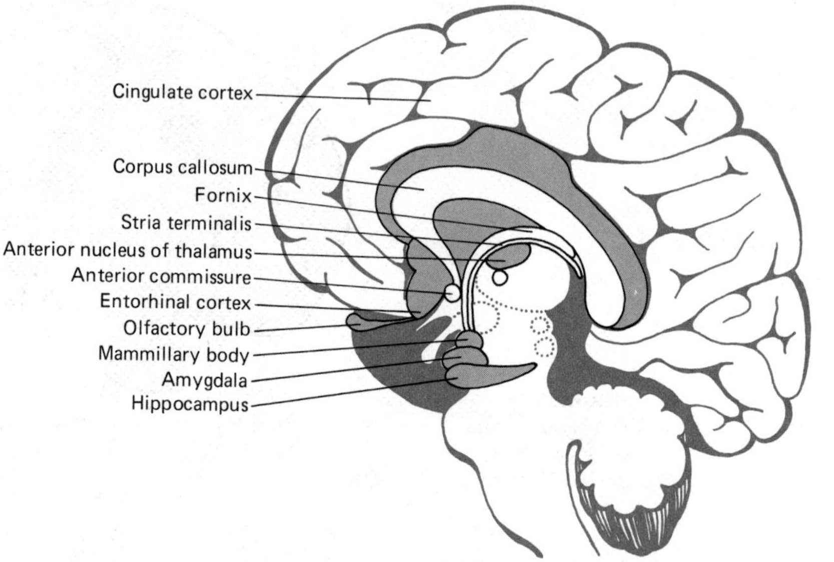

FIGURE 3.17 The limbic system with related nuclei and interconnections.

cuit, named after its discoverer, has been postulated to be the critical neuronal circuitry of emotional and instinctive responses. We shall return to these issues in Chapter 11.

Neocortex

The *neocortex* is phylogenetically the "youngest" structure of the brain. Present in well-developed form only in mammals, the neocortex accounts for 9 billion of the 12 billion neurons in the human nervous system, and one-half of the actual mass. Take away the neocortex in those organisms where it is highly developed and you are left with a vegetable, a creature incapable of volitional actions that will probably die.

Naturally, 9 billion neurons take up space, and the space adaptation through evolution is interesting. In lieu of expanding the skull and developing an enormous head, making the animal top-heavy, the cortex instead folded over the subcortical structures and developed a convoluted surface with numerous folds and valleys to accommodate the increased number of neurons. The result was that the neocortex, particularly in man, is an enormously complex mass of nuclei, the surface area being about 2 1/2 square feet if all the wrinkles and folds were unfolded.

Not only does the neocortex present a complex outward appearance;

the internal structure of the neocortex is also complicated. There are several cell types, and these types are aligned in six layers of varying thicknesses (Figure 3.18). This contrasts with the older types of cortex, which are uniform (no apparent layering), that occupy parts of the limbic system.

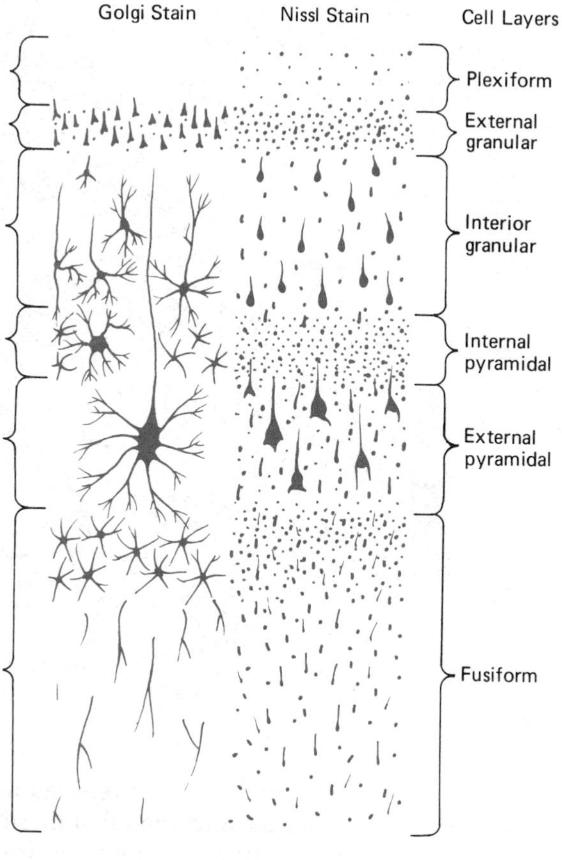

FIGURE 3.18
Laminar organization of the cerebral cortex.

The surface layer of the neocortex is composed of small cells called *horizontal cells.* The second layer consists of *granular cells*, which are small and roundish. The third layer is composed of *pyramidal cells* (so named because of their triangular shape), the fourth layer has more granular cells, the fifth layer has larger pyramidal cells, and the bottom layer has small *spindle-shaped cells.*

The density of each layer varies in different areas of the neocortex, and the surface of the cortex can be mapped using these differences in the cellular arrangements. Brodmann, a German anatomist, used this basis for mapping the cortex, and found a variety of distinct areas, which

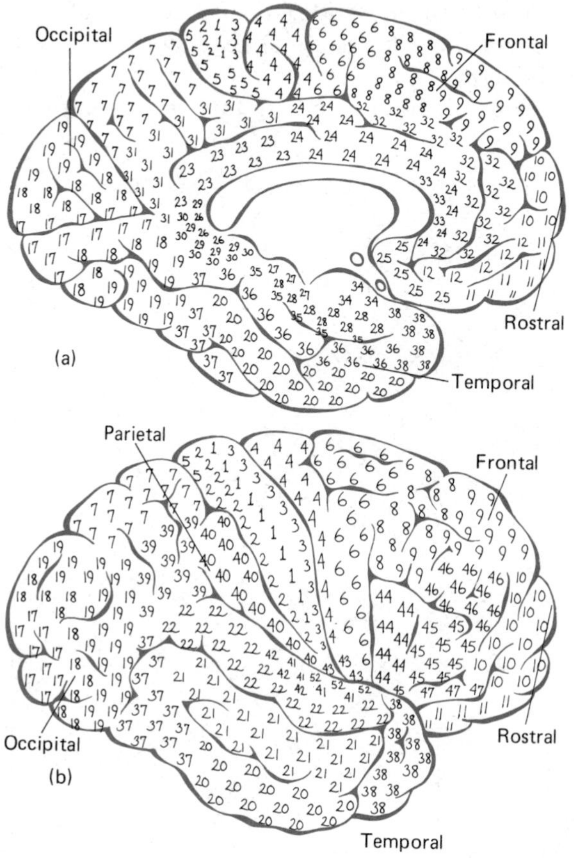

FIGURE 3.19 Brodmann's areas, a map of the cortex, often with functional significance. Part (a) represents the medial view of the left hemisphere. Part (b) represents the lateral view of the right hemisphere.

are numbered and referred to as area 7, area 29, etc. (Figure 3.19). It has since been learned that these areas, which differ in structure, also differ in function. For instance, area 17 is a visual area, and area 4 is the main cortical region of motor control.

A general statement that can be made about the cortex is that the motor areas are toward the rear, and sensory areas are toward the front. These two regions differ somewhat in their cellular composition. The sensory areas have large granular layers and small pyramidal cells, while the motor areas show just the opposite tendencies, having smaller granular layers and larger pyramidal cells.

Using the folds, made up of *gyri* (ridges) and *sulci* (valleys), for landmarks, we may divide each cerebral hemisphere into four lobes (Figure 3.20). Though the folds may look random, the brain of each species presents a similar appearance, and the folds are named, usually according

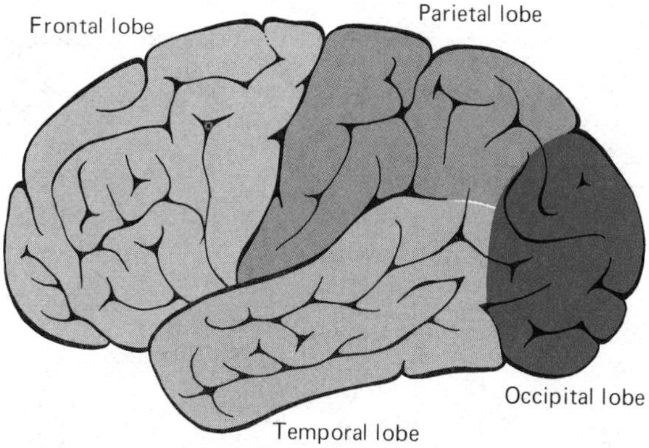

FIGURE 3.20 The lobes.

to their location. The *frontal lobe* is separated from the *parietal lobe* by the *central sulcus*. The *lateral sulcus* separates the *temporal lobe* from the frontal and parietal lobes. The posterior portion of the cortex, though not clearly separated by a single sulcus, is called the *occipital lobe*. Each of these lobes serves a different general sensory-motor function. The occipital lobe is a visual center, the temporal lobe is primarily involved with hearing, but also vision, the parietal lobe is concerned with somatosensory functions, and the frontal lobe mediates motor functions. These lobes are by no means exclusively involved with the function listed, but because sensory and motor functions are easily studied (as opposed to thought, for instance), more is known about the cortical organization of sensation and movement. Higher functions associated with particular lobes are language (temporal) and spatial ability (parietal). In addition, the frontal lobe is believed to play a role in the regulation and sequencing of behavior, but we shall discuss this in more detail later.

White Matter of the Cerebral Cortex Beneath the six layers of cells run the billions of fibers that are ascending, descending, and interconnecting the various cortical areas. Here, we are concerned with *cortico-cortical* connections, or fibers that connect one cortical area with another.

The two cerebral hemispheres, each of which contains the four lobes, are interconnected by fiber tracts called *commissures*. The two main commissures are the *anterior commissure*, which interconnects the two temporal lobes and parts of the limbic system, and the *corpus callosum*, which interconnects all four lobes of the neocortex. The commissural fibers are largely *homotopic*. That is, they arise and terminate in the same area, but in opposite hemispheres. Thus, fibers arising in the auditory association cortex (area 22) in the left hemisphere mainly terminate in area 22 in the right hemisphere.

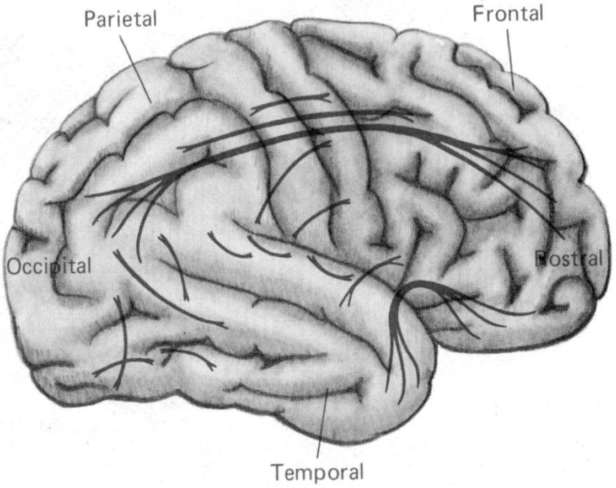

FIGURE 3.21
Intrahemispheric connections, the arcuate cortico-cortical interaction system.

In addition to the interhemispheric connections, there are cortico-cortical fibers within each hemisphere (see Figure 3.21). There are two main types of *intrahemispheric* cortico-cortical connections. The *short fibers* interconnect cells that are closely spaced. These fibers are responsible for integrating functions within a particular cell group. *Long fibers*, in contrast, are responsible for mediating functions between cell groups. Thus, while the visual functions of the occipital lobe are sustained by the short fiber connections between the cells in the occipital lobe, visual-motor integration is mediated by the long fibers between the visual areas and the motor areas.

Summary

The study of the structure and function of the human brain presents problems that are both the most complex and the most urgent to which man can address himself. It would be idle for a student of neuroscience to pretend this study will be anything but difficult. The brain is the most highly developed structure in each member of the animal kingdom, and much of the complexity in studying the human brain results from man's immense functional capabilities. Yet, there is an order to the gross organization of the brain that repeats itself with regularity not only within a species, but also within a phylum. The fundamental geometry of the nervous system that you have learned in this chapter is a necessary lesson for understanding the basic organization of brain relations in humans. Even at this gross level, one immediately confronts important issues, not only in understanding the mechanisms involved in evolutionary change, but in the role brain mass plays in human cognitive and emotional behavior.

In the stories of Grace and Ed three principles of neuroscience were illustrated. First, the hierarchy of function subserved by each general brain area was seen clearly in the case of Grace. She recovered the basic vital functions of respiration as the sedating poison left her body and the midbrain area of her brain functioned properly. The return of her ocular reflexes signaled complete return of full midbrain function, and an optimistic indication for total recovery from coma. Consciousness and the ability to sense, to process, and to respond to impulses from the outside world would be the true and final test of recovery. It was forthcoming for the vast area of cortex—frontal, temporal, parietal, and occipital—once again functionally connected to subcortical forebrain, midbrain, and hindbrain structures, produced consciousness.

The second story illustrates a specificity of function subserved by each general brain area. Dysfunction of the cerebellum produced incoordination and interruption of the smooth processing of sensory information and execution of motor commands. Specific, isolated motor acts were not lost, but the combination of several component motor parts into a complex voluntary movement, as in walking or tossing a dart, was lost.

Lost but not forever—the final principle of the structure and function of the nervous system that Ed's story illustrates is the brain's plasticity. Recovery would take time, and might never be complete, but it would progress as different remaining undamaged structures took over old functions, and damaged structures healed and reestablished new connections. Complexity abounds in the human nervous system, but there is a harmonious organization of structure and an interrelation with function that makes its study particularly exciting.

There is an urgency to this excitement; urgent not only because of the intense challenge to understand but also because of the humanitarian commitment to relieve suffering caused by mental dysfunction. Perhaps no greater illness exists than loss of cognitive or emotional or sensory-motor processes—the functions that define human life.

References

Dethier, V. G., and E. Stellar. 1964. *Animal Behavior: Its Evolutionary and Neurological Basis*. Englewood Cliffs, N. J.: Prentice-Hall.

Hoyle, G. 1975. Neural mechanisms underlying behavior of invertebrates. In: Gazzaniga, M. S., and C. Blakemore, eds. *Handbook of Psychobiology*. New York: Academic Press, pp. 3–48.

Isaacson, R. L., R. J. Douglas, J. F. Lubar, and L. W. Schmaltz. 1971. *A Primer of Physiological Psychology*. New York: Harper & Row.

Jerison, H. 1973. *Evolution of the Brain and Intelligence*. New York: Academic Press.

Lashley, K. 1950. In search of the engram. *Symp. Soc. Exp. Biol.* 4:454–482.

LeDoux, J. E., G. L. Risse, S. P. Springer, D. H. Wilson, and M. S. Gazzaniga. 1977. Cognition and commissurotomy. *Brain* *100*:87–102.

Nakamura, R., and M. S. Gazzaniga. 1977. Processing difficulties following commissurotomy. *Exp. Neurol.* 56:323–333.

Netter, F. 1974. *The CIBA Collection of Medical Illustrations*. Vol. I. Summit, N. J.: CIBA.

Thompson, R. 1967. *Foundations of Physiological Psychology*. New York: Harper & Row.

CHAPTER 4

Principles of Brain Development

To what extent did the genetic backgrounds of your parents influence the development of your brain? Are all brains alike? These questions address the controversial issue of nature vs. nurture—is development controlled genetically from within the organism itself, or do environmental factors play a part in the process? As we shall see, both nature and nurture contribute to development. The following story is one example of how nature contributes to the process of neural development, and in this case, abnormal neural development.

Allen had sought medical attention only recently. It was a reluctant search prompted by his mother, who prayed her son would be spared the agonizing disorder that affected her husband. Allen's father had been a strapping, healthy lobsterman, repeating the generational imperative of his father and his grandfather. In his fortieth year several subtle but real personality changes occurred. Always a laconic man, he became even more withdrawn, often not talking to his son or his wife for days at a stretch. And the silent period would often be punctuated by an outburst of temper in which he would destroy completely 10 or 15 lobster pots. He would find fault and complain about everything when he was not silent. Later he seemed almost to be losing his memory. The men he had dealt with since his youth were often unrecognized, and he certainly forgot their names.

The tedious and exact chores of mending the nets and the intricate wooden traps became overwhelming. Though he had once found joy in completing these chores, inattentiveness now made them a prolonged agony. The years that followed were marked by gradual deterioration of all cognitive functioning, but the progressive movement disorder made life at home impossible. In retrospect these movements were apparent even as his personality was changing. The evolution of the movements, though, was slow and almost imperceptible. At first Allen's father was considered to be fidgety or restless. Later it was determined that he suffered from Huntington's chorea.

Chorea was derived from a Greek word meaning "dance" and it referred in this case to involuntary, irregular, abrupt, jerky movements of the head, face, upper arms, and trunk. In many respects they represented a complex voluntary movement yet they were never combined into a coordinated act. Chorea accompanied all deliberate movements, and forced the old man to assume exaggerated, often grotesque, postures. Jerks of the head, facial grimacing, tongue protrusion all followed, interrupting the orderly sequence of breathing and speaking. Eventually his erratic, explosive utterances were so unintelligible that communication ceased.

This form of chorea was described by George Huntington in 1872, when he published the cases of Long Island families that his grandfather and father had studied some 50 years earlier. Huntington's major contribution was the observation that this disorder was inherited, and in fact, he called it hereditary chorea. Many studies have traced the disorder back to 1630. A vessel arrived in Boston Bay from England carrying two brothers and a third individual from Bures in Suffolk. From these men and their wives, who it is said also came from choreic stock, can be traced the evolution of the disease in Long Island, Connecticut, and Massachusetts. Old medical records indicate that by 1916 over 1000 cases could have been identified. Huntington's chorea is inherited in a dominant fashion, but it is impossible to foretell which of the offspring will be stricken in the course of years, as symptoms do not appear until the third or fourth decade. Individuals carrying the fatal genes may have died young, and Huntington himself stressed this possibility in considering apparent exceptions to his general rule that the malady "never skips a generation to manifest itself in another; once having yielded its claims, it never regains them."

Allen's mother knew the story described by Huntington because she lived with its agony. Her husband mercifully expired with pneumonia some 10 years after the onset of symptoms. He had been a wreck of a man, at the end unable to be still for even a few seconds. Sleeping and eating became as difficult as communication; exhaustion from lack of food followed. For Allen, genetics was destiny. Many promising drugs that affected the levels of different neurotransmitters were coming to the market. And maybe further study of Huntington's chorea would lead, if not to cure, at least to amelioration of the symptoms that were sure to result.

Allen's case is only one example of the relation between genetics and specific neuroprogramming. Neural development in general adheres to a genetic programming, and in this chapter we shall examine both the prescribed order of development and what happens when minor variations are introduced into that order by environmental manipulation.

The vertebrate nervous system begins development as merely a thickened area on the embryo. From these humble origins, however, emerges a complex network consisting of more than 1 trillion cells that direct the organism's every action. Neural development is naturally quite complicated, and many of the details are yet unknown. Research on neural development involves tracing the trillions of cells produced as they make their way to specific areas and selectively form synaptic connections. A particular neuron may travel through thousands of available "circuits" before forming its proper connection. Somehow, cells that appear to be the same are programmed to carry out the varied activities of brain function, ranging from maintaining basic processes, such as breathing and heart rate, to simple reflex reactions to abstract thinking and problem solving. To unfold the mysteries of this process, one must examine both the "how" and the "why" of neural development.

The question of "how" neurons progress from birth to death involves looking at the processes of proliferation, migration, and differentiation. Examining these processes provides clues concerning the answers to such key questions as "how are neurons produced?" (proliferation); "how does a neuron move from its embryonic point of origin to its terminal location?" (migration); and "how do cells form specific neuronal connections?" (differentiation).

The question of "why" cells develop in a particular way refers to the nature vs. nurture issue discussed previously. Abnormalities in genetic makeup or in environmental conditions are likely to result in variations in neural development.

We begin this chapter with a discussion of the embryonic origins of the central and peripheral nervous systems. We shall start with a description of the origin of the two types of cells found within the CNS—neurons and glial cells. Considering the "how" of neural development, we discuss the processes of proliferation, migration, and differentiation. While proliferation and migration are fairly rigid processes under genetic control, environmental factors are capable of introducing variability into the process of differentiation. Lastly, developmental variability is described in more detail, including a discussion of the anatomical, physiological, and behavioral correlates of neural plasticity.

The Embryonic Beginning of the Central and Peripheral Nervous Systems

The beginning of the nervous system in the human embryo can be seen as early as the seventeenth day after conception. This is when the thickened, elongated area called the neural plate first appears under the ectoderm on the embryonic complex (see Figure 4.1(a)). The neural plate, which represents the embryonic origin of all neural tissue, undergoes neurulation (a folding in of the edges of the neural plate). Neurulation results in the formation of the neural tube, out of which develop the central nervous system and the neural crests, from which much of the peripheral nervous system is derived (see Figure 4.1(b)). From the neural groove comes the neural tube, formed as the edges of the groove elevate further and finally meet. The three stages (plate, groove, tube) are present at the same time in different regions of the embryo. Thus, the neural groove closes first in the middle part of the embryo and proceeds to grow simultaneously in both directions, while either end is still open. The

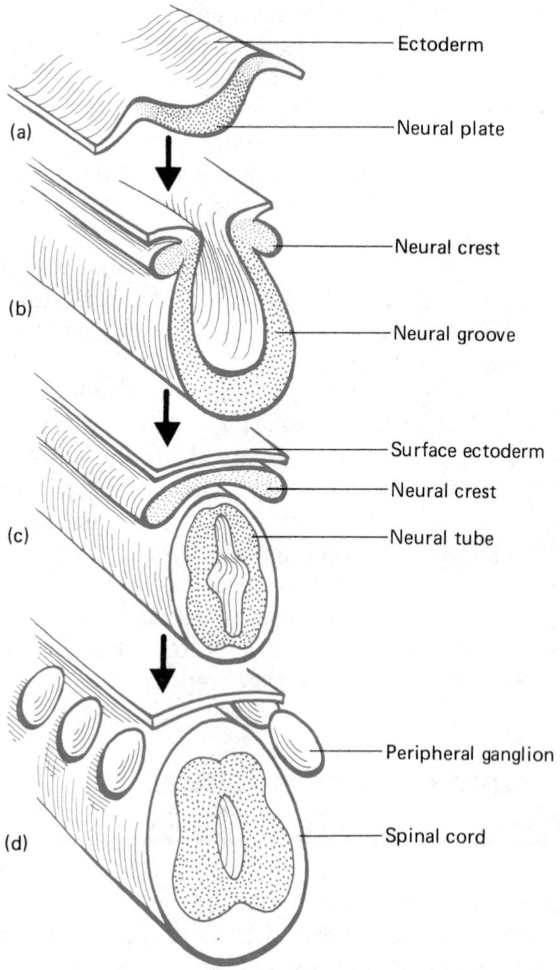

FIGURE 4.1 The developmental sequence of the neural plate as it forms to eventually develop into the spinal cord and brain, as explained in the text. (Adapted from Tuchmann-Duplesis et al., 1974.)

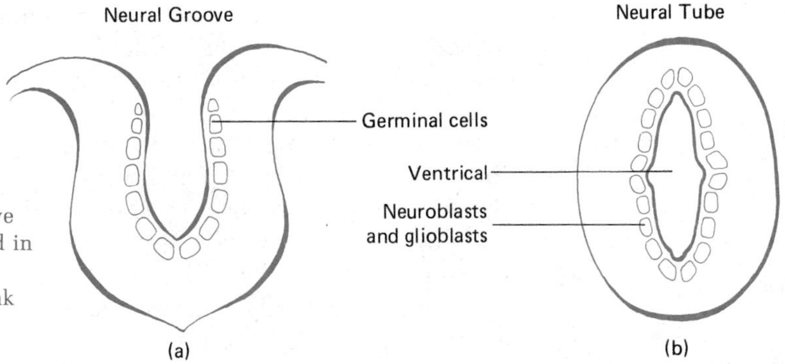

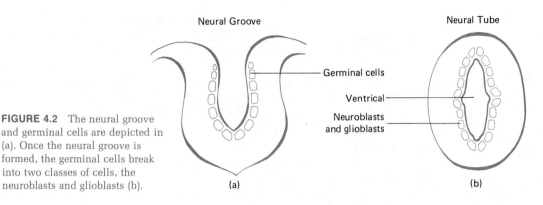

FIGURE 4.2 The neural groove and germinal cells are depicted in (a). Once the neural groove is formed, the germinal cells break into two classes of cells, the neuroblasts and glioblasts (b).

formed tube is the precursor of the central nervous system, with the wider rostral end of the tube destined to become the brain, and the caudal end developing into the spinal cord.

In addition to the neural tube, the neural crests, the cells of which give rise to parts of the peripheral nervous system, are another product of neurulation. The crests are formed as the boundary cells become detached from the region where the neural tube borders the ectoderm (see Figure 4.1(c)). The cells of the crest become lumpy and pigmented and originally form a flat band lying over the midline of the neural tube, but soon fragment. At this stage, the cells form clusters on either side of the neural tube and become the peripheral ganglia (see Figure 4.1(d)).

The Origin of Each Cell Type

The nervous system is occupied by two types of cells—neurons and glial cells. While neurons are the actual nerve cells, glial cells represent supportive tissue. Both cell types have a common origin, the neuroepithelial germinal cells. Until the neural groove closes to form the neural tube, the germinal cells are the sole occupants of the inner boundary of the neural groove (see Figure 4.2(a)). Once the neural tube is formed, the germinal cells divide to form two classes of daughter cells—neuroblasts and glioblasts (see Figure 4.2(b)). As one might guess, the neuroblasts are the precursors of neurons and the glioblasts are the precursors of glia.

Cell Proliferation

Proliferation is the process of cell production by mitosis or cell division. Germinal cell mitosis in the ventricular zone of the neural tube results in the production of neuroblasts. These daughter cells are the precursors of the neurons of the central nervous system. Cell division in the ventricular zone of the caudal (spinal cord) region of the neural tube produces thickened walls and a thin roof and floor (the dorsal side is the "roof," and the ventral side is the "floor"). From the dorsal portion, known as the alar plate, come the sensory neurons. From the ventral portion, known as the basal plate, come the motor neurons (see Figure 4.3). The sensory neurons occupy the dorsal horn area of the spinal cord, while the motor neurons occupy the ventral horns. It is the gray matter (neurons) in the dorsal and ventral horns that gives the spinal cord its characteristic butterfly appearance. Surrounding the gray matter is the marginal zone of fibers (white matter).

Mitosis in the rostral portions of the neural tube results in cells destined to become the brain. This portion of the neural tube develops with three distinct areas appearing early: the forebrain, or prosencephalon; the midbrain, or mesencephalon; and the hindbrain, or rhombencephalon. In the brain, the cell bodies (gray matter) come to occupy the areas surrounding the core of white matter. This pattern is the opposite of that found in the spinal cord.

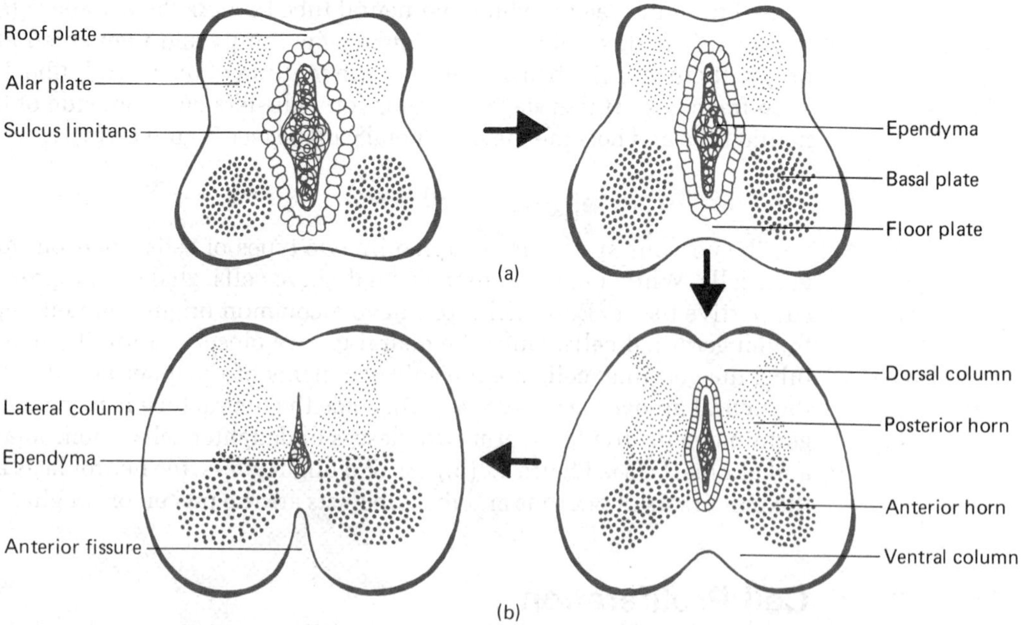

FIGURE 4.3 Part (a) is a schematic cross sectional representation of the development of the spinal cord. As the alar and basal plates begin to develop, the ventricle in the center closes in. (Adapted from Hamilton et al., 1964.) The adult spinal cord is shown in (b). See Chapter 3 for details on spinal cord organization.

The importance of proliferation in neural development is highlighted by the fact that, unlike other cell types, these daughter cells are incapable of further mitosis, thus restricting the organism's total supply of neurons to the quantity produced during embryonic proliferation. As a result a tremendous excess of neurons is produced as a safeguard against mishaps during the formation of connections. In fact, only 20 to 40 percent of the neurons produced survive as functioning cells. The remaining 60 to 80 percent die because they formed faulty or useless connections, because they were actually defective, or perhaps, according to a kind of "survival of the fittest" theory, because they were somewhat weaker than other cells.

Proliferation is an example of a developmental process under precise genetic control. There is little variation in the orderly manner in which proliferation is realized. Cells are produced sequentially, from large to small, and the basic functional cell clusters and pathways develop first, with refinements coming later. Finally, the time and place of origin of a cell determine which of the 100 or so different neuronal phenotypes will develop. The importance of space and time factors is further discussed in the next section in conjunction with studies of cell migration, another developmental process under genetic control.

Cell Migration

The migration phase of the embryonic regulation of the CNS is closely tied to both the proliferation and differentiation phases of development. Migration occurs immediately after proliferation, and the time and place of origin are significant in that they determine the destination of a migrating neuron. These same factors then affect differentiation, because the area to which a cell migrates is important in influencing what phenotype of nerve cell will develop.

The technique of autoradiography—injecting radioactive tracers into cells and following their progress (see Appendix 1)—is used to find out how a cell gets from one place to another. It is still not precisely known what factors are responsible for the migratory process. However, the following three possible explanations are being investigated: differential adhesiveness, mechanical guidance, and chemospecificity.

Migration is the process that determines the relative location of gray and white matter in the CNS. In the adult spinal cord, the white matter surrounds the gray matter. This is so because the neuroblast daughter cells produced by neuroepithelial cell mitosis in the ventricular zone of the neural tube migrate to the surrounding mantle layer (see Figure 4.4). Here, the neuroblasts become neurons and soon elaborate their axonal

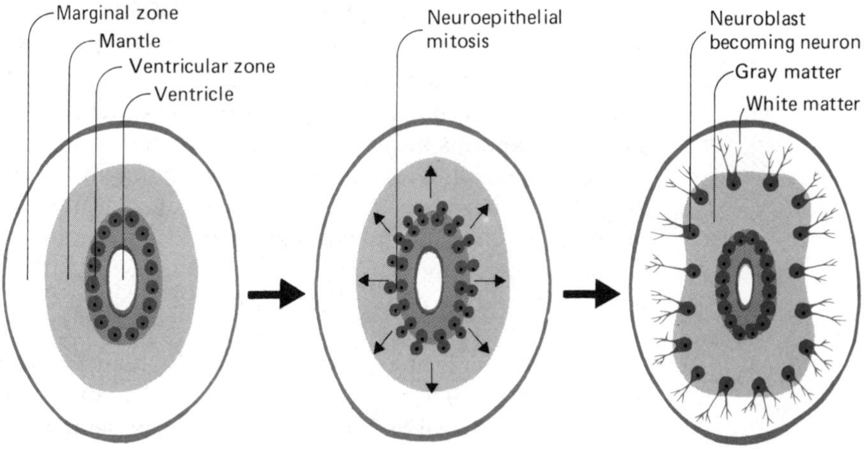

FIGURE 4.4 Migration of neuroblast daughter cells. Mitosis of neuroepithelial cells in the ventricular zone produces neuroblast daughter cells. The daughter cells then migrate to the mantle, which will become the gray matter (because it contains the cell bodies). When the neuroblasts develop into neurons, they send their fiber processes to the marginal zone, which will become the white matter (because it contains myelinated fibers).

and dendritic processes, which extend outward to the marginal layer. The end result is the beginning of the spinal cord, with white matter surrounding gray matter. Within the gray matter, neuroblasts destined to become sensory neurons migrate dorsally, while those destined to be motor neurons migrate ventrally.

In the cephalic (brain) end of the neural tube, cell mitosis in the ventricular zone produces neuroblasts that migrate outward and terminate in the most external layer. The resulting neurons send their processes inward, giving the adult brain its characteristic appearance of gray matter surrounding white matter. Autoradiographic studies of migration have shown that in the cerebral cortex of the brain, cells formed earlier are in deeper layers and cells formed later migrate through the deep layer cells to terminate more superficially (see Figure 4.5). Also, in the hippocampus, larger cells form the base, with smaller cells migrating outward to form the external layers of this structure.

In contrast to the cerebral cortex and the hippocampus, migration in the cerebellum occurs in an outside-in fashion (see Figure 4.6). This is probably due to the cerebellum's unique relation to the ventricular zone (it does not surround it). Germinal cells from the ventricular zone produce neuroblasts that migrate to the outermost layer of the cerebellum (the external granular layer). Neurons produced here migrate inward, terminating in several layers and sending their processes inward. Thus,

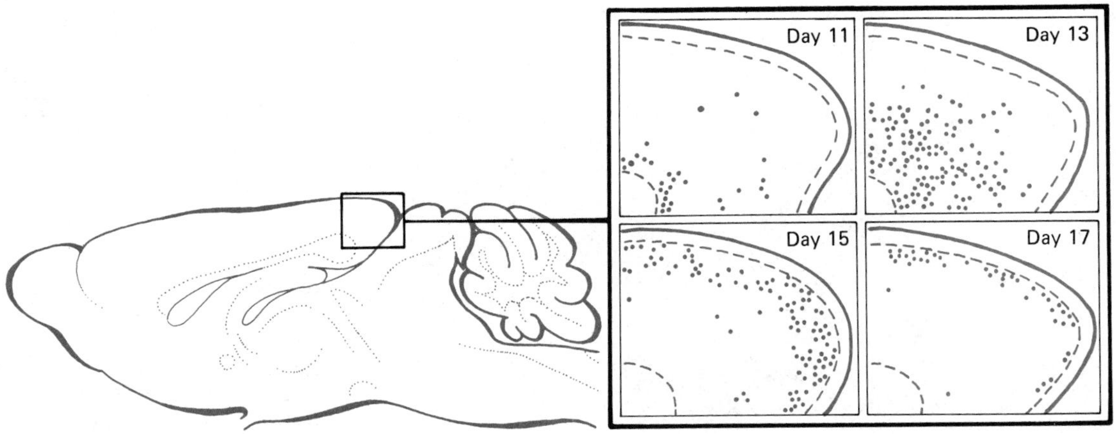

FIGURE 4.5 The results of an autoradiographic study (Angevine and Sidman, 1961), on the devlopment of mouse cortex. Each mouse received an injection of thimidine-H3 on the eleventh, thirteenth, fifteenth, or seventeenth day of gestation. The animals were killed 10 days after birth, when the radioactive neurons had reached final positions. Outer and inner borders of the cortex are indicated by the dotted lines.

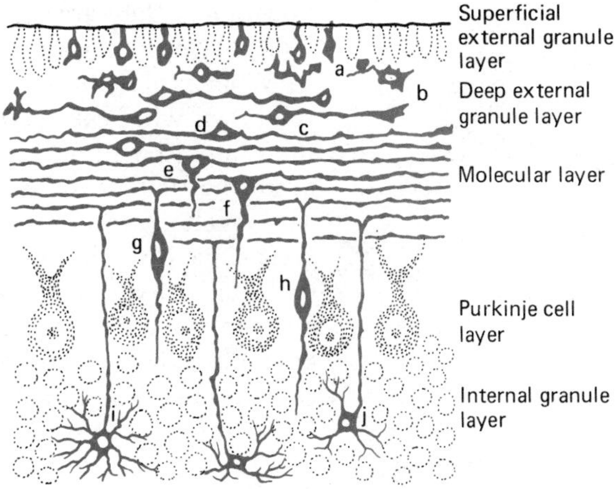

FIGURE 4.6 The phases in migration and differentiation in cerebellar granule cells (a–j). Cells move through the external granular layer, then through the molecular layer and the Purkinje layer to the internal granuler layer. (Modified from Ramon y Cajal, 1909–11.)

although migration is an outside-in sequence in the cerebellum, the gray matter is external to the white matter, as in the rest of the brain.

Interesting studies of nerve cell migration have been conducted "in vitro," that is, using the tissue culture approach. In these culture experiments, cells are removed from a developing brain. The isolated cells are

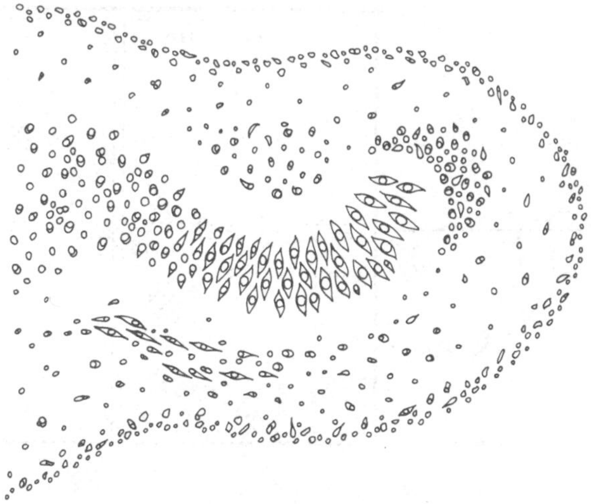

FIGURE 4.7 Drawing after the photomicrographs of Delong (1970) shows how cells aggregate after being dissociated (taken out of the mouse). The reaggregated cells resemble the adult hippocampal region of the mouse.

put in a solution and rotated for seven days. Amazingly enough, after being removed from the brain and rotated, these isolated cells reaggregate and form histotypical structures (see Figure 4.7). Studies done with cells from the hippocampal region of an 18.5-day-old mouse embryo show that the cells not only form a structure similar in shape to the hippocampus; they are also accurately aligned side by side, with the correct polar orientation.

What explanation is given for this phenomenon? It is still not precisely known what causes this cellular formation, but one can deduce that there must be some kind of alignment and orientation mechanism or agent that is distributed in a distinctive manner over the cell surfaces. The mechanism is obviously independent of the body or other brain cells since it works even with isolated cells. However, the mechanism is definitely time-dependent. Alignment is incomplete when cells are taken even half a day earlier or later. Such evidence suggests that the mechanism is a time-dependent, surface-bound chemical agent, but more research is necessary to prove the existence of such an agent.

Cell Differentiation

Differentiation of cells actually begins during proliferation, since as mentioned in the discussion of migration, the time of origin and place of origin are significant factors in determining what kind of nerve cell develops. The process of differentiation is most dramatically shown, however, in the formation of neural connections. Growth of dendritic and axonal processes has been shown to be highly specific; fibers grow along selected routes, with their final destination being specified sometimes as precisely as a particular part of a cell. Each axon sends out many branches to its target area, but only those that make appropriate synaptic connections will survive. Differentiation of dendritic processes is dependent on the availability of axonal terminals; like axons, dendrites branch out, searching for the proper connection that is specified, and only those branches that form suitable connections remain. Researchers are currently investigating what is responsible for a cell having such a high level of specificity in forming connections and what guides a migrating cell through layers of available connections without forming any connections until it reaches a certain area. Three explanations were mentioned as possible influences on migration: differential adhesiveness, mechanical guidance, and chemospecificity. Researchers are also trying to determine the degree of specificity involved. Is it so specific as to be cell-to-cell, or is it more area-to-area?

The Argument For Chemospecificity

An interesting series of studies has recently been done on the formation of connections between the eye and the brain. The optic tectum, an area of the midbrain concerned with visual function, has an orderly point-to-point correspondence with the retina. In other words, the nerve fibers leaving the retina project onto the tectum in such a way that the organization of the visual field is preserved. M. Jacobson conducted an experiment designed to show at what point the unique prespecified connections are irreversible. At early stages in a frog's development, the optic nerve can be cut and the eye inverted; the nerve will regenerate and the eye will develop normally. However, at a later stage, inversion of the eye causes the frog to have permanently inverted vision (see Figure 4.8). Thus, apparently before larval stage 29, the retinal ganglion cells are unspecified and are capable of forming connections in the tectum that are appropriate to the new position of the eye. But, within 10 hours, this capacity for connecting properly after inversion is lost, and inverting the eye of the frog after larval stage 29 will cause the frog to have permanently inverted vision, the angle of inversion depending on the angle of rotation of the eye. Actually, at larval stage 30, a mirror image is produced (one axis is correct), but at larval stage 31 and beyond, total inversion occurs. Obviously, the cells of the visual system are directed by forces within the body. Sperry, and others long before him, hypothesized that the developmental process is due to a genetic control such as a biochemical specificity acquired by each retinal ganglion cell, but no direct evidence of chemospecificity in the nervous system has yet been produced.

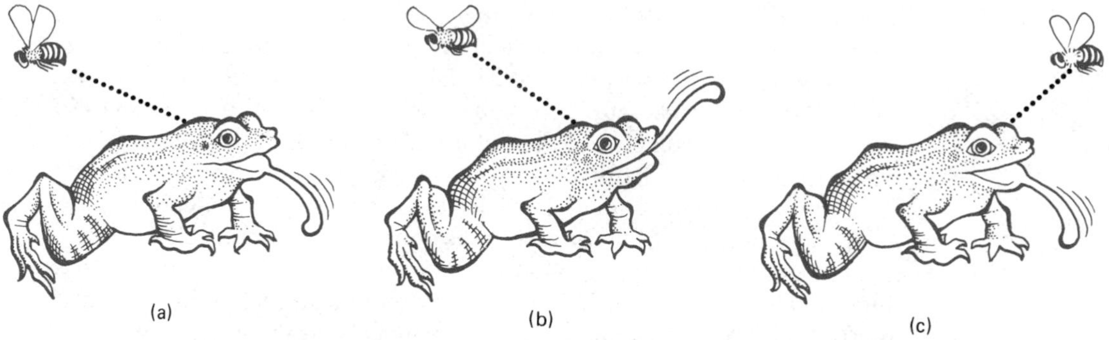

FIGURE 4.8 When the eye is rotated in various ways in the frog, the animal never compensates. (a) When the eye is rotated 180°, the animal strikes out in the opposite direction to enticing morsel of food. (b) With dorsal-ventral inversion of the eye, the animal views up as down and down as up. (c) With nasal-temporal inversion of the eye, the frog is correct with respect to the dorsal-ventral gradient, but is in error with respect to the nasal-temporal gradient. (After Sperry, 1951.)

The issue of the degree of specificity of neural connection formation has been studied in another set of experiments involving the optic tectum of fish. It should be pointed out here that the tectum in lower vertebrates consists of nine layers. Layers one through six contain most of the cells, and layers seven through nine comprise the outer, fibrous half.

A series of studies by Sperry, Attardi, and Arora demonstrated the amazing capabilities of cells when forming neuronal connections. The experiments involved cutting the optic nerve in a rough manner and removing half the retina. Then the regeneration of the fibers was traced and it was found that fibers from particular areas of the retina, according to Sperry, "connect with specific predesignated target zones in the midbrain tectum." The results of the study are shown in Figure 4.9. Consistent distinctive patterns of regeneration occurred for each type of lesion.

There was also evidence that pathways, as well as synaptic connections, were selectively determined. Fibers in some cases could have traveled through layers of the tectum with available terminals; instead, the fibers remained in the outer superficial layer, bypassing possible areas of connection in favor of their designated connections.

Sperry explained that this invariant programmed behavior was due to chemospecificity (see Figure 4.10). He postulated the general principle of chemospecific contact guidance: A growing nerve sends out an advance spray of microfilaments that seek chemical affinity in making connections. The correspondence between retinal and tectal fibers could be explained as a function of a chemical design that is assigned between the retina and the tectum on two axes, as the latitude and longitude of a map. This chemical code influences the growth path of the fiber as it

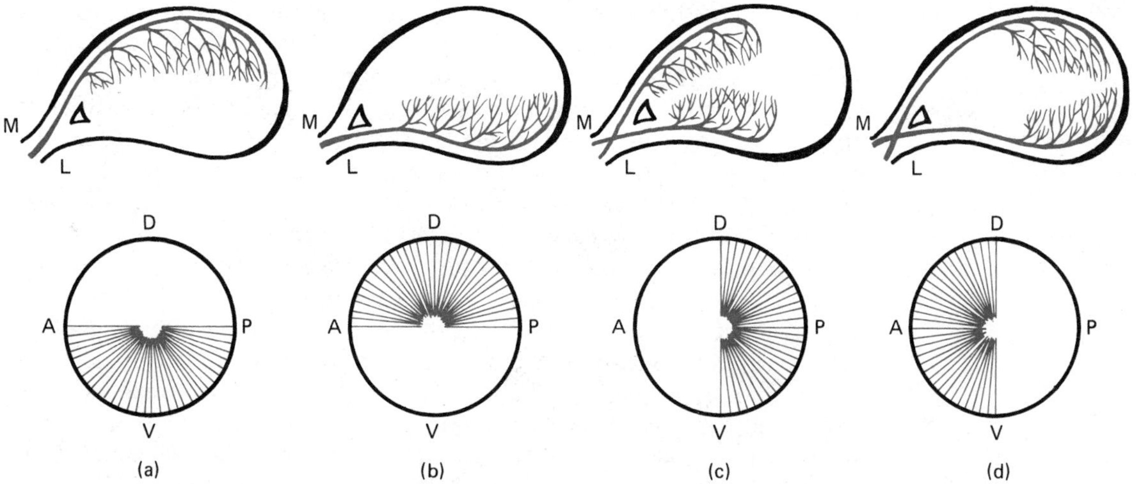

FIGURE 4.9 The degeneration pattern of the optic nerve into the tectum following nerve section and ablation of the dorsal or ventral hemiretina, respectively. The upper figures show the tectum and lower figures show the corresponding retinal lesion producing the specific tectal degeneration: (a) ventral retinal lesion, (b) dorsal lesion, (c) left hemiretinal lesion, and (d) right lesion. (After Attardi and Sperry, 1963.)

FIGURE 4.10 Schematic view of Sperry's idea of chemotactic guidance of the growing nerve fiber. Numerous alternate paths are possible, but a regenerating or freshly growing neuron specifically grows to particular points in the brain. (After Sperry, 1963.)

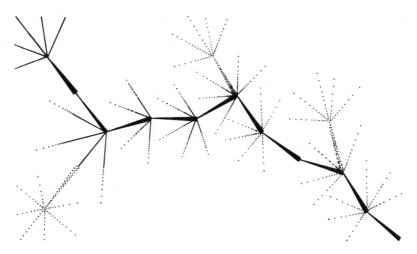

comes to each of the many hundreds of decision points in its progress from one area to another (i.e., from the retina to the tectum). The chemical specification of the two axes is apparently assigned separately; hence the results of the inverted eye experiment with the frog differ at the crucial stages between 29 and 31. At stage 29, inversion does not alter the frog's vision; at stage 30, inversion causes only one axis to be reversed (a mirror image is produced), but at stage 31, both axes are reversed and the frog has totally inverted vision.

Skin grafts on frog tadpoles give evidence supporting the idea of chemospecificity. Apparently, the central terminals of some sensory nerves are specified after the axons of the sensory neurons make contact with peripheral receptor organs. There is an amazing correlation between skin type (back or belly) and the direction of reflexes after a skin graft. Grafts were done by removing a section of belly skin and replacing it with an inverted section of back skin and vice versa (see Figure 4.11). After a few days, stimulating a point on the grafted skin evoked a response aimed at the original position of the skin: that is, touching the back skin grafted on the belly evoked a response aimed at the back. One should note, however, that these misdirected reflexes occur only *after* normal reflexes have developed. Immediately after the operation the frog will direct its reflex movement at its back if a point on

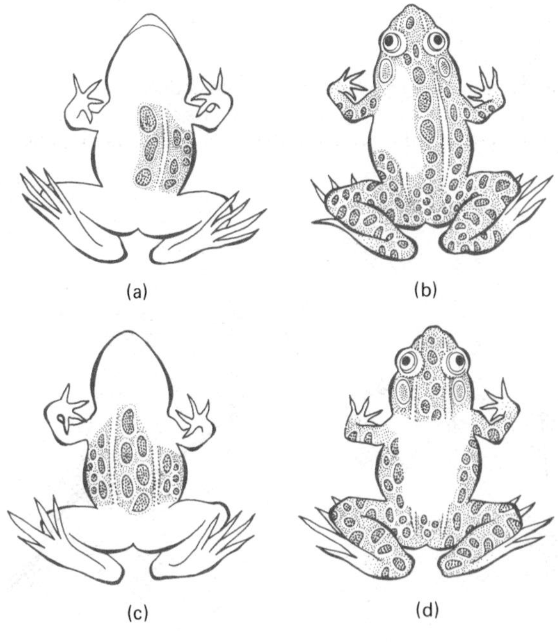

FIGURE 4.11 Frogs with a variety of skin grafts. (a) Ventral view of a frog with a back-to-belly graft; (b) the dorsal view of the frog shown in (a); (c) a view of a frog with 180° rotation of the skin on the trunk; (d) Dorsal view of the frog shown in (c). (Adapted from Jacobson, 1970.)

the grafted belly skin on the back is touched, but after a few days the frog will direct its reflex movement at the belly in the same stimulation.

This behavior may be explained as follows: When the patch of skin is removed, the cutaneous (skin) nerves are of course cut, but they soon form a connection with the new patch of skin and sensitivity is restored. The normal responses that first result come from the original central connections. After a few days, however, the nerves are somehow directed by the skin to match the reflex associations in the spinal cord to the particular type of skin (say, back) on the surface where the nerves receive information. Thus, stimulation of the grafted back skin, (grafted onto the belly in an inverted position) results in a response aimed at the back.

Time is of critical importance in this study: Grafts made *after* metamorphosis elicit only normal responses—apparently the mutability of central connections is lost after metamorphosis. Size of the graft is important also. Small grafts of less than 30 mm^2 do not elicit misdirected responses, whereas those with an area of more than 120 mm^2 elicit about 70 percent misdirected responses.

One hypothesis for explaining how the skin instructs the nerve is that "each region of the skin produces a specific biochemical change in the nerve, resulting in the formation of specific central connections." Consequently, size of the graft would be important so that enough of the central connections would be changed to affect the gross response. However, this study illustrates another problem facing those involved with research on neural connections: The results from skin grafts are based on functional behavioral responses; the anatomical conclusions are only speculative. Currently, research is concentrating on anatomical rather than functional evidence, since behavior may be influenced by many circumstances including different conditioning.

The Argument Against Chemospecificity

The problems of neural connection research are further illustrated by the somewhat contradictory experiments involving the optic tectum of fish. A series of experiments done by Jacobson and Gaze produced results that are surprisingly different from those produced by Sperry. For the first experiments, they either cut, or cut and crushed the mediolateral half of the optic nerve and removed the corresponding part of the tectum, and found that the regeneration of fibers occurred as Sperry's results predicted. Regeneration of the crushed nerve resulted in partial restoration of connections to the appropriate part of the tectum, indicating a complete lack of plasticity in the formation of connections. However, Jacobson and Gaze obtained completely different results when they moved to the rostral-caudal (front-to-back) plane of the tectum, rather than the mediolateral (side-to-side). Removal of the caudal half of the tectum combined with crushing of the optic nerve resulted in a very different result: The entire visual field projection was compressed onto the remaining half of the tectum. Gaze holds that this result argues against cell-to-cell chemospecificity. Normal cell-to-cell linkage of the retina and tectum was obviously impossible, since half of the tectum was missing, yet function was fully restored. Gaze maintains that the connection is more one of projection pattern, thus supporting a more plastic control mechanism than cell-to-cell chemospecificity. Such seemingly contradictory results may not be as confusing as they appear at first glance, however. What may be of importance here is termination pattern in the layers of the tectum. It is not yet known what is happening at the cellular level in the tectum.

The next sections will discuss other experiments that involve a degree of plasticity in the differentiation phase of the development of neural connections.

Rigidity or Plasticity?

Up to this point most of the neural cell development described has been largely under rigid control. The development of the cells studied seems to be precisely specified or "wired in" to the cells through genetic action. Jacobson has proposed that some aspects of development (e.g., differentiation) are more receptive to influence by environmental factors, while others are not. In the invariant cases, controls are activated at a certain stage in the developmental sequence and are unmodifiable. However, in the variant cases, Jacobson proposes that there are some aspects of development that, up to a point and sometimes extending into adulthood, can be changed or modified by forces outside the organism. This ability to reorganize or regenerate connections in the nervous system is called plasticity.

The cells discussed thus far can be classified as Golgi type I or class I neurons. A second type of nerve cell is the Golgi type II or class II. In contrast to type I cells, these cells are more mutable in forming connections. Often the specification of connections for type II cells must be described through functional validation. Table 4.1 summarizes the main characteristics of each type.

TABLE 4.1

Type I	Type II
1. Severely constrained genetically	1. Loosely constrained genetically
2. Rigid specification	2. Lax specification
3. Generated early	3. Continue to be generated late in ontogeny
4. Mainly macroneurons (afferent and efferent neurons with long axons; connectivity often organized topographically)	4. Mainly microneurons (interneurons with short axons)
5. Invariant connectivity	5. Variable connectivity
6. Genetic specification sufficient	6. Genetic specification not sufficient; require functional validation
7. Unmodifiable after specification that takes place early in development	7. Modifiable until specification, which may be delayed until late in development

(After Jacobson, 1970.)

Developmental Neuroplasticity

The question of whether or not development of neurons can be altered or influenced has generated much research. Evidence produced by this research supports at least a neontal period of plasticity in some areas in all animals, and there is some evidence that fish and amphibians may retain a considerable degree of plasticity even during adult life.

While it is true that genetic programming is responsible for much of the development of the CNS, changes can be induced by surgically altering neural connections, or by modifying the environment to which an animal is exposed. Plasticity is shown to a much larger extent if such changes are introduced early in life; environmental manipulation is not at all effective in changing existing neural connections.

A problem with research on plasticity, as with research on invariant development, is that many of the studies are behavior oriented. Such results cannot be as reliable as histologically oriented studies, since behavior varies from animal to animal depending on many factors. The fact that an animal after surgical manipulation is still able to perform efficiently on a particular task is not sufficient evidence for re-formation of neuronal connections; the animal may have solved the problem by using a revised strategy that did not require the connections that had been surgically altered. Behavioral evidence alone would not be sufficient to support the neonatal plasticity theory; a young animal may be more inclined to solve problems correctly simply for the novelty, whereas an older animal may have lost interest in problem solving. Thus, we shall focus on anatomical (histological), physiological, and biochemical evidence of plasticity; behavioral plasticity will be considered only as a correlate of the more direct evidence.

Surgical Alteration of Neural Connections: Anatomic Evidence

When cell bodies, or gray matter, are surgically destroyed in the CNS, the associated axons, or white matter, degenerate, as the cell body is necessary to sustain the axon. Alternatively, if axons are severed, the terminal end of the axon is isolated from the cell body and thus degenerates. The target cells of the degenerating axons therefore lose a source of afferent fibers and are said to be in a deafferented state.

The classical notion regarding deafferented cells in the CNS was that they either degenerated or survived without afferentation. However, recent data suggest that deafferented cells may reacquire synaptic input, that is, form new connections. This process is called synaptic reorganization (Lynch, 1974), and is the basis of neural plasticity.

Synaptic Reorganization Three forms of synaptic reorganization have been observed: sprouting, spreading, and extension (Steward et al., 1973) (see Figure 4.12). These processes are best explained by way of example. A simple system that can be used to exemplify these forms of synaptic reorganization is the system of afferents to an area of the hippocampus called the dentate gyrus.

The dentate gyrus is organized in a very neat and simple fashion. It has two divisions: (1) the granular division and (2) the molecular division (see Figure 4.12). The granular division contains the cell bodies, and these give rise to dendrites that extend straight up into the molecular division. Incoming axons connect to, or synapse on, the dendrites in the molecular division. These axons (afferents) are *normally* from two sources: (1) the entorhinal cortex on the same side (ipsilateral) and (2) the dentate gyrus on the other side (contralateral). The axons from the ipsilateral entorhinal cortex synapse on dendrites in the outer molecular layer, and the axons from the contralateral dentate gyrus synapse in the inner molecular layer (see Figure 4.12).

If the ipsilateral entorhinal cortex is lesioned, the molecular layer loses one of its two sources of afferents. To compensate for this loss of afferents, synaptic reorganization is initiated.

Sprouting involves an increase in the terminals in the normal dendritic target area. For example, in Figure 4.12 fibers from the contralateral dentate gyrus are shown to terminate normally in the inner molecular

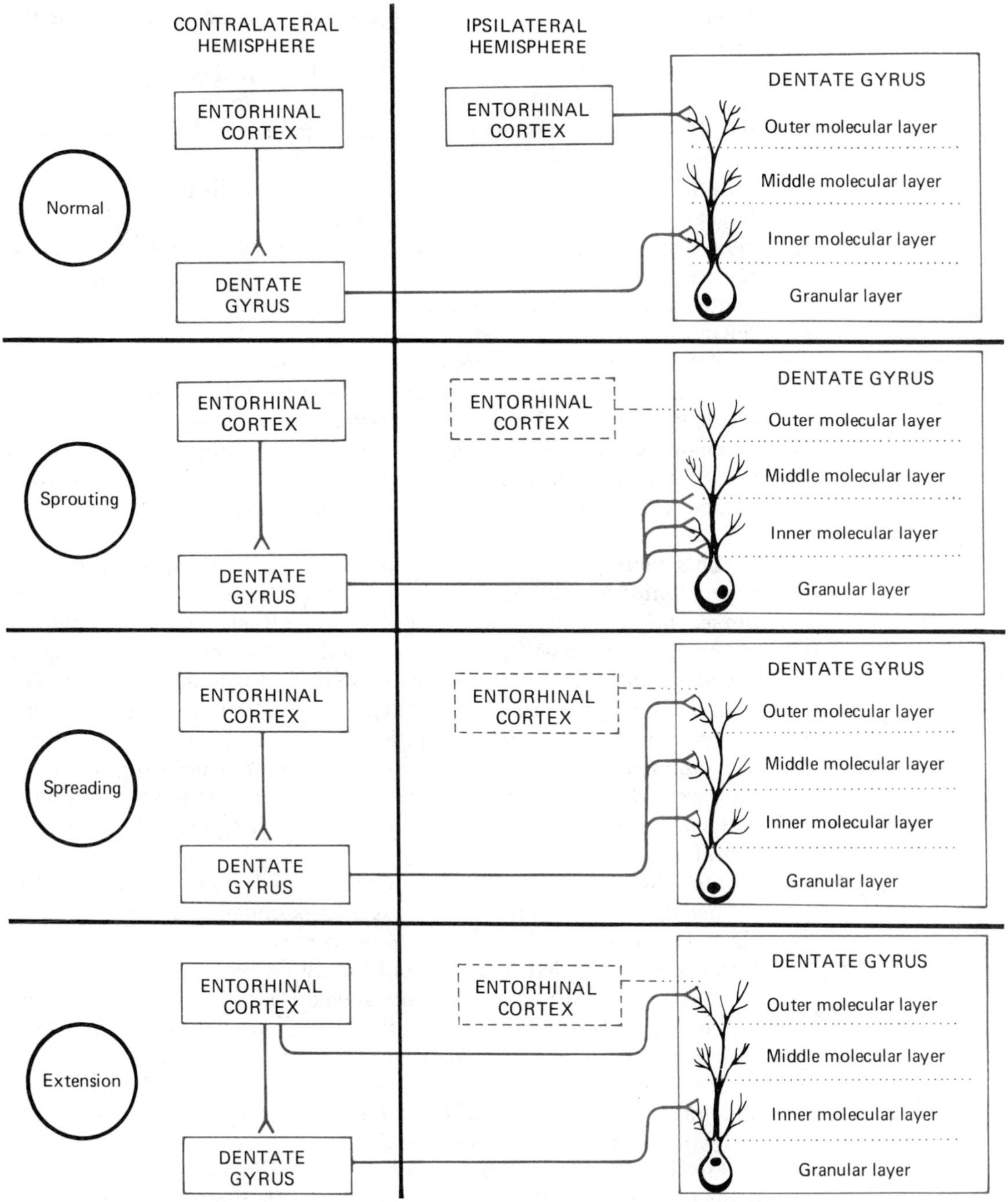

FIGURE 4.12 Types of synaptic reorganization: sprouting, spreading, and extension. See text for explanation.

layer. Sprouting occurs when there are more terminals than usual in this layer.

Spreading involves the development of terminals in new target areas, but on the original dendritic tree. This is shown in Figure 4.12 as the development of terminals throughout the molecular layer from the contralateral dentate gyrus.

While sprouting and spreading take place on cells that are the normal target of the afferent, *extension* involves the termination of afferents on cells that are not the normal target. For example, the entorhinal cortex normally gives rise to afferents forming connections with the ipsilateral dentate gyrus. In Figure 4.12, these afferents are shown extending across the midline to the contralateral dentate gyrus.

Although the synaptic reorganization of the dentate gyrus by sprouting, spreading, and extension has been shown to result in electrophysiologically functional connections, it remains to be seen whether these anomalous connections have any behavioral significance. On the other hand, a very clear example of synaptically reorganized connections correlated with behavior is presented in the following section.

This neuroplasticity phenomenon was particularly important for young Jimmy Chipps. Mr. Chipps was a fireman and Mrs. Chipps was a nurse, and they looked forward to their three-week vacation of camping in the Maryland woods. This year would be a special, new experience because their youngest boy Jim was five and he would come along. The night before leaving was filled with hectic packing, so when Jimmy appeared more irritable than usual no one noticed. He was stringing several words together now and usually both parents would stop anything they were doing to listen and talk to him. But they were planning to leave at 5 A.M. *the next day and there was still so much to do; Jimmy would just have to wait.*

Just after 11 P.M. *the details were finished, and even Jimmy had calmed down. He had his usual glass of milk and quickly dropped off to sleep. His parents followed, only to be awakened at 3* A.M. *by his cries. Mrs. Chipps struggled in and found Jimmy awake and quite upset. He seemed to be in pain, but he did not speak. He had no temperature and was quickly reassured by his mother's presence. Whatever had happened, and nothing was evident at this point, had passed, and all returned to bed. A nagging suspicion remained with Mrs. Chipps. Jimmy had not awakened in the middle of the night for over a year, and she had an instinct that something was wrong.*

Five o'clock came all too soon and the children were carried asleep to the waiting car. All loaded, the Chipps family proceeded to the Maryland woods. Soon the three other children were awake and restless for breakfast. Jimmy remained drowsy, and would not speak. Mrs. Chipps, the memory of the prior evening still fresh in her mind, was panic-stricken. Now halfway through Pennsylvania, she called her physician in New York who advised them to seek attention for the child immediately. It was now clear that Jimmy's reluctance to talk was because he could not; it had nothing to do with his sleepiness.

By noon they had returned to New York and the condition of their frightened 5-year-old was quickly evaluated. Jimmy was aphasic (could not speak) and hemiparetic (slightly paralyzed on the right side only). It seemed unlikely, but he had suffered a cerebrovascular accident. For some reason Jimmy had experienced a slight stroke in the temporal lobe of the left hemisphere. The cause of the stroke remained a mystery. He had not suffered any bad trauma. There was no evidence of heart disease, or of tumor, clotting abnormality, or arteriovenous malformation; further, there was no sign of infectious inflammation or metabolic dysfunction.

Although there was no clear cause for a vascular incident in this small boy, prognosis for recovery was much greater than in the usual case of stroke with aphasia in an adult. That he had no seizures was also a good prognostic sign, and Mr. and Mrs. Chipps could hope for much recovery of the paresis and complete return of speech. For this Mr. Chipps was grateful. He recalled the day his grandfather suffered a stroke. From that day on, normal speech was impossible for the elderly man. He never recovered the use of the right side of his body, and the debilitation of morale that resulted from the paralysis and lack of speech finally led to a sad death of the old man. Things were different for young Jimmy, however. In fact, three months later he was speaking clearly; sentences of several words were again flowing from his mouth. The paresis in his arm had completely cleared, and all that remained of that frightening experience was a memory.

Neural Plasticity and Behavior It is generally accepted that early brain damage is less devastating than lesions occurring later in life. This is believed to be true because the developing nervous system is capable of greater plasticity than the mature system. As pointed out before, however, in research on the nervous system, behavioral evidence of plasticity is not enough; the experiments by Schneider discussed below present the anatomical evidence that can be correlated with behavioral results. Schneider has shown that neonatal removal of the optic tectum of hamsters results in spared visual functioning in adulthood, that is, visual functioning survives, but similar lesions in an adult result in no sparing. In the process of examining the neural basis of these spared functions following neonatal lesions, Schneider has conducted several interesting experiments that well illustrate the functional relation between neuronal plasticity and behavior. He approached the problem of the neural basis of spared function by comparing the histological details of the visual system of normal hamsters with those of the hamsters that sustained neonatal lesions of the superior colliculus. Normally, axons from the retina terminate in the superficial gray layer of the colliculus. However, after removal of the superficial layers, retinal fibers were found to terminate in the remaining layers of the colliculus. This is another example of *spreading*.

The spared behavior that Schneider correlated with these anomalous retinal projections was visually elicited turning. Normal hamsters turn to the appropriate spot in the visual field when presented with a sunflower seed. Adult hamsters with bilateral removal of the superficial gray layers of the colliculus do not respond. Adult hamsters that sustained normal superficial gray lesions responded to presentations in certain parts of the visual field, but not in other parts. For example, animals with anomalous connections in the medial part of the residual tectum responded to seeds in the lower, but not upper, visual field; animals with anomalous connections in the lateral part of the remaining tectum responded to seeds in the upper, but not lower, visual field.

This experiment demonstrates that although the normal target area of retinal fibers is removed, the retinal fibers possess sufficient plasticity to relocate by spreading to the remaining layers of the colliculus. Furthermore, these fibers reorganize in a manner that is virtually identical to their original organization in the superficial gray layer—the upper visual field is represented in the lateral tectum, and the lower field is represented in the medial tectum. Thus, neural variability is superimposed upon an invariable framework.

Neural Plasticity, Maladaptive Behavior, and Restoration of Function In further experiments, Schneider made unilateral colliculus lesions in neonatal hamsters. In this case, he found that the retinal projections not only spread to the remaining layers of the tectum, but also extended to the contralateral tectum. As adults, these hamsters were found to make inappropriate turning responses when presented with seeds in certain locations in the visual field. Schneider went on to show that if these anomalous connections were then severed, normal turning behavior was restored.

Differential Sensory Experience: Environmental Brain Surgery

An animal reared normally is exposed to a variety of stimulus conditions. By artificially manipulating these conditions, researchers have effected anatomical, biochemical, and physiological changes in the nervous systems of animals. General studies were done with rats, but the most frequent subjects in these studies were kittens, because they have been found to have an immature cortex at birth that continues to grow and develop for a period of about three months. Changes in a cat's visual system have been induced by, for example, exposing a kitten to light only in a completely striped (either totally vertically or totally horizontally) enclosure. A cat reared under such conditions (say, exposed only to vertical lines) lacks any response to horizontal lines. Normal development of the visual system has also been changed from binocular to monocular by depriving one eye of vision. Results are presented in the following sections.

Anatomical and Biochemical Effects of Differential Experience In a series of studies carried out at the University of California at Berkeley it was found that raising rats in either enriched or deprived environments induced substantial and lasting changes in the nervous system. In the enriched condition, the rats lived in groups of 10 in a large cage supplied with many "toys" (ladders, boxes, wheels, etc.), while rats in the impoverished conditions lived alone in quiet, dimly lit, empty cages. When the brains of the enriched and deprived rats were compared, three major differences were found: (1) the enriched rats had heavier brains; (2) although the number of neurons was not found to be different, the enriched rats were found to have more glial cells; (3) the enzyme contents of the brains of the two groups were different.

In another series of studies, it was found that rearing animals in total darkness resulted in changes in the anatomical organization of the visual cortex. The most prominent of these changes were a decrease in the size of the neurons and an alteration of the length of dendrites (of type II cells) and the number of synapses on the dendrites (of type I cells).

Although these changes demonstrate that differential experience can alter the nervous system, the observed changes were very general. In the following section, specific physiological changes highly correlated with differential experience are shown.

Physiological Effects of Differential Experience Another example of neuronal plasticity has been demonstrated in recent years with a series of experiments using environmental manipulation to alter the visual system of cats. Two factors have made this type of study feasible. First, techniques for recording from single cells have been developed in the last few decades—a must for studying how the nervous system works, since each cell is extremely specialized. Second, the visual system offers a relatively easy to follow, direct pathway from the retina through the geniculate to the striate cortex.

Single-cell recording has produced precise mapping of how visual cortex cells respond. The cells respond quite selectively: Each cell re-

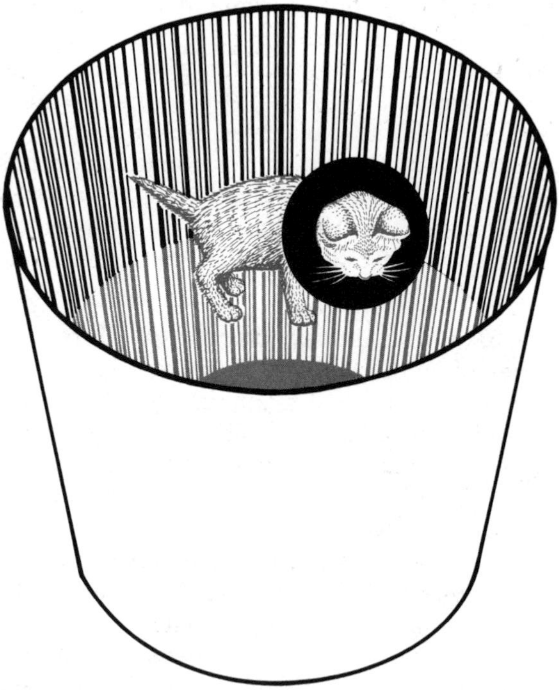

FIGURE 4.13 The visual display used to test the cats consists of a drum with vertical black and white lines. See text for explanation. (Adapted from Blakemore and Cooper, 1970.)

sponds to a particular stimulus in the receptive field, usually some kind of straight-line stimulus with a range of orientation of about 10° to 30°. The cells appear to be grouped together in columns and function as units that respond to a straight line with a particular angle of orientation (say, 45°). About 80 percent of the cells in the cortex receive input from both eyes; the other 20 percent receive input from only one eye.

Using the information recorded from visual cortex cells that had developed under normal conditions, experimenters began to alter the conditions for development and measure the effects for comparison. Cats were raised with selective visual experience, that is, they were raised in a dark room with their mother, and were exposed to light only in an environment that consisted entirely of either vertical or horizontal lines (see Figure 4.13). Analysis of visual cortex cell recordings revealed that the vertically deprived cat did not respond to vertical lines, but instead responded to horizontal lines (see Figures 4.14 and 4.15). The horizontally deprived cat exhibited no response for horizontal lines. Then further experiments were done using monocular conditions: A mask with horizontal lines over one eye and vertical lines over the other eye was worn by the kittens whenever they were exposed to light. When one eye was deprived vertically and one eye was deprived horizontally, record-

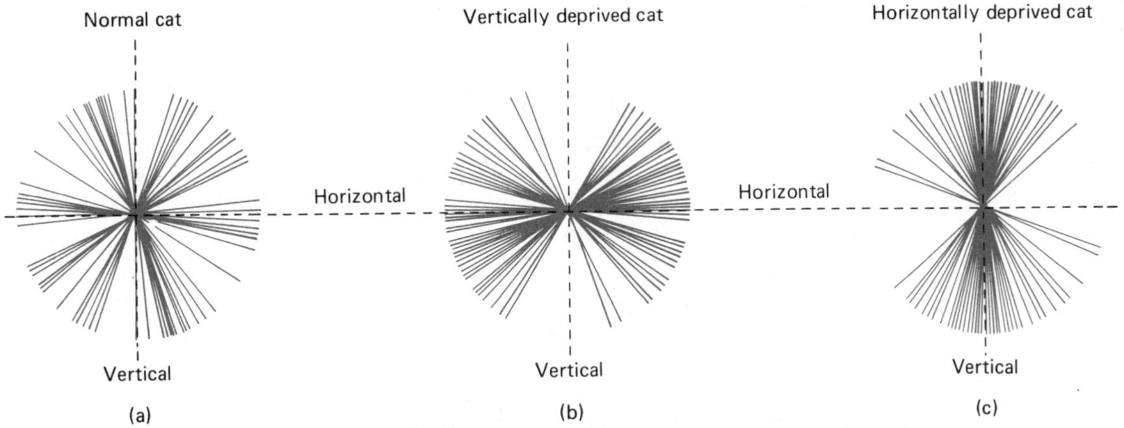

FIGURE 4.14 In (a) is seen the distribution of optimal orientation of the 34 cortical cells from a normal cat; in (b), the distribution of neuron responses of a cat brought up in a visual world containing only horizontal stripes; (c) shows cells recorded from a cat exposed only to vertical lines. (From Blakemore and Mitchell, 1973).

FIGURE 4.15 (a) This cat was raised in an environment with only vertical white lines appearing on a black background. (b) This cat saw only horizontal lines. After a few months, the horizontally deprived cat can see and navigate only around vertical obstacles. The converse is true for the vertically deprived cat.

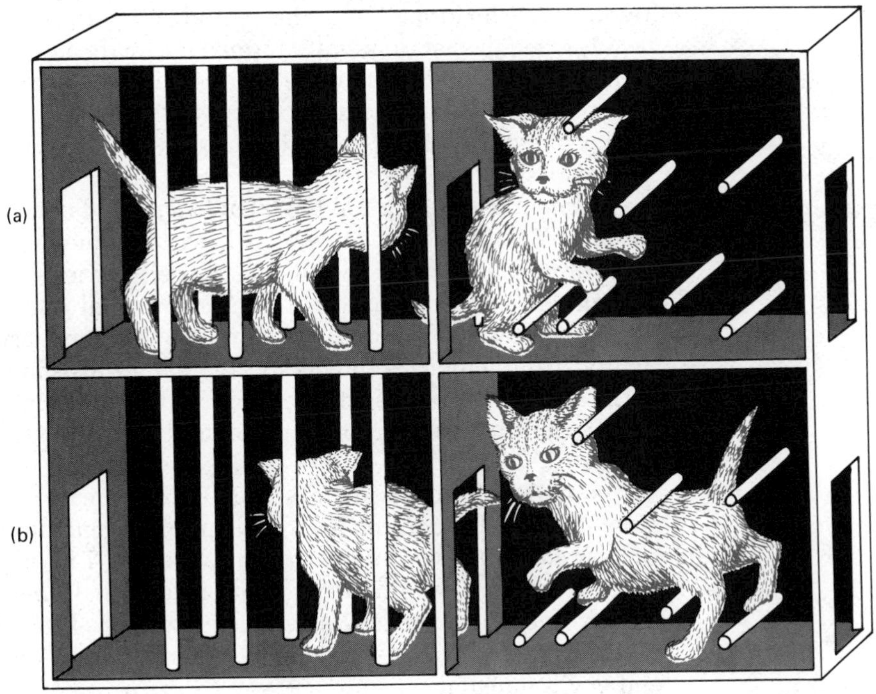

ings from the cells of the striate cortex showed that most cells responded to only one eye (under normal conditions 80 percent of the cells receive input from both eyes) and cells responded quite selectively—the cells from the eye that was trained vertically responded only to vertical lines, while the cells from the eye that was trained horizontally responded only to horizontal lines. Recordings from units of cells in the cortex showed the shape of the visual field as being either vertically or horizontally elongated, or in some cases, diffuse.

Further manipulation of cells was achieved by depriving one eye of light completely. The effect produced by this monocular occlusion was found to be worse than if *both* eyes were deprived during the developmental period. In the monocular occlusion case, none of the cells received input from the eye that had been closed—it was essentially blind. However, kittens raised in the dark were able to receive input from both eyes. Obviously, the visual system is based on binocular stimulation, and an imbalance in stimulation fails to functionally validate the right connections.

Summary

The complex adult nervous system is the end product of neural development. The formation of the central and peripheral nervous system begins when the *neural plate* is formed late in the third week of fetal life. This region of ectodermal tissue is only a single cell layer thick. It undergoes rapid proliferation and becomes stratified. Because the growth rate at the margins exceeds the growth rate in the midline, a process of neurulation results.

The neural plate folds at the lateral edges and develops into the neural tube. This tube later closes, for it will become the brain and spinal cord, or central nervous system. On the cellular level, both the neurons and glia have a common origin—neuroepithelial germinal cell mitosis. Two classes of daughter cells are produced: Neuroblasts (precursors of neurons) and glioblasts (precursors of glia). Mitosis in the cephalic end of the neural tube represents the proliferation of the brain, while mitosis in the more caudal portion represents the proliferation of the spinal cord.

As proliferation is being executed under genetic control, migration, also under genetic control, begins. Neuroblasts and glioblasts in the ventricular zone migrate outward (in most cases). The migrating daughter cells further divide, producing neurons and glial phenotypes. Finally, the developmental process is completed with the formation of interneural connections. This last process (differentiation) is under both genetic and environmental control.

The expression of genetic control is among the most fundamental questions in all neuroscience if not all biology. Allen's story illustrates the relentless expression of an aberrant genotypic heritage. Chorea and cognitive dysfunction are the features of this genetic abnormality of neural development. This disorder represents a fundamental defect in programming the structure and function of the nervous system.

Plasticity in neural development can be demonstrated through nature's own experiments. The story of little Jim Chipps represents cerebral dysfunction and remarkable recovery. Because of an acute decrease in blood supply, developing neurons were damaged. Reorganization then proceeded on a structural and functional level.

Plasticity in neural development can also be demonstrated more experimentally through surgical alterations, or environmental manipulations. In the former instance, lesions of the CNS result in deafferentation, which is the signal for the reorganization of connections to the deafferented area. *Sprouting, spreading,* and *extension* are the three forms of synaptic reorganization that have been observed. Neural plasticity (synaptic reorganization) has been correlated with spared function, novel maladaptive functions, and restored functions.

Environmental manipulations add dimension and power to the surgical experiments. One focus of these energies is to create treatment paradigms in response to nature's experiments. Another focus, just as pressing, is to understand the fundamental nature of humans.

References

Angevine, J. B., and R. L. Sidman. 1961. Autoradiographic study of cell migration during histogenesis of cerebral cortex in the mouse. *Nature 192*:766–768.

Attardi, G., and R. W. Sperry. 1963. Preferential selection of central pathways by regenerating optic fibers. *Exp. Neurol. 7*:46–64.

Blakemore, C., and G. F. Cooper. 1970. Development of the brain depends on the visual environment. *Nature 228*:477–478.

Blakemore, C., and D. E. Mitchell. 1973. Environmental modification of the visual cortex and the neural basis of learning and memory. *Nature 241*:467–468.

Cajal, S. Ramon y. 1909–11. *Histologie du Systeme Nerveux de l'Homme et des Vertebres.* Trans. by L. Azoulay. Reprinted by Instituto Ramon y Cajal del CSIC, Madrid, 1952–55.

Curtis, B. A., S. Jacobson, and E. M. Marcus. 1972. *An Introduction to the Neurosciences.* Philadelphia: Saunders.

Delong, G. R. 1970. Histogenesis of fetal mouse isocortex and hippocampus in reaggregating cell cultures. *Develop. Biol. 22*:563–583.

Gaze, R. M. 1970. *The Formation of Nerve Connections.* New York: Academic Press.

Globus, A., and A. B. Scheibel. 1967. Effect of visual deprivation on cortical neurons: A Golgi study. *Exp. Neurol. 19*:331–345.

Hamilton, W. J., J. D. Boyd, and H. W. Mossman. 1964. *Human Embryology.* Cambridge, England: Heffer and Sons.

Hirsch, H. V. B., and M. Jacobson. 1975. The perfectible brain: Principles of neuronal development. In: M. S. Gazzaniga and C. Blakemore, eds. *Handbook of Psychobiology*. New York: Academic Press.

Hirsch, H. V. B., and D. N. Spinelli. 1970. Visual experience modifies distribution of horizontally and vertically oriented receptive fields in cats. *Science 168*:869 – 871.

Hirsch, H. V. B., and D. N. Spinelli. 1971. Modification of the distribution of receptive field orientation in cats by selective visual exposure during development. *Exp. Brain Res. 12*: 509 – 527.

Hubel, D. H. 1972. Effects of distortion of sensory input on the visual system of kittens. In: D. Singh and C. T. Morgan, eds. *Current Status of Physiological Psychology: Readings*. Belmont, Calif.: Wadsworth.

Hubel, D. H., and T. N. Wiesel. 1959. Receptive fields of single neurons in the cat's striate cortex. *J. Physiol.* (London) *148*:574 – 591.

Jacobson, M. 1970. *Developmental Neurobiology*. New York: Holt, Rinehart and Winston.

Kerr, F. W. L. 1975. Structural and functional evidence of plasticity in the central nervous system. *Exp. Neurol. 48*:16 – 31.

Lynch, G. 1974. The formation of new synaptic connections after brain damage and their possible role in recovery of function. *Neurosci. Res. Prog. Bull. 12*:228 – 233.

Lynch, G., B. Stanfield, and C. W. Cotman. 1973. Developmental differences in post-lesion axonal growth in the hippocampus. *Brain Res. 59*:155 – 168.

Rosenzweig, M. R. 1970. Evidence for anatomical and chemical changes in the brain during primary learning. In: K. H. Pribram and D. E. Broadbent, eds. *Biology of Memory*. New York: Academic Press.

Schneider, G. E. 1974. Anomalous axonal connections implicated in sparing and alteration of function after early lesions. In: E. Eidelberg and D. G. Stein, eds. Function recovery after lesions of the nervous system. *Neurosciences Research Program Bulletin 12* (2).

Sidman, R. L. 1970. Cell proliferation, migration, and interaction in the developing mammalian central nervous system. In: F. O. Schmitt, ed. *The Neurosciences: Second Study Program*. New York: Rockefeller University Press.

Sperry, R. W. 1951. Mechanisms of neural maturation. In: S. S. Stevens, ed. *Handbook of Experimental Psychology*. New York: Wiley, pp. 236 – 280.

Sperry, R. W. 1963. Chemoaffinity in the orderly growth of nerve fiber patterns and connections. *Proc. Nat. Acad. Sci. 50*:703 – 710.

Steward, O., C. W. Cotman, and G. S. Lynch. 1973. Re-establishment of electrophysiologically functional entorhinal cortical input to the dentate gyrus deafferented by ipsilateral entorhinal lesions: Innervations by the contralateral entorhinal cortex. *Exp. Brain Res. 18*:396 – 414.

Tuchmann-Duplessis, H., M. Aroux, and P. Haegel. 1974. *Illustrated Human Embryology: Nervous System and Endocrine Glands*. New York: Springer-Verlag.

Wiesel, T., and D. H. Hubel. 1963. Single cell responses in striate cortex of kittens deprived of vision in one eye. *J. Neurophysiol. 26*:1003 – 1017.

CHAPTER 5

The Chemical Basis of Experience and Behavior

"Better living through chemistry" is a commercial slogan that typifies the era in which we live. Chemical additives preserve our bread, flavor our processed food, make up our toothpaste, and compose our cosmetics. Even the clothes we wear are often synthetic products of a chemical reaction that results in fabric. In the midst of a trend to protest the extensive use of chemicals, perhaps it is worth noting that the human body is itself composed of chemicals, and in fact, natural chemistry plays an essential role in determining our behavior. Understanding the chemistry of neuromuscular function was where a lot of our present understanding of modern biological chemistry started.

All neuromuscular transmission depends on a chemical reaction. It was in the 1930s that the chemical basis was formulated. Researchers found that the release of a certain chemical (acetylcholine) into the gap between the neuron and the muscle was necessary for muscular function to occur. Release of enough acetylcholine led to changes in membrane conductivity and propagation of an action potential that finally resulted in a movement of the muscle. It was this basic discovery that eventually led to successful treatment of disorders such as Stephan's, described below.

Stephan, a robust 32-year-old, had worked the North Atlantic shipping routes since quitting school 10 years ago. He was a reticent Nordic type with fine features and an extremely charming manner. He loved the sea and the seafarer's life, so it was only through absolute insistence of the company president that he consented to an in-hospital evaluation. Stephan had experienced double vision (diplopia) often, but this condition had occurred only when he had been in port and usually after much celebration. Now diplopia troubled him frequently while he was on ship, and the episodes were lasting longer and interfering with his navigations. They occurred mostly in the late afternoon, and during one attack he even noticed his left eyelid drooping. The more frustrated he became with the double vision during a single attack and the more he tried to fuse the images, the worse it became. Improvement did seem to occur after rest. He never felt sleepy or lost consciousness during these attacks, and he was always better the following morning. In the last three months he had made major sacrifices by abstaining from alcohol and taking the morning vitamins the ship's first mate suggested.

When he entered the hospital he had a fluctuating or episodic weakness of his eyelids and the yoke muscles of his eyes (the muscles that rotate the eye). There were no changes in his visual acuity (ability to distinguish objects) or in his visual fields (the areas within which objects can be seen by the eye when fixed on a point). There were also no changes in his body muscle strength. The fact that the muscles of the eye were sometimes able to function correctly implied that Stephan's disorder lay in variable factors that affected muscular transmission. In other words, the variable weakness of the eye muscles implied an important physiologic rather than structural change, and this change was probably located at the neuromuscular junction.

Stephan was suffering from a neurochemical disorder called myasthenia gravis, a malady described first in the seventeeth century but more completely 200 years later. Myasthenia gravis particularly affected his extraocular muscle function. Muscles of facial expression, mastication, swallowing, and speech are also frequently affected in patients with this disease, but they were spared in Stephan. In the most advanced cases muscles of the diaphragm, abdominal wall, and intercostal wall are affected, and when a patient is so debilitated, respiratory paralysis often occurs.

The neurochemical basis of this disease offers a rationale for treatment. Patients suffering from myasthenia gravis can be treated with chemicals that prevent certain enzymes from breaking down the neurotransmitter; improvement in muscular power often results. Edrophonium, a representative of a class of drugs that inhibits the activity of the degrading enzyme acetylcholinesterase, prevents the breakdown of acetylcholine at the neuromuscular junction. As the concentration of the enzyme transmitter, acetylcholine, remains higher, the probability of initiating muscular movement increases.

Stephan's clinical condition provided no exception to the typical improvement of muscle power when anti-acetylcholinesterase drugs were used. His drooping eyelids (called ptosis) became apparent only after blinking 20 times in rapid succession; otherwise, the drooping eyelids were completely cleared, as was his double vision.

It is almost common knowledge that certain other aspects of human behavior, such as sexual drive or state of arousal, are also under chemical influence. What we wish to present in this chapter, however, is the mounting evidence that chemical processes play a fundamental role in all aspects of human behavior. Changes in such behavioral variables as mood, emotion, attention, and motivation all appear to correlate, at least to some extent, with underlying changes at the biochemical level.

The Implications of Chemical Transmission

It is now recognized that nerve cells interact with other nerve cells by means of chemical processes at synapses—points of functional contact between neurons. These processes are a normal and integral part of brain functioning: Chemicals not only affect the brain, but are inherent in its operation. It is, in fact, through actions similar to normal brain biochemistry that drugs such as psychotogenics (e.g., LSD) induce their characteristic effects.

The implications of chemical control of neural transmission are enormous. Biochemical processes must play a fundamental role in learning, thinking, and other complex and significant aspects of human behavior. These processes may very well be intimately linked with a great many behavioral problems and mental illnesses and deficiencies. It is quite conceivable, for instance, that we will eventually understand such puzzles as why humans experience both subtle and radical changes in mood without observable cause from the environment.

Integrating the Microscopic and Macroscopic

The microscopic processes occurring at synapses have been elucidated only recently through the use of very sophisticated techniques. Our knowledge of synaptic transmission is still not complete, though enough is known to enable us to understand the importance of the biochemicals serving as transmitters in these junctions. Through increasing our knowledge of the role of neural transmitters in synapses, we also gain insight into the reasons for the effects of certain externally administered drugs on the central nervous system.

We are faced essentially with the integrative problem of understanding the relationship between a drug acting on a simple neuron, causing it to fire or not, and the incredible diversity of effects on the nervous system as a whole. This relationship between processes at the microscopic level and behavior at the macroscopic level is what the field of neuropharmacology painstakingly and slowly uncovers.

Distinguishing Biochemistry Unique to the Brain

Since all living cells involve a great variety of chemical processes, it is necessary to distinguish what it is about the biochemistry of the brain that is unique to brain cells. All cells are involved in certain metabolic activity necessary for energy production, growth, and reproduction. This includes, for example, respiration and the synthesis of proteins. We are not, however, concerned with these more or less universal characteristics of cellular chemistry.

The biochemical uniqueness of the brain appears to be in the chemistry of neural transmitters. Almost all drugs affecting mental functioning and behavior do so by either facilitating or interfering in any of a number of ways with these transmitter substances. There are also several drugs that seem to affect the rate of transmission along a single nerve fiber (rather than across synapses) by acting directly on the axonal membrane. In any case, the chemistry with which we are concerned inevitably involves the control of the transmission of information in neural pathways.

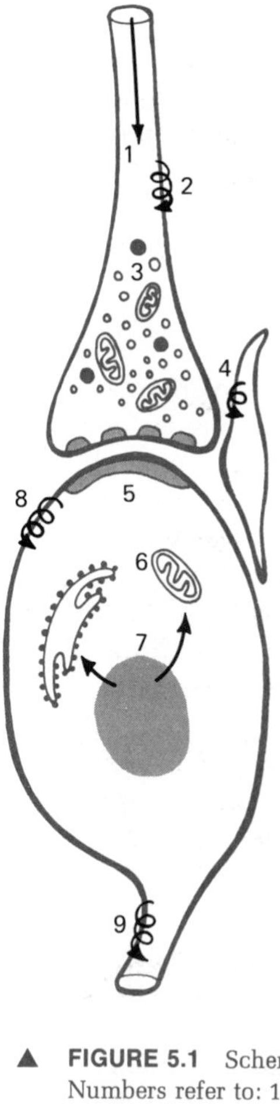

Synaptic Transmission in Action

In an earlier chapter, we described the process of synaptic transmission (see Chapter 2). In order to understand the ways in which biochemicals, or more specifically, neuropharmacological agents, can affect this transmission, it is necessary to delineate all the steps involved. Figure 5.1 is a schematic diagram of an axon of one neuron terminating on another neuron. Events on the axon side of the synapse are termed presynaptic, and events on the other side are postsynaptic (see Chapter 2).

The events are summarized as follows: The transmitter moves down the axon and is stored in the vesicles of the bouton. Any leakage of the transmitter from the bouton is destroyed by an enzyme in the glial cells and postsynaptic cell. When an action potential (spike) travels down the axon to the bouton, the chemical transmitter is released into the synapse. The membrane spike potential actually triggers an inward movement of calcium ions into the bouton, a movement which in turn somehow triggers release of the transmitter. When the transmitter reaches the chemical receptor in the postsynaptic membrane, a change in the membrane results in a postsynaptic potential. This can be either an excitation, moving the membrane potential toward spike threshold, or an inhibition, which moves the membrane potential further away from spike threshold. A spike potential will develop in the postsynaptic cells if any one or a combination of presynaptic action potentials release enough transmitter to cause depolarization of the postsynaptic cell to reach threshold level. Each release of transmitter is inactivated by a breakdown enzyme at the postsynaptic membrane, immediately after its contribution to changing the polarization (see Figure 5.2).

▲ **FIGURE 5.1** Schematic diagram of a synapse. The steps involved in transmission are summarized in the text. Numbers refer to: 1. Transport of transmitter down axon to bouton. 2. Action potential in axonal membrane. 3. Organelles and enzymes involved in synthesis, storage, release, and reuptake of transmitter. 4. Exterior enzymes for catabolizing excess transmitter. 5. Postsynaptic receptor triggered by transmitter. 6. Organelles that respond to trigger. 7. Interaction between genetic mechanism and organelles responding to trigger. Nerve cell membrane, which integrates successive postsynaptic potentials and produces an action potential. 9. Continuation of information flow down axon of postsynaptic cell via action potentials. (From Cooper et al., 1974.)

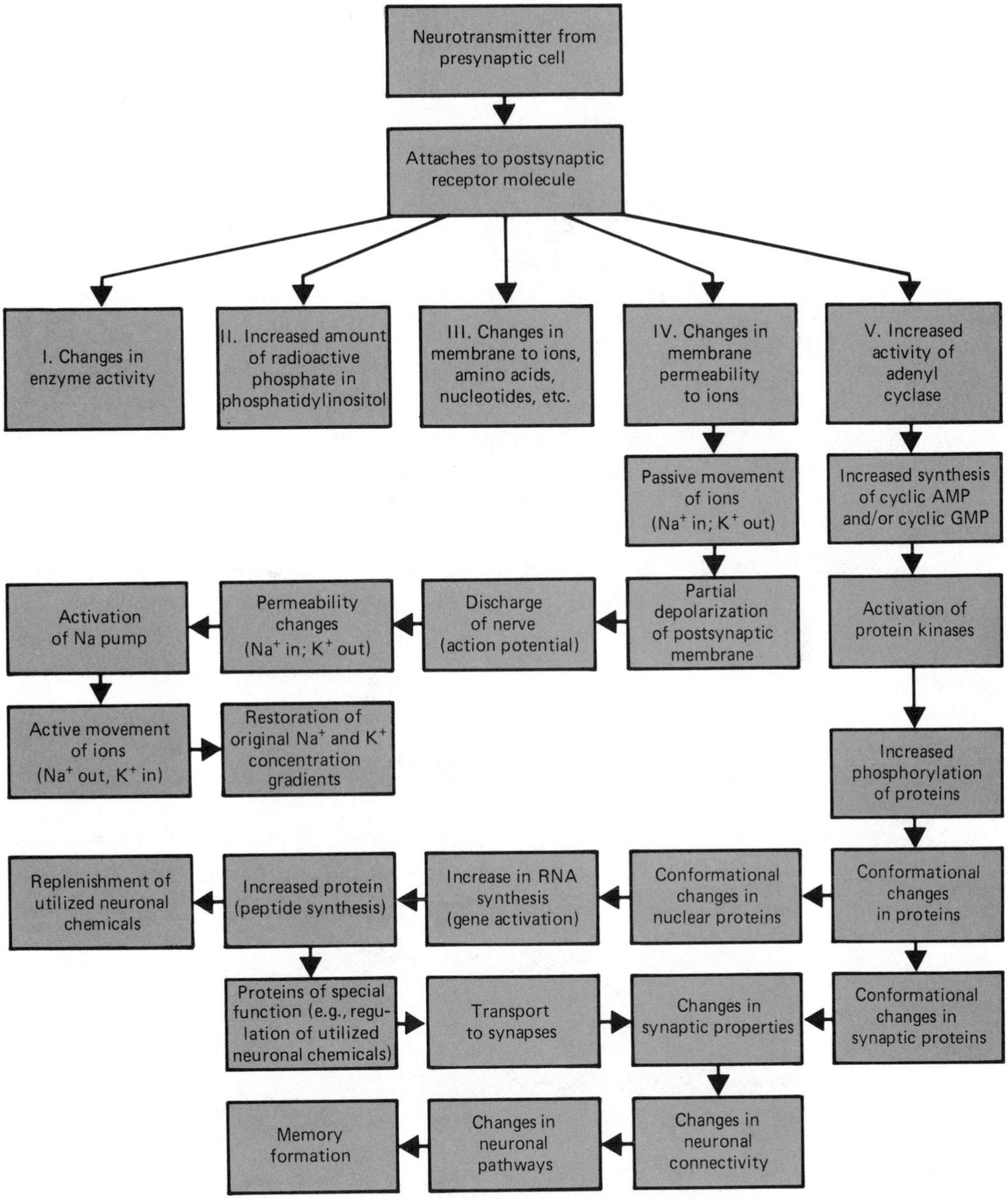

FIGURE 5.2 Some chemical events following the attachment of a neurotransmitter to a postsynaptic cell. The steps in the lower portion of the diagram are thought to lead to more permanent changes in neural interaction following repeated transmitter action. (From Glassman, 1974.)

Synaptic Transmission and Drugs: Complex Interactions

Although there are a few drugs that affect neural transmission by affecting the generation and propagation of the action potential along the axonal membrane, most drugs affect the central nervous system through their actions at synapses (see Figure 5.3). Drugs that affect synaptic transmission can do so in a number of ways, a fact that should not be surprising now that we have reviewed the complex processes involved in any transmission across a synapse.

Synaptic transmission can be affected by any of the following categories of drugs:

receptor agonists
receptor antagonists
inhibitors of transmitter synthesis
false transmitters
inhibitors of transmitter inactivation
depleting agents
displacing agents

Receptor agonists and *antagonists* mimic or antagonize the action of the naturally occurring transmitter at postsynaptic receptor sites. *Inhibitors*

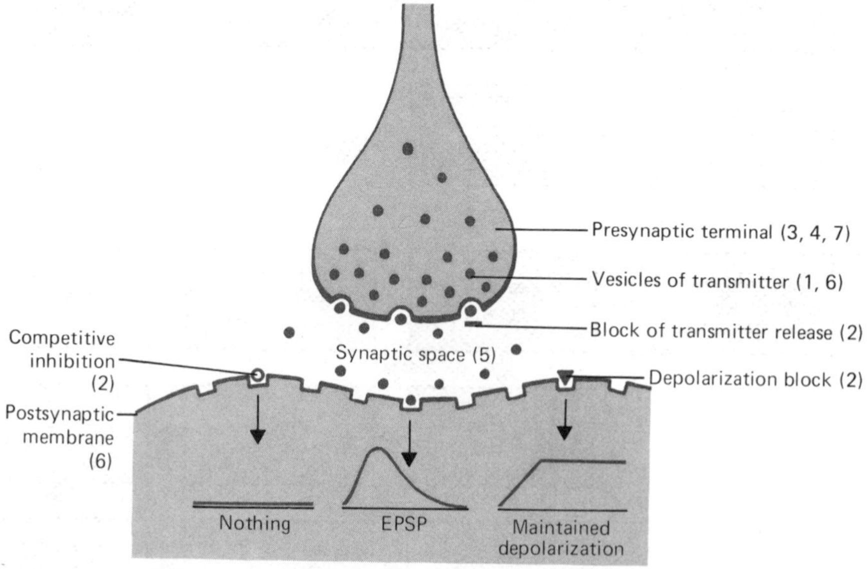

FIGURE 5.3 Schematic of where drugs can affect synaptic transmission. (1) Receptor agonists (e.g., acetylcholine), (2) receptor antagonists (e.g., botulinus toxin, curare, decamethonium), (3) inhibitors of transmitter synthesis (e.g., α-methyl p-tyrosine), (4) false transmitters (e.g., α-methyl dopa), (5) inhibitors of transmitter inactivation (e.g., anticholinesterase), (6) depleting agents (e.g., tricyclic antidepressants), (7) displacing agents (e.g., tyramine, ephedrine).

of transmitter synthesis are substances that depress synaptic transmission by blocking the normal replacement of the transmitter in the presynaptic terminal; that is, they prevent its biosynthesis. *False transmitters* are substances that are taken up and stored in presynaptic terminals and released in place of the naturally occurring transmitter. These substances depress synaptic transmission because they are usually less effective in stimulating the postsynaptic receptors. *Inhibitors of transmitter inactivation* interfere with the mechanisms normally responsible for terminating the actions of a transmitter at the postsynaptic receptor site. As a consequence, the transmitters' action is potentiated and prolonged. *Depleting agents* block the normal storage of a transmitter in synaptic vesicles and, as a consequence, create a long-lasting block in transmission in neurons using the transmitter. *Displacing agents* cause an indirect stimulation of postsynaptic receptors by releasing the naturally occurring transmitter. The transmitter is released because these agents displace it from its normal neuronal storage site.

Examples of these different types of drugs are summarized in Table 5.1.

TABLE 5.1 Some Commonly Used Drugs and Their Actions on Transmitter Systems

	Transmitter System			
Type of Action	**Noradrenaline**	**Dopamine**	**5-Hydroxytryptamine**	**Acetylcholine**
Receptor stimulant (+)[a]	Isoprenaline Clonidine	Apomorphine	Tryptamine	Oxotremorine Arecoline Carbachol
Receptor antagonist (−)[b]	Propranolol Chlorpromazine Phenoxybenzamine	Chlorpromazine Pimozide Clozapine Haloperidol	Lysergic acid-diethylamide Methysergide	Scopolamine Atropine Benztropine
Inhibitor of uptake (+)	Cocaine Amitriptyline Desipramine	Cocaine Amphetamine	Chlorimipramine Imipramine	— —
Inhibitor of metabolic breakdown (+)	MAO inhibitors: pheniprazine, iproniazid, pargyline, tranylcypromine, phenelzine			Di-isopropylfluorophosphate (DFP) Physostigmine
Inhibitors of biosynthesis (−)	α-Methyl-p-tyrosine Disulfiram	α-Methyl-p-tyrosine	p-Chlorophenylalanine	Hemicholinium
Displacing agent (+)	d-Amphetamine	d-Amphetamine l-Amphetamine	—	—
Precursor (+)	L-Dopa	L-Dopa	L-5-Hydroxytryptophan	—
False transmitter (±)	α-Methyl-*m*-tyrosine α-Methyl dopa, metaraminol			
Depleting agent (−)	reserpine, tetrabenazine, and related substances			

(Adapted from Iversen, 1974.)

[a](+) = stimulates or enhances actions of transmitter.
[b](−) = antagonizes or decreases actions of transmitter.

Neurotransmitter Pathways: Biochemical Anatomy

Our knowledge of chemical transmission in the central nervous system is far from complete. We do not yet even have a complete list of all the substances involved as transmitters, not to mention a comprehensive knowledge of the particular transmitters used in particular pathways in the CNS. A few neurochemicals have been confirmed as transmitters. In addition, a greater understanding of the functional importance of some of these has been acquired as the result of the discovery that specific neurochemicals occur in specific regions of pathways in the brain.

Chemical pathways can be defined in the sense of describing connections of neurons using some particular transmitter. In other words, certain transmitters are utilized in different areas of the brain. It may be that a particular transmitter is connected with a specific function, and it is hoped that by tracing the route along which the transmitter is found, more will be learned about how the brain functions. To find the pathways, special techniques to selectively stain neurons that contain certain transmitters are used, yielding a semiquantitative picture of the distribution of a particular transmitter in a section of the brain (Figure 5.4).

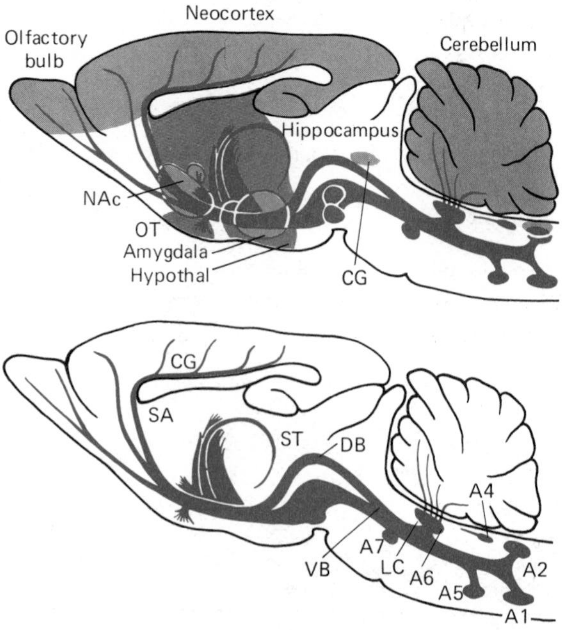

FIGURE 5.4 Schematic diagram of the major pathways of the catecholamine transmitters in rat brain. Abbreviations are defined as follows: NAc, nucleus accumbens; OT, olfactory tubercle; Ht, hypothalamus; DB, dorsal bundle; VB, ventral bundle; LC, locus ceruleus; ST, stria terminalis; CG, cingulate gyrus; $A_{1,2,4,5}$ are pontomedullary collections of norepinephrine containing neurons. (From German and Bowden, 1974; modified from Ungerstedt, 1971b.)

The Participants: Known Neurotransmitters

The present list of central nervous system transmitters is as follows:

acetylcholine (ACh)
noradrenaline (NA) also known as norepinephrine (NE)
dopamine (DA)
5-hydroxytryptamine (5-HT) also known as serotonin
gamma-amino butyric acid (GABA)
glycine

There are several other substances, such as the amino acids glutamate and aspartate, that seem likely to be transmitters, but this has not been confirmed. It is almost certain that there are other transmitters. Transmitters used by many neurons in most sensory pathways, for instance, do not appear to be any of the above. There are several contending biochemicals that may play a role in sensory pathways, but each strict criterion that establishes a substance as a neurotransmitter must be met.

The chemical structures of some of the transmitters are shown in Figure 5.5. The transmitters ACh, NA, and DA are all *amines*, com-

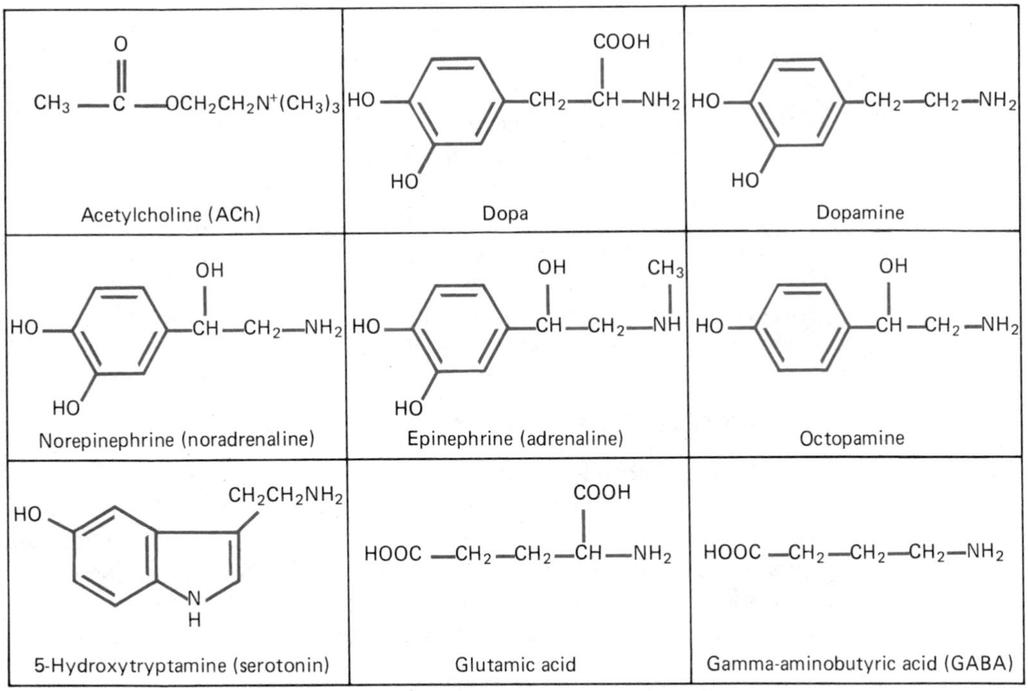

FIGURE 5.5 Chemical structures of some neurotransmitters.

pounds derived from ammonia. They are also the transmitters studied in most detail so far. Of these, DA and NA are collectively referred to as catecholamines, having a catechol nucleus in common (see Figure 5.6).

Terms such as "adrenergic" are used at times to refer to terminals involved in the release of nor*adrenal*ine (NA) or related amines. Similarly, "cholinergic" refers to terminals involved in the release of acetyl*choline* (ACh).

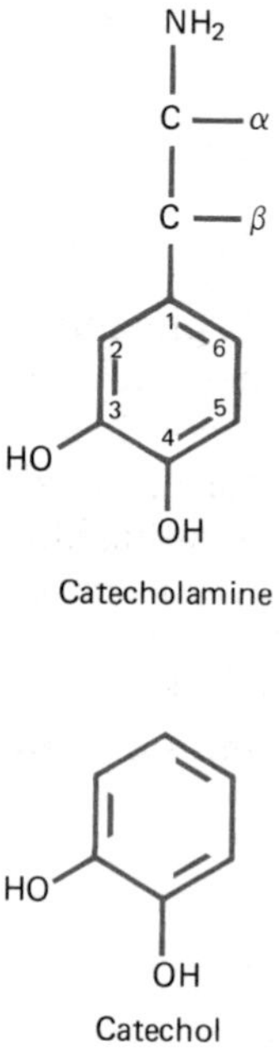

FIGURE 5.6 Catechol and catecholamine structure. The catecholamine is a catechol nucleus (benzene ring with two adjacent hydroxyl groups) and an amine group. Catecholamine usually refers to dopamine (DA) and its metabolic products noradrenaline (NA) and adrenaline.

The Biosynthesis of the Neurotransmitters

Like most substances, transmitters must be synthesized in the body. Rarely is the body able to assimilate food or other elements without first at least breaking them down into simpler compounds, and often not without further processing these compounds to form still another compound. The neural transmitters are no exception. They are formed through a process of biosynthesis. It is only in recent years that details of this process have been specified. We have just begun to crack the chemical code of the brain, and there is much more to be done to unravel all of its mysteries.

It is important to understand a little about the biosynthesis of the transmitters—that is, the steps in their formation. A great deal of control of transmitter action is dependent on the control of transmitter precursors (substances involved in transmitter synthesis), since deficiencies in certain transmitters may be due to a deficiency of necessary precursors. For example, dopamine is formed in the brain when a chemical compound called L-dopa is synthesized. Thus if there is a shortage of L-dopa (the precursor), there will be a shortage of dopamine.

Figure 5.7 shows the biosynthesis of DA, NA, and 5HT. Note especially the role of L-dopa in the formation of dopamine. This precursor of DA was critical in the discovery of the role of DA in Parkinson's disease, and also in devising therapy for the disease. Dopamine is itself a precursor for another transmitter—noradrenaline.

The Question of Transmitter Function

In turning now to studies of the functional significance of specific transmitter systems in the brain, it is important to realize that the substrates for behavioral control probably involve *interacting* neurochemical systems most of the time. There do appear, however, to be some aspects of behavior that correlate directly with single transmitters in specific pathways. The reason that a great deal of research has concentrated on establishing relations between single neurochemicals and behavior is the emergence of new experimental techniques. The actual and undoubtedly more complicated picture should eventually evolve from test-

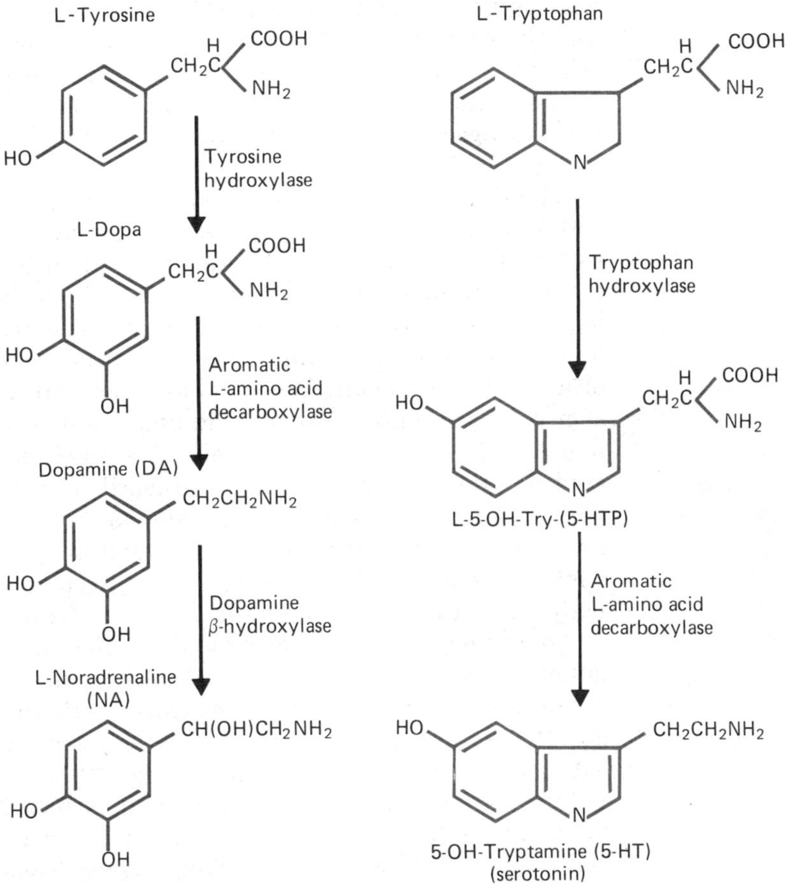

FIGURE 5.7 Biosynthesis of the monoamine transmitters dopamine (DA), noradrenaline (NA), and 5-hydroxytryptamine (5-HT, or serotonin). (From Iversen and Iversen, 1975b.)

ing and refining the original and somewhat simplistic assumptions. We shall approach the question of function both in terms of single transmitters and their role, and in terms of certain behaviors that seem to have interacting transmitter systems as their substrate.

Functions of Some Specific Neurotransmitters

Noradrenaline Before the discovery of specific anatomical pathways of transmitter-specific neurons, there was a great deal of conflicting evidence for the role of a particular transmitter, due to the "blunderbuss approach" of systemic injection. General administration of NA into the central nervous system, for example, would show inhibitory effects on certain behaviors, and yet, at times, would cause behavioral arousal. Such seemingly contradictory actions made it rather difficult for investigators to come up with a role for NA and other neurotransmitters.

The situation has improved recently, through the manipulative skill and knowledge of experimenters, and through the realization that a transmitter system with such varied projections to different parts of the brain as NA does not have to operate as a single entity. Furthermore, it has also been shown that the effects of manipulatory drugs on a transmitter system, and consequently on the organism, are dependent on the level and type of ongoing behavior (Kelleher and Morse, 1966). For instance, amphetamine is thought to produce its stimulating effects by a release of NA (and DA), and its effectiveness is determined by the level of activity of the organism. It will hardly affect an animal trained to perform a response task at a high rate, yet it will enormously increase low rates of responding. These differential drug effects that are dependent on behavioral states also contribute to some of the conflicting experimental results, especially those seen in the psychiatric clinics.

Some attempt has been made to determine the role of specific transmitters in certain behaviors. Noradrenaline, for example, seems to be involved with learning to avoid an aversive stimulus (avoidance behavior). But learning induced by positive reinforcers also seems to involve NA. It has been shown (Lewy and Seiden, 1972) that lever pressing for water in rats is normally associated with an increased NA turnover in the brain. Further, there is a correlation between levels of NA in the brain and stress. Electrical shocking, overcrowded living conditions, and forced activity all deplete NA levels in the forebrain.

Dopamine

Dopamine (DA) has been implicated in certain forms of motor control, including the "level of readiness" of motor response mechanisms and aspects of spontaneous motor activity.

Figure 5.8 shows the major DA concentrations and pathways in the rat brain. The most studied pathway is that projecting from the substantia nigra to the corpus striatum. These structures are considered extrapyramidal motor structures, and the pathway involved is known as the nigro-striatal pathway.

One of the classic discoveries of neuropharmacology was that a loss of DA from this pathway is associated with Parkinson's disease. Parkinson's disease is characterized by extrapyramidal motor symptoms, including akinesia, rigidity, and tremor. Treatment with L-dopa, a precursor for DA synthesis, produced remarkable improvement in the patients,

FIGURE 5.8 Distribution of dopamine (DA) pathways (neurons containing DA) in rat brain. Areas 8, 9, 10 represent the substantia migra, a major local concentration of DA in the brain. (From Livett, 1973; modified from Ungerstedt, 1971a.)

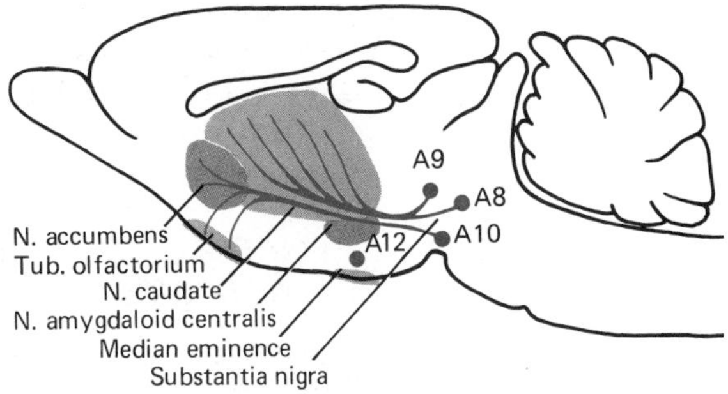

except for the tremor symptom (the tremor is thought to be due to some connected malfunction in the thalamus). Dopamine was therefore implicated in certain forms of motor control.

To determine more specifically the role of DA in motor control, techniques involving both pharmacological blocking of DA receptors and overstimulation of these receptors were used. The drug chlorpromazine, a DA antagonist, depresses locomotor activity, and also induces extrapyramidal motor symptoms such as those of Parkinson's disease. Stimulation of DA receptors also results in abnormal extrapyramidal motor activity and demonstrates the normal role of DA mechanisms in holding motor mechanisms in balance.

Reward-Punishment and the Role of Transmitters

Over 20 years ago, the phenomenon of intracranial self-stimulation (ICSS) was discovered. Laboratory rats were observed to return to the same place where they had previously received electrical stimulation of the septal area of the brain. It was subsequently discovered that rats would quickly learn to press a lever to stimulate their own brains, indicating that the stimulation was pleasurable or comparable to conventional positive reinforcement. Since then, ICSS has been found in many species, including man. Stimulation of ICSS loci in man is commonly associated with verbal reports of intense pleasurable sensations.

Studies have been conducted to determine relationships between ICSS sites and transmitter pathways in the brain. One fairly substantial hypothesis claims that activation of central catecholamine (NA and DA) systems is essential for ICSS (German and Bowden, 1974). Brain sites that support ICSS in the rat (ICSS sites in the human brain appear to overlap with the sites supporting ICSS in the rat) were found to be highly correlated with electrodes in the DA systems and the NA system. In keeping with these data, lesion studies have shown suppression of ICSS proportional to the degree of lesion damage to the DA and NA systems. Also, drugs that influence ICSS seem at the same time to affect NA and DA synapses.

The Relationship Between ICSS and Reinforcement

"Positive reinforcement" and "reward" have come to be used synonymously to denote stimuli that increase the probability of preceding behavior occurring again. Since many stimulation sites seem to be positively rewarding (they can be used as reward in training animals), it follows that there could be a relationship between pathways involved in ICSS and those involved in mediating "normal" rewards such as food or water.

The relationship between the satisfaction or feeling of satiety (or the fulfillment of other needs) and the reward of ICSS is not really understood. There is evidence that certain chemical pathways are common to both. As we have said, the distribution of positive ICSS sites in the rat brain corresponds quite closely to the distribution of the NA and DA systems.

ICSS responding may be a corollary of several different neural systems. One such function is possibly reinforcement mediated by NA terminals (of the perifornical region). We have mentioned the role of NA in feeding and satiety. It has been suggested that ICSS mimics immediate reinforcement by stimulating those systems normally involved in behavior associated with reinforcing behavior, such as feeding. Researchers (Stein and Wise, 1969) have reported that ICSS in the hypothalamus and amygdala is associated with release of NA. The ascending NA system to the hypothalamus and limbic system is thought to have a role in coding reinforcing stimuli. The DA-containing nigro-striatal pathway has also been shown to mediate a form of ICSS (Crow, 1972).

Interaction Between Reinforcement and Punishment

It has been suggested (Iversen and Iversen, 1975a) that an ACh mechanism in the hypothalamus may be responsible for the interaction between reinforcing and punishing contingencies. Anatomical connections utilizing the ACh transmitter exist between the anterior and ventromedial portions of the hypothalamus. The ventromedial hypothalamus is known to respond to reinforcing stimuli and also to be involved in punishment mechanisms. A neural interaction via ACh pathways could perhaps explain how sensitively behavior is able to reflect the constantly changing influence of reinforcement and punishment.

Schizophrenia

It can be argued that the highest priority in linking specific human behavior to particular neurochemical events lies with the aberrant behavior of the mentally ill. Schizophrenia is a major mental illness with many profound consequences, both social and scientific. We have mentioned several techniques used in animal research to ascribe behavioral effects to one or another transmitter pathway or system in the brain. Most such direct techniques are not available for exploring the neurochemical substrata of altered behavior in man. In the case of disturbed psychiatric patients, animal models are never really adequate. Despite this, attempts are being made to evaluate the roles of brain biochemicals in the pathophysiological mechanisms in schizophrenia.

Adding to the difficulty of this enterprise is the uncertainty as to whether the disease is a single entity or a cluster of illnesses. Psychiatrists make diagnoses by relying upon certain arbitrarily selected clinical symptoms. There is general agreement that "classic" schizophrenia is determined by a prominent genetic component. The "fundamental" symptoms (Bleuler, 1911) of schizophrenia include a peculiar thought disorder, a disturbance of feeling or "affective" responses to the environment and "autism," a withdrawal from meaningful interactions with other people. Hallucinations and delusions are thought to be secondary symptoms because they are not constant or essential to the disease though they are what is most popularly attributed to it.

DRUG-INDUCED PSYCHOSES AS MODELS

For two years Georgia had suffered from narcolepsy, a neural disorder characterized by an uncontrollable desire to sleep. Falling asleep at work had cost her one job, but she finally landed another. Her narcolepsy had become so severe that even with careful spacing of naps and pharmacologic stimulant she could not stay awake. In this new job she had her own cubicle, so if she dropped off to sleep no one noticed.

Following the course of Georgia's narcolepsy is a frightening experience. The condition began after Georgia graduated from college when she experienced attacks of uncontrollable sleepiness. What probably began as boredom and decreased attention during lectures was occurring several times a day irrespective of activity.

In the next two years the complete tetrad of symptoms, so vividly described by Kinnier Wilson in 1916, unfolded. Assaulted by her uncontrollable desire to sleep, her eyes closed, her muscles relaxed, and she had the appearance of dozing. A slight stimulus aroused her from these 15 to 30 minute episodes. Moreover, periods of extreme emotion, whet-

her laughing or crying, led to temporary paralysis of all her muscles and she often fell to the floor; this was cataplexy. She never lost consciousness when she experienced cataplexy. Periods of brief somatic paralysis also accompanied her falling asleep at night or waking in the morning.

The fourth symptom of narcolepsy—hypnogogic hallucinations—gave her the most trouble. Hypnogogic hallucinations, the perception of visual or auditory stimuli that are not really present, sometimes occurred at the beginning of the period of sleep paralysis. Georgia, however, was reporting that the hallucinations had become more frequent and were occurring throughout her waking hours. Hearing voices several times a day led to inevitable and obvious personality changes. These became profound. She slowly withdrew into the world of her auditory hallucinations and constructed a complicated paranoid delusional system around them. She believed that these voices were intruding into her head and controlling her will. In fact, she began believing that all her thoughts were public knowledge and that anyone could read exactly what she was thinking. Before long her friends noted her extreme withdrawal, and when they interacted she seemed strange and emotionally inappropriate. They brought her to the hospital emergency room.

It was clear that Georgia was in the throes of a serious thought disorder most like schizophrenia. The reasons for this break became clear only when the nurses emptied her purse. They found enough amphetamine to supply an ordinary narcoleptic for several months. Unknown to her doctors, Georgia's need for amphetamine—dexedrine—had increased beyond all reasonable limit. While dexedrine was appropriate pharmacologic regimentation considering Georgia's narcolepsy, she had begun taking more than her doctor prescribed. Taking upwards of 200 mg a day, though, was unquestionably dangerous, and the chronic ingestion of such a dose of amphetamine commonly causes behavioral changes such as Georgia was undergoing. Hallucinations, often visual as well as auditory, delusions, then thought disorder, personal withdrawal, and inappropriate affect all characterize the spontaneous disorder called schizophrenia. Here the disorder was drug induced with chronic amphetamine overdose.

The amphetamine dosage was decreased slowly, to ease the pain of her withdrawal symptoms. As the dosage level was lowered, Georgia's thought disorder cleared and so did the hallucinations. It took several more months of careful therapy to adjust her amphetamine dose in order to control the narcolepsy. She returned home not cured, but with a better understanding of the dangerous medicine crucial to her life.

One approach has been to investigate the neurochemical action of drugs that elicit psychoses similar to the behavioral symptoms of schizophrenia. Some of the psychedelic drugs were tested in this sense for a while, but a much better candidate seems to be amphetamines.

Many cases of amphetamine psychosis, such as Georgia, have been misdiagnosed as acute paranoid schizophrenia (until clinicians learned of the drug use). Amphetamine is generally thought to act in the brain via the transmitters DA and NA. It has obvious similarities to these brain catecholamines and is a potent inhibitor of their uptake mechanism in synapses. It must be kept in mind that we are discussing the actions of a drug that mimics schizophrenia. Whether it reflects the same physiology through which the disease manifests itself is not known; the evidence is only suggestive.

Antipsychotic Drug Implications

Phenothiazine and several other drugs that alleviate the symptoms of schizophrenia have been found to have one thing in common—an effect on the DA systems of the central nervous system (see Figure 5.9). It is debatable, however, whether these drugs actually act upon something fundamental to schizophrenia, or whether they are merely some sort of supersedative. As mentioned, in discussing DA, it has been suggested that certain drug-induced motor dysfunctions (stereotypy) can be used as animal models for some human psychoses.

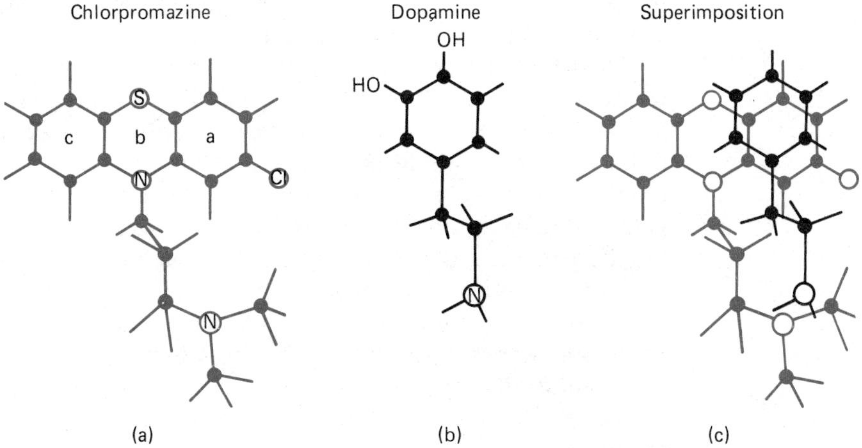

FIGURE 5.9 Molecular models of the conformations (as determined by x-ray crystallography) of (a) chlorpromazine, a phenothiazine drug, (b) dopamine, and (c) their superimposition. This is suggestive of a molecular mechanism whereby phenothiazines might block dopamine receptors at synapses in a feedback system that would cause greater release of dopamine as a result. (From Snyder, 1974; adapted from Horn and Snyder, 1971.)

Although these connections are not conclusive, they are further evidence of the subtlety of interactions brain researchers are discovering in attempting to integrate behavioral function (and dysfunction) with brain function. For instance, linking schizophrenic symptoms with some symptoms of motor dysfunction raises questions about the traditional view of what "motor" is and what role brain structures supposedly involved in motor behavior such as the basal ganglia play in some of the very subtle and integrated aspects of behavior. We mention this not because evidence from research on schizophrenia is so strong, but because there are many parallel discoveries implicating such structures as the basal ganglia in roles supposedly anomalous to their assumed functions.

Summary

Interest in the functional basis of behavior has focused in recent years on the action of chemical transmitter substances in the central nervous system. This is not because other aspects of brain anatomy, physiology, and chemistry are not important in influencing behavior, but rather because the study of chemical transmission offers powerful methods with which to explore the interrelationships between physiologic events in the nervous system and behavior. Biochemical reactions are important in every organ of the human body, yet the use of chemical transmitters is a biochemical function unique to the brain.

Identifying transmitters and understanding transmitter pathways are far from complete. Although it is generally recognized that communication between neurons involves the presynaptic release of chemical transmitters, which leads to propagation of an electrical impulse, the exact identity of the transmitter at various points in the central nervous system pathway remains obscure. Only a partial list of all the substances that function as transmitters is possible. Further study proceeds by affecting synaptic chemical transmission by any one of several categories of drugs, or by administration of the actual transmitter or transmitter precursor. Careful observation of the effects on behavior allow some understanding of the relation between dynamic structure and function. Certainly Stephan's problem with acetylcholine transmission is an example.

It is much more difficult, however, to understand the processes determining complex behavior, partly because the behavior in turn may affect the underlying biochemical events. The thought disorder that Georgia experienced while taking too much amphetamine mimicked a disease of behavior called schizophrenia. Whether the increased chemical neurotransmission caused by the amphetamine use is the functional basis of that group of behavioral disorders remains a mystery. Evidence, especially clinical trials with drugs that change certain aspects of chemical neurotransmission, suggests a complex relation between behavior and underlying brain process.

In any case, the role of neurotransmitters is stressed because they directly reflect the information flow in neural networks, and as such, appear to be the most immediate chemical substrate of behavior. The unavoidable separation and distinct treatment of certain psychological functions as "aggression" or "avoidance" in an attempt to establish connections between physiology and function is necessarily an oversimplification. It is not clear to what extent these aspects of psychological function are independent of one another, just as the accompanying physiologic mechanisms may not be independent. These artificial divisions of behavior undoubtedly contribute to the problems and anomalies constantly rising in the endeavor of relating physiology and behavior.

References

Bleuler, E. 1911. *Dementia Praecox or the Group of Schizophrenias.* Trans. by J. Zinkin, 1950. New York: International University Press.

Bunney, B. S., G. K. Aghajanian and R. H. Roth. 1973a. L-Dopa, amphetamine and apomorphine: Comparison of effects on the firing rate of rat dopaminergic neurons. *Nature 245:* 123.

Bunney, B. S., J. R. Walters, R. H. Roth, and G. K. Aghajanian. 1973b. Dopaminergic neurons: Effect of antipsychotic drugs and amphetamine on single cell activity. *J. Pharmacol. Exp. Ther. 185*:560.

Crow, T. J. 1972. A map of the rat mesencephalon for electrical self-stimulation. *Brain Res. 36*:265–273.

German, D. C., and D. M. Bowden. 1974. Catecholamine systems as the neural substrate for intracranial self-stimulation: A hypothesis. *Brain Res. 73*:381–419.

Goodwin, F. K., D. L. Murphy, H. K. H. Brodie, and W. E. Bunney, Jr. 1970. L-Dopa, catecholamines and behavior; a clinical and biochemical study in depressed patients. *Biol. Psychiat. 2*:341–366.

Horn, A. S., and S. H. Snyder. 1971. Chlorpromazine and dopamine: Conformational similarities that correlate with the antischizophrenic activity of phenothiazine drugs. *Proc. Nat. Acad. Sci. 68*:2325–2328.

Iversen, S. D. 1974. 6-hydroxydopamine: A chemical lesion technique for studying the role of amine neurotransmitters in behavior. In: F. O. Schmitt and F. G. Worden, eds. *The Neurosciences: Third Study Program.* Cambridge, Mass.: M. I. T. Press.

Iversen, S. D., and L. L. Iversen, 1975a. Chemical pathways in the brain. In: M. S. Gazzaniga and C. Blakemore, eds. *Handbook of Psychobiology.* New York: Academic Press.

Iversen, S. D., and L. L. Iversen. 1975b. Central neurotransmitters and the regulation of behavior. In: M. S. Gazzaniga and C. Blakemore, eds. *Handbook of Psychobiology.* New York: Academic Press.

Kelleher, K. T., and W. H. Morse. 1966. Determinants of the specificity of behavioral effects of drugs. *Ergebnisse der Physiol. 60*:1–56.

Lewy, A. J., and L. S. Seiden 1972. Operant behavior changes norepinephrine metabolism in rat brain. *Science* 175:454–455.

Schildkraut, J. J., and S. S. Kety. 1967. Biogenic amines and emotion. *Science* 156:21–30.

Stein, L., and C. D. Wise. 1969. Release of norepinephrine from hypothalamus and amygdala by rewarding medial forebrain bundle stimulation and amphetamine. *Comp. Physiol. Psychol.* 67:189–198.

Ungerstedt, V. 1971a. On the anatomy, pharmacology and function of the nigro-striatal dopamine system. *Acta Physiol. Scand.* (Suppl. 367).

Ungerstedt, V. 1971b. Stereotaxic mapping of the monoamine pathways in the rat brain. *Acta Physiol. Scand.* (Suppl. 367) 82:1–48.

Ungerstedt, V. 1971c. Adipsia and aphagia after 6-hydroxydopamine induced degeneration of the nigro-striatal dopamine system in the rat brain. *Acta Physiol. Scand.* (Suppl. 367) 82:95–122.

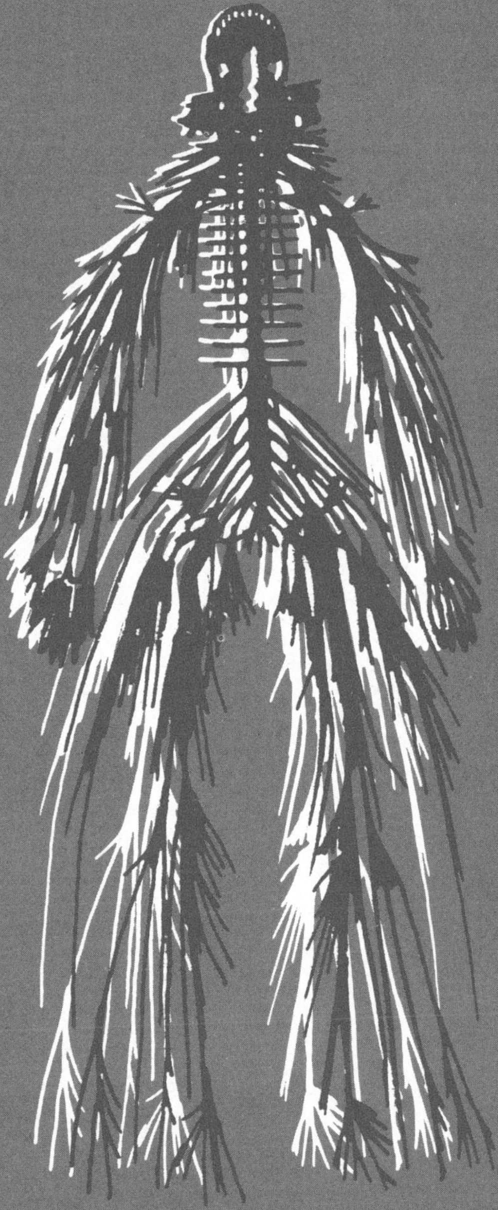

PART III The Senses and Beyond

CHAPTER 6

Visual Processing

When thinking of vision it is natural to think first of the eye, where light is received by the organism. Important transformations of visual information occur in the eye, but they are only the beginning of a complex series of processing stages that carry visual information to the higher centers of the brain.

In this chapter, we shall examine information processing along the visual pathway. This pathway begins at the retina, the structure lining the rear of the eyeball that contains the photoreceptor cells. Surprisingly, a significant amount of activity occurs at the retinal level before the visual impulses are transmitted to the brain by way of the optic nerve. Once in the brain, the impulses follow one of the two main routes. They may be conducted along the retino-cortical pathway, which leads from the retina to the thalamus to the cortex, where the highest level of processing is done, or they may travel along the retino-tectal path, which goes from the retina to the tectum (see Figure 6.1). The effects of disruption of these distinct paths will be considered in this chapter, especially the visual malfunction occurring from damage to the cortical areas.

The Retina: The Pathway Begins

The retina, the first site of visual processing, is not a part of the eye that we normally see. We see only the iris, which is the colored part of the eye, the sclera, which is the mass of fibrous white tissue surrounding the iris, and the pupil, which is the opening in the center of the iris, through which light must pass if it is to enter the eye. The pupil is the first controlling mechanism of vision, allowing more or less light to enter the eye by dilating or contracting (see Figure 6.2). Once inside, the

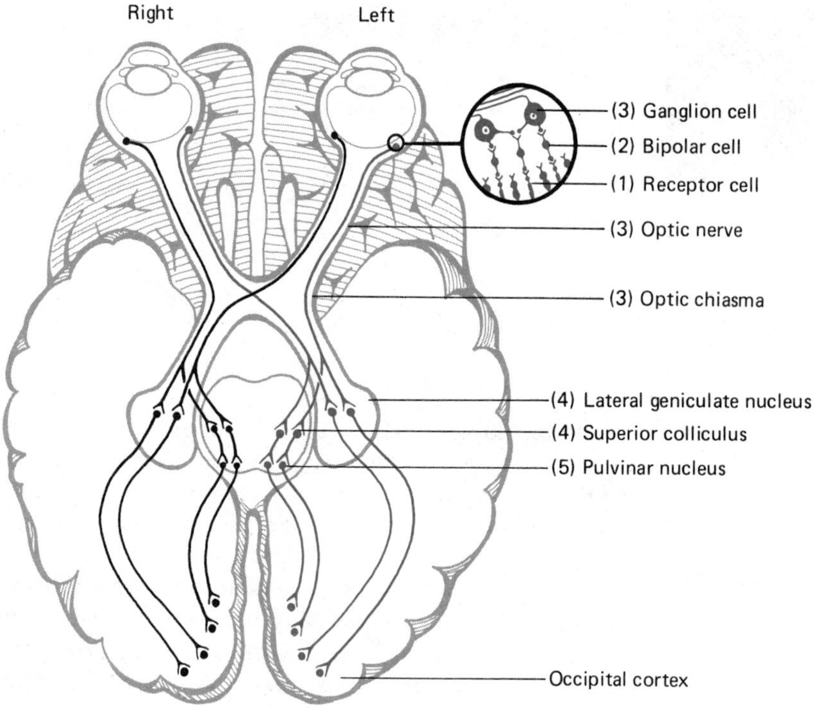

FIGURE 6.1 The basic visual pathways from the retina to the brain.

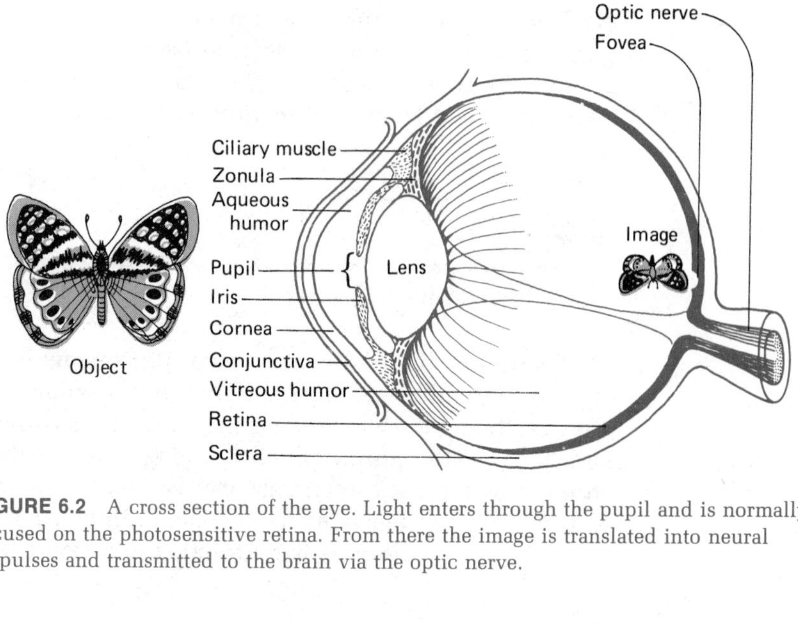

FIGURE 6.2 A cross section of the eye. Light enters through the pupil and is normally focused on the photosensitive retina. From there the image is translated into neural impulses and transmitted to the brain via the optic nerve.

light strikes the retina, the photosensitive surface within the eye. The image projected onto the retina is actually upside down, with right and left reversed because of the bending of the light rays by the lens of the eye. However, our perceptual processes are designed to take into account this reversal, and interpret the actual orientation of the retinal image.

The retina consists of three layers of cells, each of which plays an important role in the processing of visual stimuli. As in other sensory systems, the layer that first receives the stimuli consists of receptor cells, here called *photoreceptors*. Interestingly, in the retina, the receptor cells are behind the other two layers of cells (see Figure 6.3). Thus light coming in through the pupil must pass not only through a network of blood vessels that supply nutrients to the eye, but also through two additional layers of cell bodies and axons. Despite these obstructions, light does manage to get through, and normal visual acuity is not disrupted. The center of the retina, called the *fovea*, is responsible for fine visual acuity since there is a more or less clear path from the pupil to the center of the retina.

The Receptors

Animals with color vision have two types of receptors: rods and cones. *Rods*, which outnumber cones by at least a 16:1 ratio (Rodieck, 1973), are inoperative in bright light and function optimally at night, or wherever illumination is low. *Cones*, on the other hand, work best in bright light and have the pigments and neural connections that allow for the perception of color. In addition, it is the cones that allow for detail vision, or high visual acuity. We could not read, for example, without cones. Although concentrated in the center of the retina, called the fovea, cones are also scattered in the surrounding retina. Rods are distributed evenly throughout the retina, excluding the foveal region.

The Transduction Process: Neural Energy Conversion

Rods and cones, like the receptor cells of other sensory systems, are the cells that actually receive physical energy from environmental stimuli and convert it into a graded potential, which, if sufficiently large, is then transformed into a neural impulse. This transduction process in both rods and cones occurs in reaction to light (electromagnetic energy), which results in a change in the chemical composition of the cell. The chemical constituents of each cell are "retinal," which is a substance with a structure similar to vitamin A (actually an aldehyde of vitamin A) and the proteins of the class opsin. In the rods, retinal combines with opsin to form the chemical element rhodopsin, and in the cones, retinal

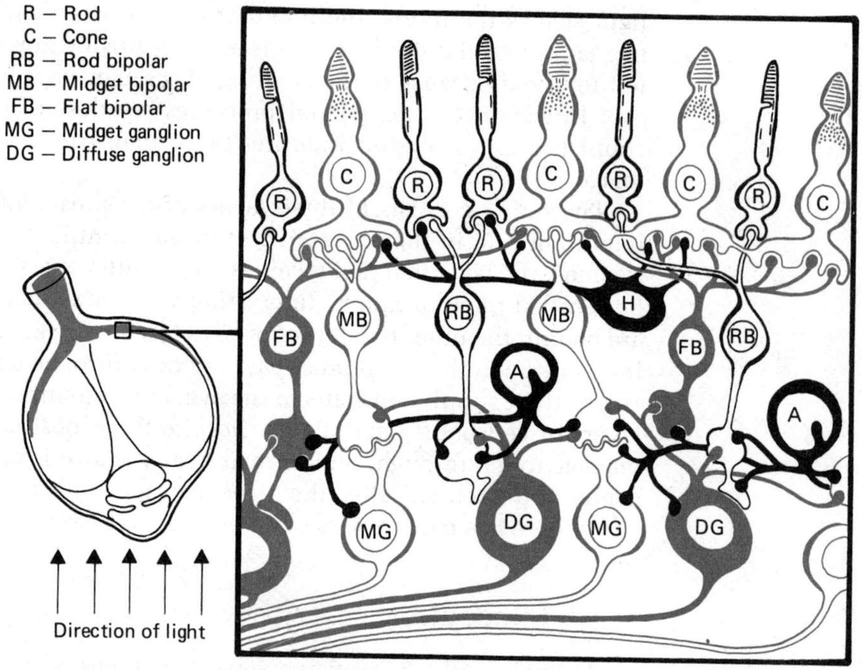

FIGURE 6.3 Dowling and Boycott (1966) have been able to distinguish between various types of bipolar cells and their variety of synaptic connections.

combines with another opsin, photopsin, to form iodopsin. Because cones are believed to operate on a three-color coding scheme, the protein in the cones is thought to differ slightly in each of the three color-detecting types of cones, forming a pigment that is more sensitive to either red, blue, or green light (Stiles, 1959).

Although rods and cones function in essentially the same way, there are basic differences in their anatomy and physiology. One obvious difference (from which their names are derived) is in their shape: Rods have a thicker, longer outer segment than cones, which are slightly pointed. The outer segments of both rods and cones are connected to the cell body by a thin stalk called the cilium, through which nutrients such as proteins are transported to the outer segment. Both rods and cones are composed of flat disks formed by an enfolding of the membrane of the outer segment, and the bottom disks are continuous with the membrane of the outer segment. Cones, however, have a finite number of disks, all formed by a continuous enfolding of the membrane, while rods have some free-floating disks near the end of the segment (Young, 1967, 1969).

Cones maintain their disks by transporting protein and nutrients

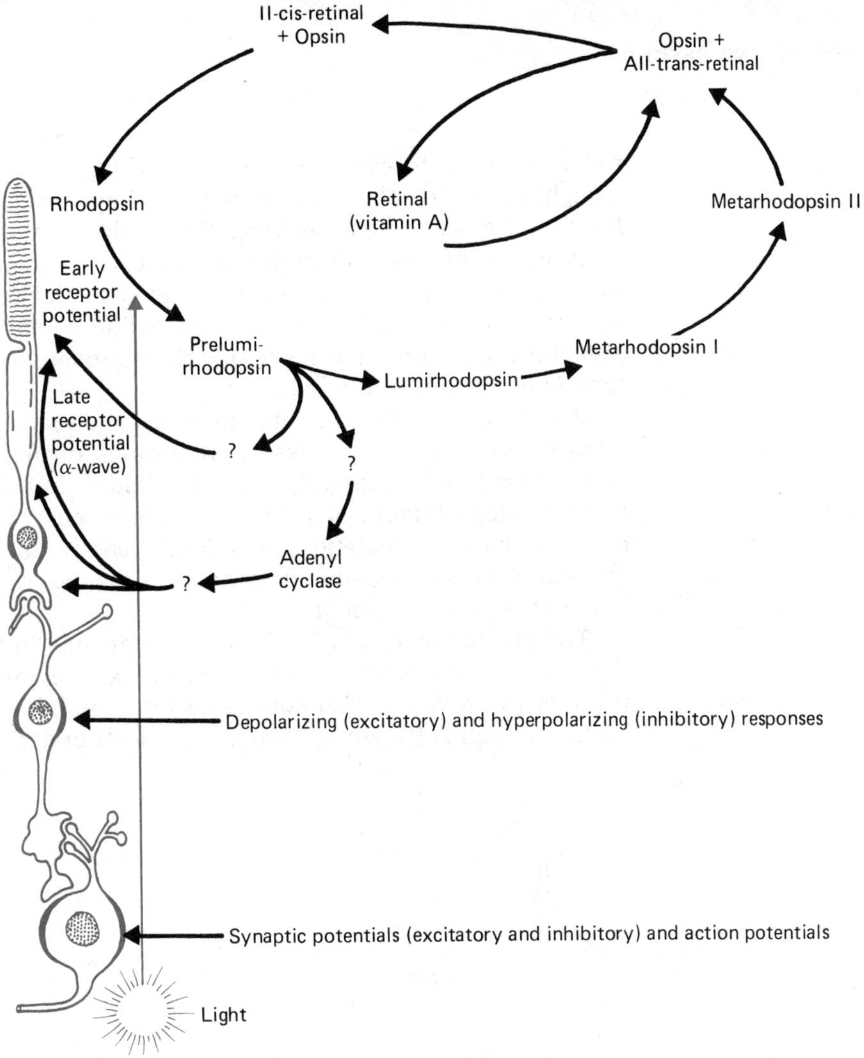

FIGURE 6.4 Basic cellular elements of the retina and the chemical process that take light energy and transfer it into electrical impulses.

through the membrane, but rods have a better maintenance system. They are able to manufacture new disks, discarding the old ones and letting them degenerate. The cones' lack of such a renewal process may account for the inevitable weakening of detail vision, mediated by cones in the foveal region, that is part of the aging process.

Despite these differences in composition, rods and cones react to light in similar ways. Exposure to light causes a chemical reaction that instantly generates electrical impulses, or generator potentials. A close look at rods (which are more readily studied, since there are few animals with cones) explains the electrical process. The structure of retinal when combined with opsin is normally twisted and bent (Wald, 1968). When a rod is exposed to even one quantum of light, the protein assumes a straight form. Somehow, the change of shape produces within 25-millionths of a second an electrical charge that is transmitted within 2-thousandths of a second to the bipolar cell, a second-order neuron in the visual system (see Figure 6.4). If the generator potentials combined add up to a level sufficient to fire the action potential, then the action potentials begin their journey along the optic nerve (cranial nerve II) to the higher centers of the brain.

Both rods and cones are able to renew their supply of rhodopsin or iodopsin very quickly, as fast as thousands of molecules per second (Wald, 1968). In bright light, however, rhodopsin may be broken down by absorption of light faster than it is able to renew itself; thus it is in a constant state of depletion in a bright environment. This so-called "bleaching effect" is gradually reversed as the rods dark-adapt by renewing their supply of pigment.

The process of adaptation is only in part due to the chemical reactions in the receptor cells; there is considerable evidence that the sensitivity of the retina is also controlled by neural feedback mechanisms within the retina (Dowling, 1967). The effects of dark-adaptation can be

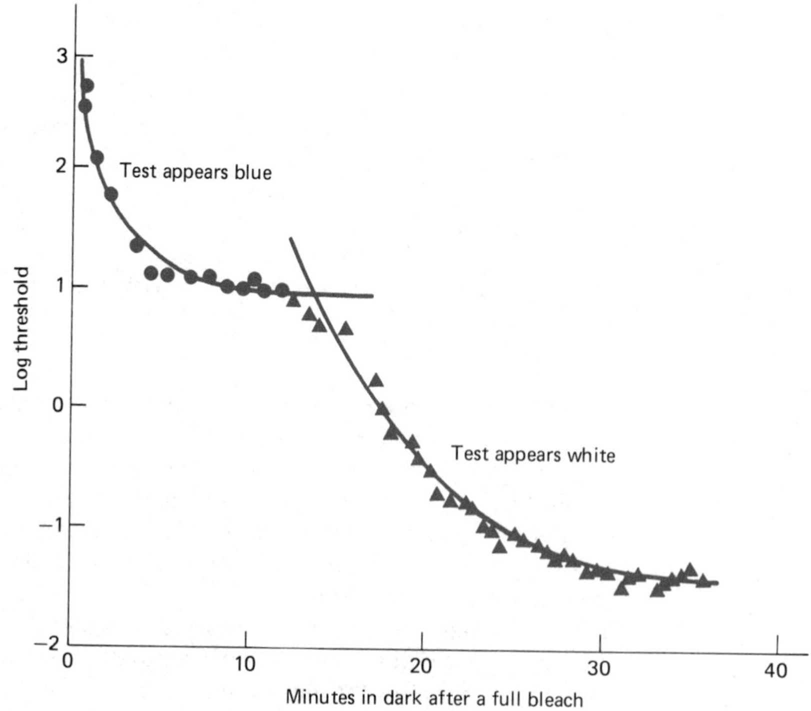

FIGURE 6.5 The dark-adaptation curve has a crisp break at the rod-cone junction.

ascertained by measuring the sensitivity of the eye under different illumination conditions. When this is done, it is found that cones dark-adapt and return to optimal sensitivity in about 6 minutes, while rods require approximately 30 to 40 minutes to dark-adapt (see Figure 6.5). Pilots flying at night are thus cautious not to expose their eyes to bright stimulation, because it takes so long for the rods to return to optimal performance.

Beyond the Receptors: The Bipolar and Ganglion Cells of the Retina

The receptor potentials generated at the receptor level by the rods and cones are transmitted to the second layer of retinal cells, the *bipolar cells*. This second stage of visual processing shows both convergence and divergence of visual impulses. Convergence occurs most frequently, with most bipolar cells receiving input from many receptors. However, divergence is also seen in that some receptors connect to more than one bipolar cell. Additionally, in the foveal region of the retina, where cones are concentrated, there is sometimes a one-to-one relationship between cones and bipolar cells, illustrating neither convergence nor divergence, but allowing a "private line" for each cone to mediate fine visual acuity in the fovea (Figure 6.6). The bipolar cells are connected to each other by the horizontal cells, which convey both excitatory and inhibitory impulses from one bipolar cell to another.

Further convergence takes place at the third retinal level, the ganglion cells. Each ganglion cell receives input from many bipolar cells, but one should not get the idea that things are getting simple just because the output from 115 million to 130 million receptor cells has been somewhat condensed. The number of ganglion cells is still quite impressive—one million. The ganglion cells are interconnected by the *amacrine cells*, which, like the horizontal cells of the bipolar level, serve both excitatory and inhibitory functions.

Two processes, lateral summation and lateral inhibition, are mediated by the amacrine cells. Lateral summation is the convergence of impulses that is necessary to fire higher-order cells. While one quantum of light is sufficient to stimulate a rod, generally at least six receptors must be excited to trigger the firing of a ganglion cell. However, the firing of a ganglion cell, though dependent on lateral summation, may be decreased by the process of lateral inhibition. This process will be discussed in more detail later.

The axons of the one million ganglion cells band together to form the optic nerve, which carries all impulses from the eye to the brain. The spot on the retina where the optic nerve leaves the eye is called the optic disk, and because the retina is organized in an outside-in fashion, that

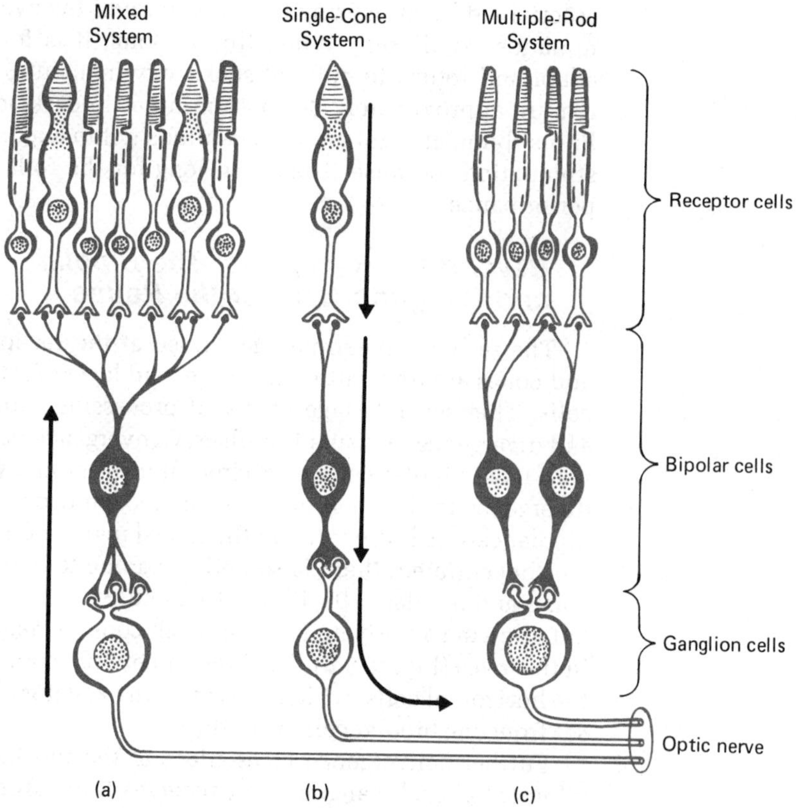

FIGURE 6.6 There are three main types of retinal connections: (a) There is the mixed rod and cone system with both types of cells synapsing on one bipolar cell; (b) in the fovea one finds the single-cone system, which is largely responsible for our crisp daylight acuity and color vision; (c) the last is the multiple-rod system, which is very active in night vision.

is, the ganglion cells and bipolar cells are in front of the receptors, the axons of the ganglion cells leaving the retina preclude any receptors being in that spot. Hence, the *optic disk* forms a *blind spot,* which you can easily find by closing your right eye, looking straight ahead at a small object, and then shifting your gaze slowly to the right. The object will seem to disappear at about 15°, but will reappear once the 15° point is passed. Normally, however, the effect of the blind spot is not noticeable, since any portion of the visual field that happens to fall on the blind spot in one eye will usually be seen by the other eye (see Figure 6.7). Sometimes, however, in certain abnormal conditions, the effect of the blind spot formed by the optic disk is quite noticeable.

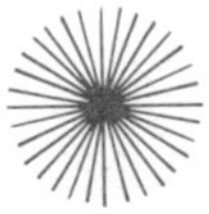

FIGURE 6.7
How to find blind spot.
Look at central "X," with your right eye. What happens?

Frequently patients from the neurological clinic can be instructive when carefully analyzed. Often their disorders are not related to a specific sensory system. Multiple sclerosis, for example, produces a diffuse array of sensory abnormalities, but each sensory system abnormality can be isolated and analyzed. Laura's story is such an example.

Laura was a graduate student working in a productive virology and immunology lab. Several important discoveries had come from this group, and Laura had contributed substantially to each. She was simply a brilliant young investigator. In fact, she had just visited The Hague, in the Netherlands, where her paper received plaudits from an international group of scientists. Since her return, however, she was not feeling well. Fatigue, lack of energy, even weight loss were all attributed to the excitement of foreign travel and her success, but all these symptoms persisted.

She also refused to complain about the frequent paresthesias, the numbness and tingling, that she experienced in her right leg. Even when the paresthesias progressed to involve simultaneously her left arm and right leg, she continued her experiments. The months passed and it was no secret around the lab that the specific symptoms were more limiting than the general fatigue and malaise. When the paresthesias were bothering her it was as though her arm or leg had been deafferented—that is, had lost all sensory input—because she retained full motor control but had no proprioception or sense of the position of her arm or leg. The arm or the leg became clumsy in responding to the external stimuli, and holding a pipette or a pencil became insurmountable chores.

Finally the acute impairment of vision forced her to seek medical attention. Examinations of her eyes in the context of her background led to only one conclusion: multiple sclerosis. This part of her story unfolded over two days. When she appeared at the hospital she felt as though a veil had been placed over her right eye. It had waxed and waned on the first day, and since she had been poring over the microscope, she concluded it was eyestrain. On the second day, with no microscope work, the haze became fixed and she could not see out of that eye. She lost all acuity in her central field of vision. Furthermore, she had no color vision. In Laura the optic nerve was inflamed and the disk margins were elevated, blurred, and surrounded by small hemorrhages. This condition, called papillitis, is common in multiple sclerosis; so is the pro-

gressive loss of color vision and acuity that left Laura perceiving only form and motion.

Of the patients with multiple sclerosis and optic neuritis, one-third recover completely, one-third improve considerably, and one-third show little or no improvement. Laura fell into the first group, and two weeks after the sudden loss of vision all her symptoms began to disappear. Four months later she had a complete recovery of vision, both acuity and color, and further, her paresthesias and clumsiness were gone. On examination a temporal pallor existed in both retinas when seen through the opthalmoscope, but the disk margins were sharp again and the hemorrhages had regressed. It had been a terrible nine or ten month ordeal, and although it was over, she could have no assurance it would not recur since recurrences were always possible. Still, once again she was able to enjoy the privileges given those who can see, and the effect of her "blind spot" had retreated to its normally unnoticeable state.

The Retina: The First Order of Processing

Significant transformations of visual information from light waves to specific neural impulses occur at the retinal level. The receptors essentially work in the same way that a computer does when it "reads" a picture. An object or scene is sensed as a pattern of light and dark spots. This pattern of spots is then transmitted to deeper layers of the retina and up the visual pathways for further processing.

In this section, we shall examine the nature of retinal processing. We shall consider first the receptive field concept. This is a basic principle that will reappear at various points throughout this and other chapters. Next, we shall examine the selective firing of retinal neurons, lateral inhibition in the retinal cells, the role of retinal cells in color vision, and finally, stabilized retinal images.

Receptive Fields

Receptive fields are usually defined retinotopically (in terms of areas of the retina) but could as easily be defined in terms of areas of the visual field, since points on the retina correspond topographically to points in the visual field. Generally, receptive fields get larger as one moves higher up the visual pathway and even those neurons with larger receptive fields retain the pattern of retinotopic organization, with adjacent neurons receiving input from adjacent areas of the retina. Receptive fields of cells at the cortical level are the largest of all, but the retinotopic organization is still evident (see Figure 6.8).

To facilitate detail vision, foveal cells sometimes have a one-to-one

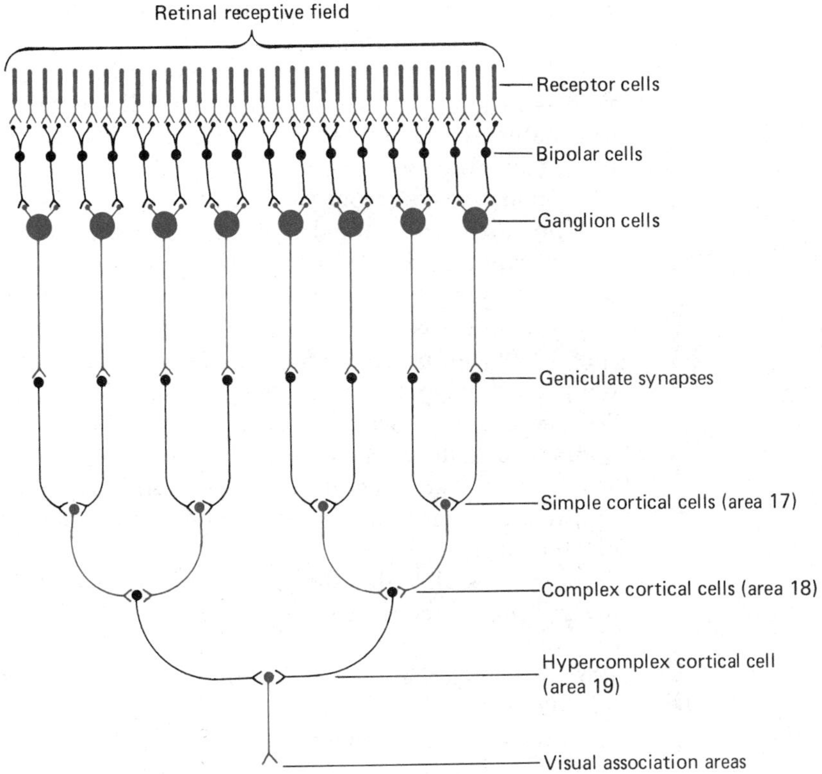

FIGURE 6.8 The size of perceptive fields changes as one goes from the retina to the cortex. (After Hubel and Wiesel, 1965.)

relationship with a ganglion cell, so input is not summed as in other areas, but retains a more specific pattern. Obviously, ganglion cells serving the fovea have small receptive fields, whereas ganglion cells connected to the receptors of the more peripheral regions of the retina will have large receptive fields. The extent of a receptive field of a ganglion cell is verified by selectively stimulating receptor cells in the retina and recording responses at the ganglion cell level. The receptive field of a ganglion cell encompasses all the connecting receptor cells.

Neurons in the Visual System: Selective and Specific

Perhaps one of the most important organizational features of visual neurons is their ability to respond selectively to particular patterns of light. This phenomenon occurs even at the retinal level. A given retinal ganglion cell does not fire indiscriminately when light occurs in the receptive field. For example, some cells fire only if the center of the receptive field is illuminated; others fire only if the center of the receptive field is dark and the surrounding area is illuminated. Further up the visual pathway, receptive fields become larger as the information from many cells converges and at the same time the stimuli required for firing the higher visual neurons become increasingly more specific.

The cat is one animal that has concentric receptive fields; within each circular field is an area that responds selectively either to light or dark, or in some cases, to a flashing light (see Figure 6.9). Such cells have been classified as *on* cells, *off* cells, and *on-off* cells, respectively (Hartline, 1940; Kuffler, 1953). More recent work has shown that the receptive fields often have an antagonistic organizational pattern, with a central "on" area, and a surrounding "off" area. That is, one neuron may have both an inhibitory (off) area of the receptive field, which if stimulated will prevent the firing of the neuron, and may also have an excitatory (on) area of the receptive field, which if stimulated will trigger the firing of the neuron.

Some speculate that the summation of these two impulses will result in the firing of the neuron only if the excitatory area is more stimulated than the inhibitory area of the receptive field (Rodieck and Stone, 1965a, 1965b). The excitatory and inhibitory area are often dome-shaped and may overlap.

Somewhat surprisingly, especially to those who believe in the notion of the evolutionary scale, frogs have been found to have considerably more complex retinal ganglion cells than the cat. Not only does a frog have cells that respond selectively to light and dark, but this lowly creature of the swamp also has ganglion cells that respond only to

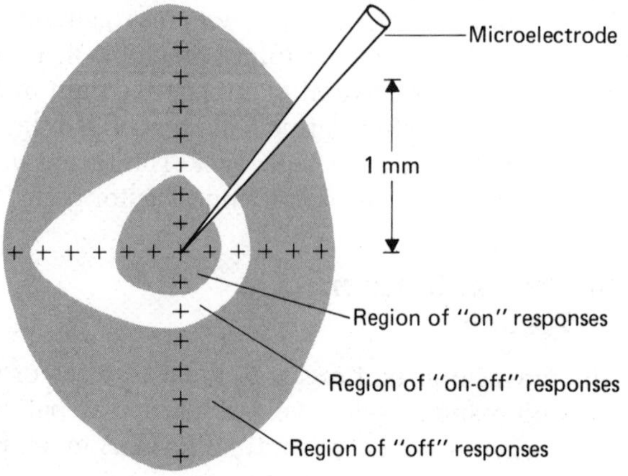

FIGURE 6.9 A typical receptive field in a cat retina cell is seen here. In this ganglion cell, the central portion of the cell fires to a light or "on" stimulus. There is a midregion of "on-off" responses, and overall surrounding field of "off" responses. (After Kuffler, 1953.)

movement, to curved edges, and to changes in contrast. Thus, the eyes of the frog are quite well adapted to catching flying insects, and in some sense, are more advanced then the retina of the human!

Whereas the cat has retinal cells that respond in a general fashion, the frog has more specific stimulus requirements. Given that a cat is considered "more intelligent" than a frog, that is, more advanced on the phylogenetic tree, one explanation for this apparent inconsistency is that animals with lesser capabilities for higher processing (i.e., smaller brain size), often have greater capabilities at lower levels. That is, cats can send information to the cortex for processing, but since frogs have no cortex, they have more need for processing at lower levels.

Further experiments with other animals (pigeons, rabbits, and squirrels) have revealed specialized retinal ganglion cells that respond best to stimulation such as verticality and horizontality or fast movement. These specific criteria for optimum response of a cell are called trigger features, since it is that particular stimulus which elicits, or triggers, the response of the cell. Although trigger features of the retinal ganglion cells seem to vary according to the particular needs faced by an animal in a particular environment, the list of trigger features may be condensed into a few basic properties:

1. contrast or edge
2. movement
3. direction of movement
4. convexity of size
5. orientation of edge
6. overall illumination

A seventh element, though not applicable to all animals, is color (from Blakemore, 1975a).

Visual cells may also be classified by characteristics other than trigger features. For example, the retinal ganglion cells of the cat have been classified on the basis of such features as their cell body size and the speed of conduction of their axons. These cells have been termed X, Y, and W cells, and their projection along the visual pathway has been mapped.

Lateral Inhibition: An Aid to Selectivity

The selective responding of retinal cells governed by trigger features is by no means the only way retinal cells code visual stimuli; contours and areas of contrast are emphasized by the process of lateral inhibition. This process occurs through a "keeping up with the Joneses" type of activity among ganglion cells. That is, the firing response of some retinal cells is affected by the activity of the neighboring cells, the effect being communicated at the ganglion level through the intricate network of

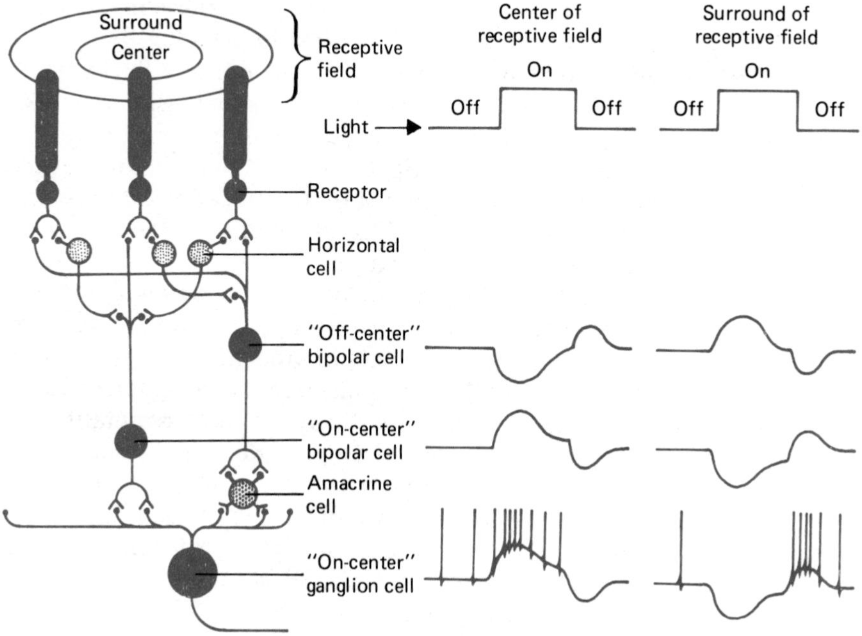

FIGURE 6.10 Some of the characteristics of lateral inhibition.

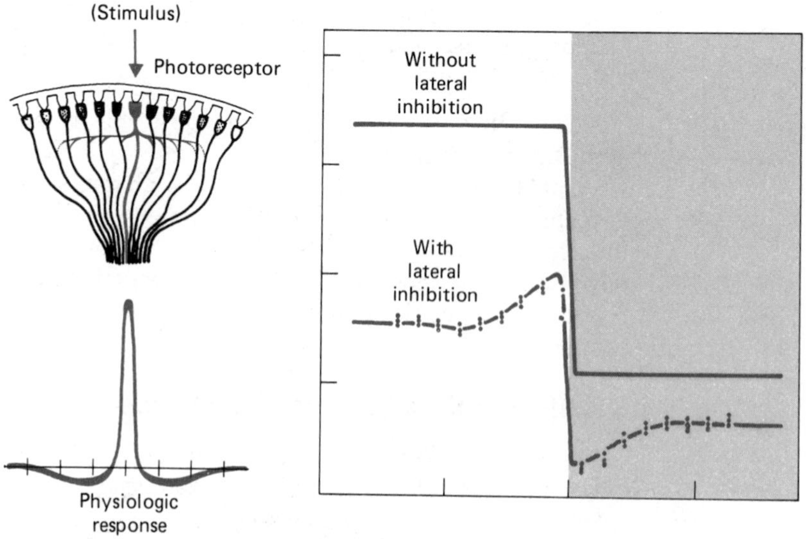

FIGURE 6.11 Lateral inhibition is studied in the horseshoe crab because of its special and simple organization. Without lateral inhibition, the responses would look like a "square wave" response, whereas in fact when the response is plotted, it shows how laterally connecting cells enhance the response at the light-dark border.

amacrine cells, which link ganglion cells to each other (Figure 6.10).

The usual effect is that the cell that fires exerts an inhibitory effect on the cells surrounding it; likewise, if instead the surrounding cells are firing, they exert an inhibitory effect on the center cell. Contrast is emphasized by a stronger firing response at the point of contrast, because a cell whose neighboring cell or cells are not firing, and thus are not exerting an inhibitory effect, has a relatively stronger response than those cells that are surrounded by firing neurons. This increased response, which occurs at areas of contrast, enhances perception because it accentuates edges and borders, the elements of a visual stimulus that usually give the most information about the object. Figure 6.11 gives a schematic depiction of neural responses that occur at an edge. In general, the stronger the firing response of the visual neuron, the stronger the inhibiting effect communicated to the next cell.

Another Dimension: Color Vision

A third form of visual coding at the retinal level is color coding. Color vision, however, is not common to all animals, and although it is possible for humans to function seeing things only in black and white, color adds a dimension to the world that only humans, primates, and surprisingly, some animals such as birds, fish, reptiles, and certain insects experience.

An understanding of color vision is based on knowledge of the color spectrum. Light itself is but a small segment of the entire electromagnetic energy spectrum, which ranges from very short cosmic rays to long-wavelength radio waves. Visible light is well between these two extremes, ranging from about 400 to about 700 nanometers (billionths of a meter), from violet to red. Thus, white light is actually made up of light of many different colors, because the spectral colors differ from each other in wavelengths, and white light includes a broad range of wavelengths. This can be easily verified by using a prism and separating the white light into its component colors. Each particular color corresponds to a particular wavelength of light.

The eye is not equally sensitive to all colors (different wavelengths), and more energy is needed to detect a pure red or a blue light than to see a green light. An additional fact to note is that any three colors can be mixed in varying proportions to form virtually any color. Thus, the trichromatic (or three-pigment) theory of color vision is based on these basic premises: that white light is composed of light (wavelengths) of many colors, that the eye is not equally sensitive to all wavelengths, and that any three colors can be mixed to form any other color.

As mentioned earlier, the cells necessary for color vision are the cones, which function best in bright light. There are three types of cones, each having a pigment that responds to a particular wavelength of light. That is, one pigment responds best to red light, another to blue light, and a third to green light (Figure 6.12). However, this does not mean that these are the only three colors that can be perceived. Because of the fact that any three colors mixed in varying amounts can form any other color, neural responses to these color pigment mixtures apparently allow all other colors to be perceived. Rather than having a particular cell to respond to each of the infinite variations of color found in the spectrum, and thus a number of seldom-used cells, the eye has three types of color cells that through a process of algebraic summation of neural impulses can produce the sensation of any color. If you are looking at a brown shirt, for example, each of the three types of cones will fire in varying amounts, producing in some still-mysterious way your personal sensation of the color you know as brown.

Yet nothing is simple in the brain. While the trichromatic theory of color vision is generally accepted as the way receptors code color, it does

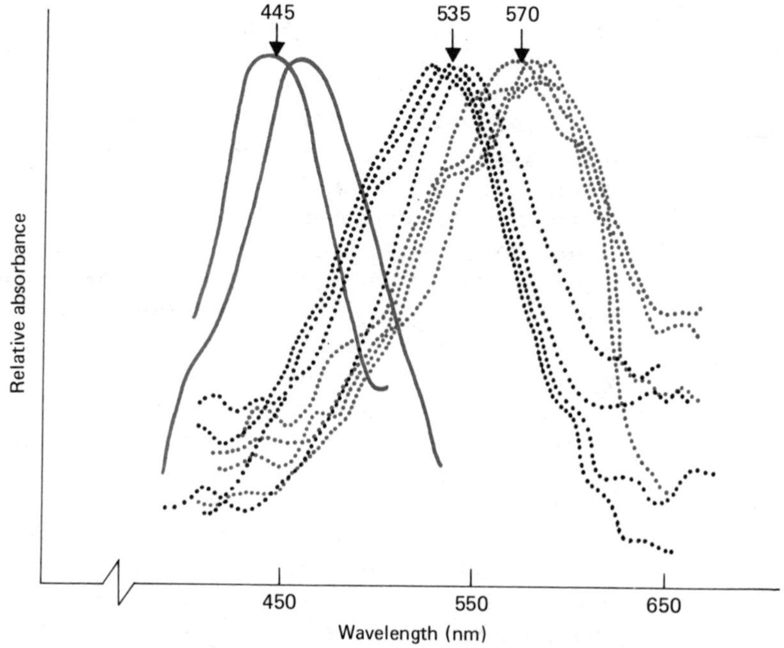

FIGURE 6.12 The absorption spectra for primate cones, showing the different peaks for blue, yellow, green, and red. (After Marks, Dobelle, and MacNichol, 1964.)

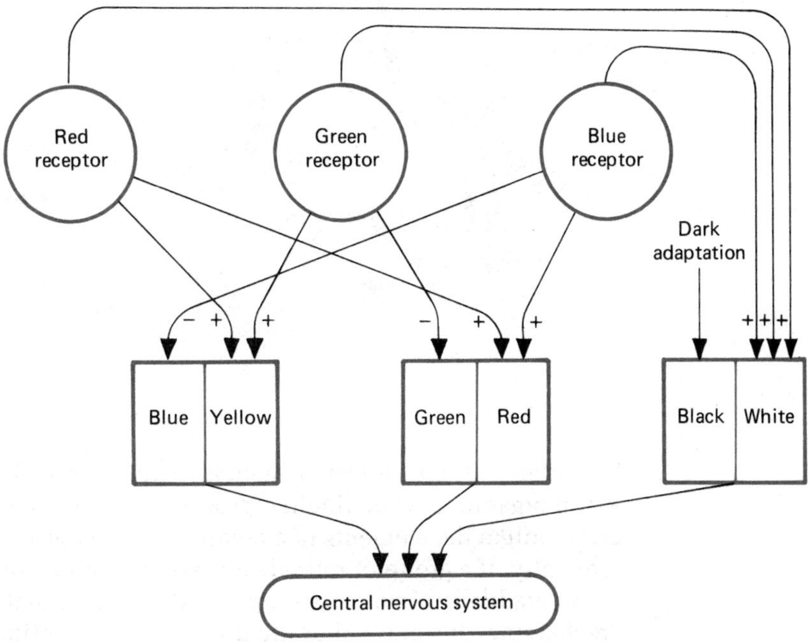

FIGURE 6.13 A sketch of a possible neural mechanism that could convert a trichromatic photoreceptor system to an opponent system. (After Hurwich and Jamison, 1957.)

not seem to be true at higher levels of processing. In fact, the coding of color even at the bipolar level is believed to be different. At higher levels such as the cortex, the pattern of activity is described as the opponent theory: The signals from the three different color receptor cells are transformed into two opposing signals that also, when combined algebraically, transmit the correct color sensation to the visual cortex. Blue and green responses are registered by one type of cell; red and yellow responses are registered by another. This opponent form of coding is not inconsistent with the trichromatic theory. Basically, the two forms work in the same way, through algebraic summation, the main difference being that the trichromatic coding process utilizes three input factors, whereas the opponent coding process uses only two color factors (Figure 6.13).

Stabilized Images and Psychological Theories of Perception

Visual processing at the retinal level is, as mentioned before, often compared to a computer scanning a visual pattern and producing a corresponding system of black and white dots. Although the analogy is not

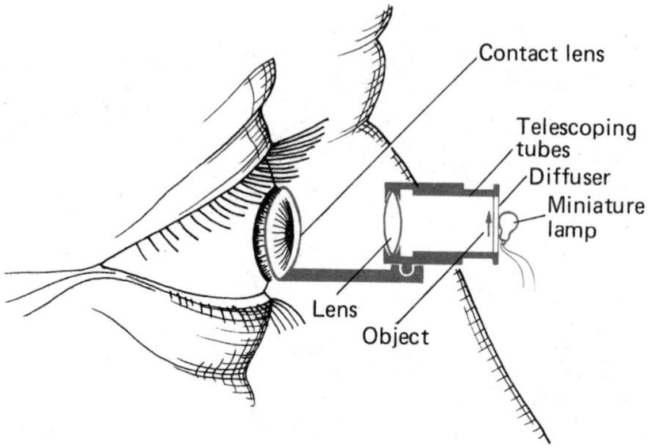

FIGURE 6.14 A stabilized image system. An image, the "object" in the telescope, is focused sharply on the retina. When the eye moves, the image remains fixed on the retina because the telescope is carried along with the eye.

too farfetched, one fallacy of such a comparison is that it does not allow for an organic nonmachinelike process that occurs in the retina. Retinal cells, unlike the elements of a computer, are subject to fatigue, and consequently, if a group of retinal cells are forced to fixate on an object, the object gradually seems to disappear. Although retinal cells are capable of "recharging" instantly, they are not capable of continuous firing without some short period of time for renewal. Fortunately, the eye is never completely still, and unless conditions are artificially manipulated, it is impossible for the same group of retinal cells to be stimulated continuously (Figure 6.14). Even when you are staring intently at an object, and think your eyes are immobile, they are constantly shifting and jumping back and forth in tiny movements called saccades. Thus a different set of receptors is stimulated with each movement, and the picture does not fade from view. Interestingly, it seems that the eye is relatively insensitive to stimulation during the jump or movement, so the brain does not receive a confusing series of blurred, fast-moving images; rather, it receives a series of sharp images that are seen during the period when the eye is stable.

However, there is an artificial way to fixate the same set of receptors on a particular object. A special contact lens with an attached object is put on the eye; thus, if the eye moves, the object moves, and no other receptors are stimulated. As expected, since the image is stable, the object gradually fades from view. What is of interest here, however, is that the object gradually comes back into view.

Differences in the way subjects report how simple and complex objects reappear suggest certain theories of perception. A simple figure rapidly disappears, leaving a blank gray field, which gradually darkens until it is black. After a short time, the simple figure then reappears in its complete form. Given a more complex figure, however, subjects report that the image disappears and then is reconstructed in parts that are "meaningful" units, that is, they are logical divisions of the figure and convey significant information about the figure. For example, a face might be reconstructed by first seeing the eyes, next the nose or mouth, then the ears, and so on, until eventually the parts come together to form the complete image of the face. Even nonsense patterns gradually acquire recognizable divisions, and they, too, reappear bit by bit. However, it is also true that meaningless figures tend to be regularized—that is, made more symmetrical or compact.

These two distinct ways of reconstruction illustrate two different theories of perception: the wholistic or gestalt theory, and the cell-assembly theory. According to gestalt theory, perception is an innate process. We are able to look at something and capture that image as a whole simply because we have an inherent ability to assimilate the form we see. In opposition to the gestalt theory, however, is the cell-assembly theory (Hebb, 1949), which holds that perception is a *learned* process. We either recognize the form after an unconscious synthesis of parts, or break it down into meaningful units (those elements of the figure with which we may already be familiar), such as corners, angles, and so forth. Further evidence for the cell-assembly theory might be construed from observing the eye movements made by persons scanning various objects or works of art. Invariably, each person consistently followed a certain pattern of eye movements when observing a particular picture. Although the pattern varied from person to person, any one person tended to repeat his own particular pattern, thus suggesting an attempt to synthesize parts rather than to get a wholistic picture. Gestalt theorists, however, might argue that such a process is segmenting the object into separate wholes. Hence, the two theories may not be as disparate as they seem, and the process of perception is probably a combination of the two processes.

Central Mechanisms of Vision

Given such phenomena as trigger features, lateral inhibition, and color coding, it is obvious that visual processing is under way even at the retinal level. However, the system is complex, and perception requires higher processing by the visual centers in the brain. Therefore, we must follow the visual pathway up into the brain.

Retinal impulses are transmitted via the optic nerve (cranial nerve II), which is formed by the axons of the retinal ganglion cells. The optic nerve from each eye projects toward the brain to a spot just below the frontal lobes, called the optic chiasma. At this point, the fibers from the

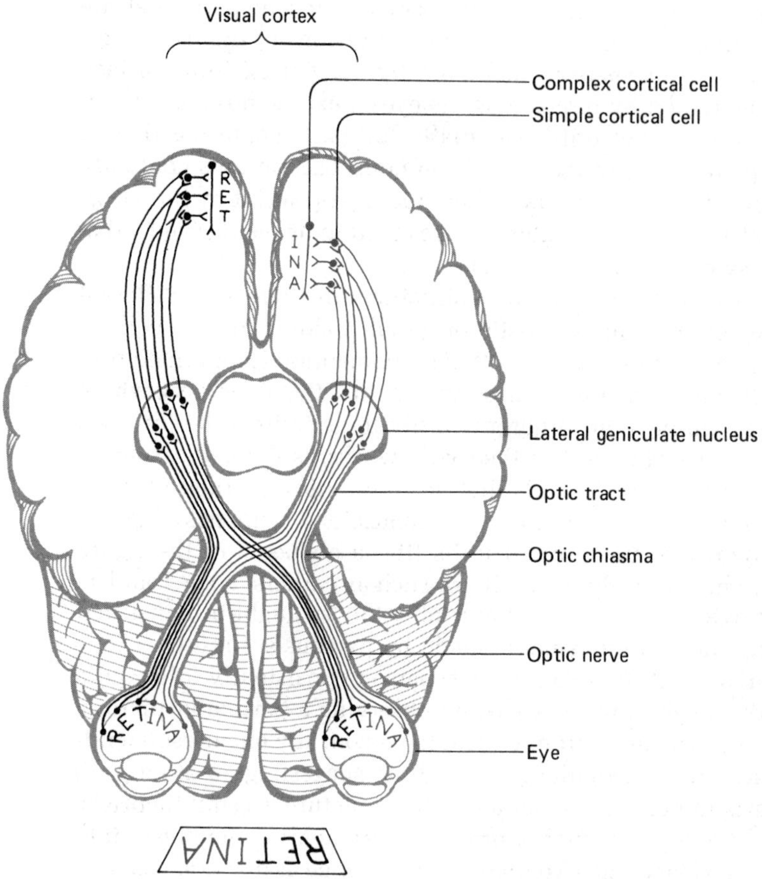

FIGURE 6.15 Visual information from the nasal retina of the left eye and the temporal retina of the right eye projected to the right hemisphere and vice versa.

nasal (inside) and temporal (outside) halves of each eye split up. While the fibers from the temporal hemiretina of the left eye project to the left hemisphere, fibers from the nasal hemiretina cross the midline in the optic chiasma and project to the opposite hemisphere (Figure 6.15). The same is true for the right eye—temporal fibers project ipsilaterally (to the right hemisphere) but nasal fibers project contralaterally (to the left hemisphere).

The temporal and nasal fibers from different eyes projecting to one hemisphere make up the optic tract. Thus, while the optic nerve contains fibers from one eye going to different hemispheres, the optic tract, which begins at the optic chiasma, is composed of fibers from different eyes going to the same hemisphere.

Visual space can be segmented into a left and right visual half-field, commonly referred to as the left and right visual fields. When the eyes are fixated (not moving), all of the visual information in the right field of vision is seen by the temporal hemiretina of the left eye and the nasal hemiretina of the right eye. Similarly, stimuli falling in the left visual field are seen by the right temporal hemiretina and left nasal hemiretina. As a consequence of this scheme, in conjunction with the projection pattern of the nasal and temporal fibers, the left visual field is seen by the right hemisphere and the right visual field by the left hemisphere (Figure 6.15).

Does the foregoing mean, then, that the right side of the brain "sees" only the left visual field, and the left half of the brain sees only the right visual field? Hardly. While it is true that *direct* input to the right side of the brain is only from the left visual field, and vice versa, the two halves of the brain communicate through bridges of fibers called commissures. Thus, through these fiber connections, we have what is called bilateral vision, meaning that each hemisphere of the brain receives visual input from both visual fields.

All of this is really a foreshadowing of things to come. Our real interest at this point is to look at the termination in the brain of the optic tract. As it turns out, while most of the tract fibers (75 percent) in humans project to the lateral geniculate nucleus (Brindley et al., 1969), the remaining fibers mostly terminate in the superior colliculi of the midbrain tectum. Though the geniculate projection is part of the mechanism by which we determine "what" it is we see, the tectal projection is believed to mediate "where" in visual space we direct our attention. We shall consider the retino-tectal pathway first.

Pathway to the Brain: Retino-Tectal Connections

Some retinal fibers leave the optic chiasma and travel to a structure in the midbrain called the superior colliculus (Figure 6.16). The superior colliculi (plural form) are two small "bumps" (one on each side) on the

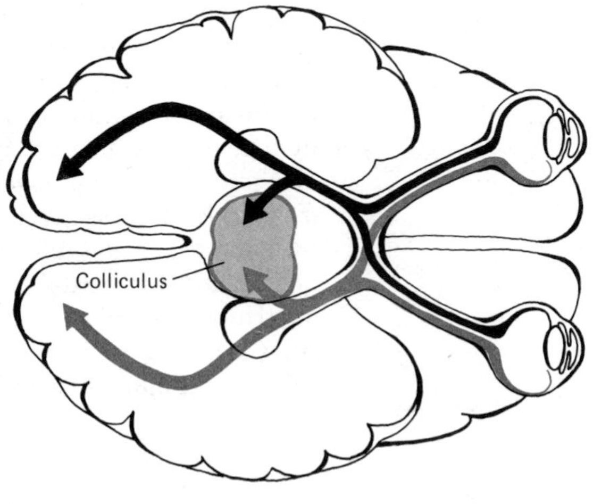

FIGURE 6.16 Retinal projections from the eye also go to the midbrain colliculus. Its functions are different from those of the cortex.

upper surface of the tectum. Each receives visual input both directly (from the retina) and indirectly (from the cortex) (McIlwain and Fields, 1971). In mammals, these nuclei serve the function of coordinating head and eye movements, essentially "telling" the eye where to look (Bizzi, 1971). In the cat, for example, the neurons of the colliculi do not have complex, rigid trigger features, but at least 75 percent of them are particularly direction-sensitive (Norton, 1974). Thus, the cells of the superior colliculus are well adapted for *locating* stimuli, though not particularly well adapted for *identifying* stimuli.

These collicular neurons are attuned to moving stimuli, especially in the periphery of the visual fields. Because these cells (like those of most of the other parts of the brain involved in visual processing) are topographically organized, a stimulus received in the colliculus can alert the animal that some object is in a certain part of the visual field. As a consequence, the animal can, on the basis of collicular input, move its head so that the moving stimulus will be seen in the center of the visual field, thus expediting the use of the more detailed vision attributed to the foveal region of the retina.

In nonmammals, that have a minimal forebrain visual representation, the superior colliculus is the main visual processing center. In mammals, however, the superior colliculus does not process information much beyond the location of the stimulus. So it is as if mammals have two visual systems: the retino-tectal or collicular system tells "where" to look; the retino-cortical system (discussed below) tells "what" is being seen (Schneider, 1969). However, current research is showing that one should be cautious about making too rigid a distinction between the retino-tectal and retino-cortical visual systems, for the colliculi receive input from the cortical areas, and may play some role in pattern vision (Sprague et al., 1970; Butter, 1974).

Processing Station: The Geniculate Relay

As we have said, the first stop for most of the fibers of the optic nerve is the lateral geniculate nucleus (LGN) of the thalamus. As you will recall from Chapter 3, the thalamus consists of three types of nuclei: the extrinsic projection or sensory relay nuclei; the extrinsic association nuclei; and the intrinsic nuclei. The LGN is one of the sensory relay nuclei, and its function is described by its category: It relays sensory information (in this case, visual) to higher parts of the brain. The LGN does little to change the information transmitted; it serves mainly as a channel for carrying neural signals from the retinal ganglion cells to the cortex (Hubel and Wiesel, 1961). In the cat, 90 percent of the LGN cells receive input from only one ganglion cell, or if there is convergence, from a few ganglion cells with similar fields. Most of the LGN cells are X or Y,

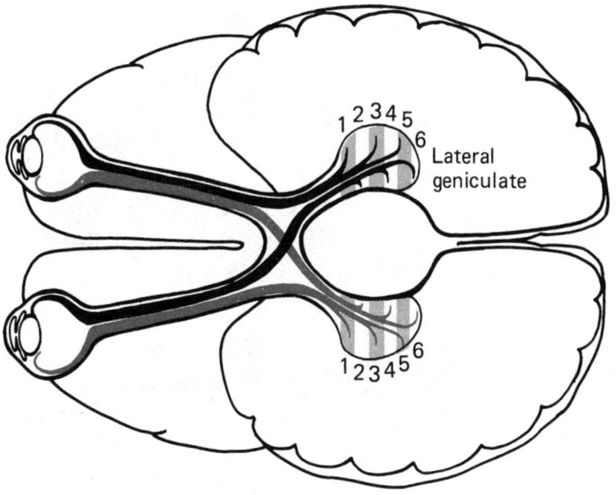

FIGURE 6.17 The lateral geniculate is uniquely organized into layers. Alternate layers respond to stimulation from the ipsilateral eye.

and their output is accordingly either slow or fast, as with the X and Y cells of the retina.

Due to the crossing of fibers at the optic chiasm, both eyes are represented in each LGN. However, the signals from each eye remain anatomically and physiologically independent (Bishop, 1965) (Figure 6.17). Alternate layers of the six layers of the LGN respond to stimulation of the ipsilateral eye (same side) while the other layers respond to stimulation of the contralateral (opposite side) eye. That is, each cell is anatomically connected to only one eye; there are no individual cells that can respond to stimulation of *either* eye. It is only in the cortical areas that we find binocular vision.

Arrival: The Visual Cortex

The highest level of visual processing takes place at the cortex, for it is here that the visual inputs from the two eyes, as well as from the two visual fields, are integrated, and that patterns of light and dark signaled from the retina begin to be interpreted and associated with psychological meaning.

Several areas of the cortex are involved with visual processing. The primary visual area is the striate cortex, so called because of the striped appearance of its cellular arrangement. Surrounding the striate area is the circumstriate belt, which is a secondary visual area (Zeki, 1969). Both the striate and circumstriate areas are largely in the occipital lobe, though the circumstriate belt extends slightly into the parietal lobe. The final visual cortical area is the inferior temporal cortex. As its name implies, this region is in the temporal lobe.

Striate Cortex

A story about a physics teacher's dilemma illustrates the function of the striate cortex and begins the complicated mechanism of integrating the parts into a perceptual whole.

Carole taught physics at the high school. Unusual as it was to have a woman teaching physics, she was excellent. This excellence and the excitement she imparted during class effectively quashed all chauvinistic or even semichauvinistic statements.

Carole's one severe problem was migraine. She had experienced these vicious headaches since sophomore year in college, much the same onset as her mother and sister before her. Her attacks occurred about five times per year. They were unilateral over the right side of her head. The throbbing began behind her right eye and spread so that the entire right hemicranium pulsed with pain. On these days she had to leave school. Her symptom complex included increased irritability, nausea, and vomiting, and when those started, it felt to her as if her head would blow off.

The symptoms that bothered her the most were visual. Early in the process of her migraine she often had a warning or a prodrome other than pain. This period existed for an hour or two before the full-blown pain manifested. Presumably, her doctor told her, this was the phase during which the arteries supplying blood to her brain constricted. Her experience was one of seeing wavy lines that became organized horizontal and vertical lines in her left visual field. Whether she closed her right or left eye the lines, organized so that they looked like the top of a fort, were always in the left side of her visual field. These so-called "fortification spectra" scintillated for about an hour.

During this period she rushed to the cabinet to take the specially prescribed drug that would prevent the well-known subsequent events. For after this stage of migraine, thought to reflect cerebral vessel vasoconstriction, vessel vasodilatation would follow and the excruciating throbbing headache would commence. Often she could abort the stepwise progression of attack at the stage of visual fortification spectra. She was comforted somewhat by the rare incidence of any permanent visual problem with disorder. She also learned to live with the medicine and to abort the attacks.

The striate cortex, like other cortical areas, has six layers. It is also the site of Carole's disorder. Input from LGN terminates in layer IV, providing the striate cortex with a complete topographic representation of the retina (Talbot and Marshall, 1941; Daniel and Whitteridge, 1961). In layer IV, as in the previous way stations in the retinocortical pathway, input from the two eyes remains segregated. If one records from single neurons in this layer, cells will respond to stimulation of one eye or the other, but not to both (Hubel and Wiesel, 1962). In contrast, if the electrode is either raised or lowered, so that cells in the surrounding layers are recorded from, it is possible to find cells that respond to stimulation of either eye. These cells represent the first point of binocular interaction (convergence of input from the two eyes) in the geniculo-cortical system. It is binocular interaction that accounts for the fact that each hemisphere sees a single, complete visual half-field (Hubel and Wiesel, 1965). The left visual field, it will be recalled, is seen by the temporal part of the right eye and the nasal part of the left eye, and all of this is projected to the right hemisphere, where these two representations of the left half-field are put together by binocular cells in the striate cortex. In a similar way, the left hemisphere sees the right visual half-field. Again, prior to the occurrence along the pathway of the binocular cells in the striate cortex, the input from each eye remains separate.

Visual processing in the striate cortex is quite complex, involving cells with intricate processing features. Accordingly, cortical neurons are more sophisticated than cells of the visual pathway below, having much more selective trigger features than retinal or lateral geniculate neurons. Whereas retinal cells respond to local contrast, that is, areas of light or dark, cortical cells require a specific orientation of a line, bar, edge, or some other specific stimulus feature, as determined by the complexity of the cell (Figure 6.18) (Hubel and Wiesel, 1974; Blakemore, 1975b). Although the trigger features are more specific than in the lower centers, the receptive fields are wider than in the lower centers, thus complying with the convergence principle stated earlier, and retinotopic organization is still preserved.

Cells of the striate cortex can be classified in terms of functional complexity (Hubel and Wiesel, 1965, 1968). Simple cells receive their input from LGN neurons, and like cells in the LGN and the retina, have on-off type receptive fields. Complex cells, on the other hand, are generally thought to receive input not only from the LGN, but also from cortical cells (simple cells). Thus, binocular integration in the striate cortex takes place in complex cells by way of convergence of input from simple cells representing the same contralateral visual half-field, but from different eyes (Hubel and Wiesel, 1962). Unlike simple cells, complex cells have no on-off zones; instead, these cells respond best, for example, when a bar is at a particular angle across the receptive field. A third type of cortical cell, the hypercomplex, is a point of further convergence, receiving input from complex cells and possibly some direct thalamic input (Dreher and Cotter, 1974). The hypercomplex cells are quite orientation selective, and demonstrate highly specific stimulus requirements. Because hypercomplex cells are a further point of convergence, their

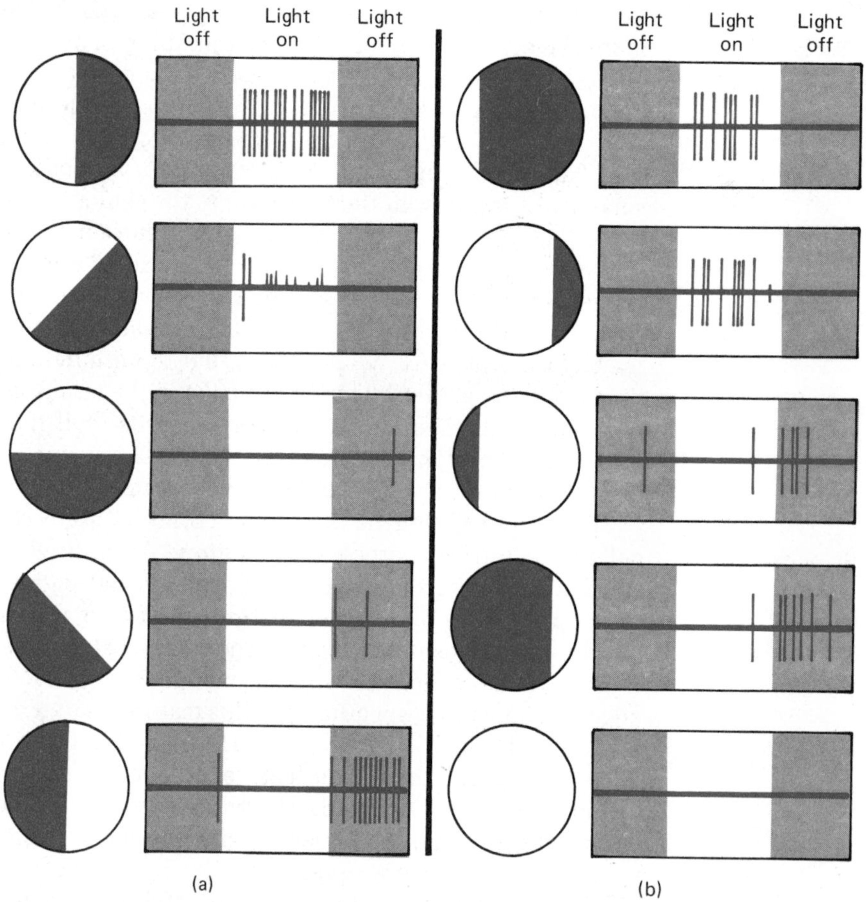

FIGURE 6.18 The varied responses of a single "complex" cell. In (a) the stimulus was presented in different orientations, and in (b), no matter where in the visual field the stimulus seemed there was a response. However, when a light covered the whole field, the cell failed to respond. (After Hubel and Wiesel, 1966.)

receptive fields are larger than the receptive fields of cells previously encountered along the geniculo-cortical pathway.

The striate cortex is organized in columns of cells with similar stimulus requirements (Hubel and Wiesel, 1962). Closely placed cells in the visual cortex have been shown to be functionally similar. These related cells are stacked on top of one another in columns. These columns are in the shape of a cylinder with walls perpendicular to the cortical surface (Figure 6.19).

Two independent but overlapping systems of columns have been identified: orientation and ocular dominance columns (Hubel and Wie-

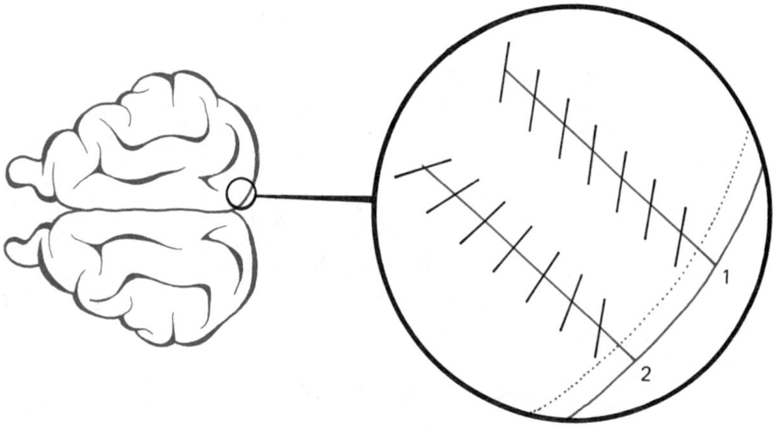

FIGURE 6.19 The original data for columnar organization of the visual cortex was electrophysiological. In electrode penetration one, all cells recorded from had an identical sensitivity. In penetration 2, the electrode hit several different columns. (After Hubel and Wiesel, 1963.)

sel, 1968; 1974). Cells in the ocular dominance columns respond primarily to stimulation of one eye or the other. These columns subdivide the striate cortex into a mosaic of alternating left and right eye strips. The orientation columns contain cells that respond primarily to the angle of stimulus presentation. Approximately 18 to 20 distinct angles of orientation have been identified with columnar organization.

The cortical column is generally believed to arise from the need to portray more than two variables on a two-dimensional surface (Hubel and Wiesel, 1974). The two dimensions of cortical surface are used up by the topographic representation of visual space. This is the primary representation. For each spatial position, there is circuitry for each possible stimulus orientation and for each eye. These secondary representations are made possible by columnar arrangement.

After the Striate, Is There More?

The circumstriate belt, which surrounds the striate cortex, contains several topographic representations of the retina (Zeki, 1974). These representations are in general less precise (have wider receptive fields) than the retinotopic organization found in the striate cortex. In primates, cortico-cortical fibers link the striate cortex to the circumstriate belt (Kuypers et al., 1965), and thus provide for the representations of the contralateral visual field in this area. However, the ipsilateral visual field is also represented in the circumstriate belt. The ipsilateral input is from the circumstriate belt in the opposite half-brain, and arrives by way of the corpus callosum, the large fiber tract that connects the two hemispheres. It is by way of these interhemispheric connections that the two visual half-fields seen by different hemispheres are brought together. Thus, although each hemisphere sees only the contralateral visual field directly, it sees the ipsilateral half-field by way of the callosal sensory window (Berlucchi et al., 1967; Hubel and Wiesel, 1977; LeDoux and Gazzaniga, 1977).

Having considered the anatomical and physiological bases of the visual system, we look now at a couple of examples of how this anatomical substrate is related to behavior.

Spatial Frequency

Hubel and Wiesel's method of studying visual neuronal responses (particularly of cells in orientation columns) is to use a bar as a stimulus aligned a certain way. An alternative method of measuring visual sensitivity is to ascertain how sensitive the visual system is to variations in contrast. It must be remembered that "real-world" stimuli, such as lines presented in various degrees of orientation, also contain infinite subtle variations in contrast. Thus, an appropriate stimulus for measuring contrast detection is a contrast grating, which is a pattern of light and dark bands varying on two dimensions: the amount of contrast between one band and another, and the number of contrasting bands occurring horizontally (Figure 6.20).

Humans have been found to differ from other animals in their sensitivity to various spatial frequencies. Cats, for example, are more sensi-

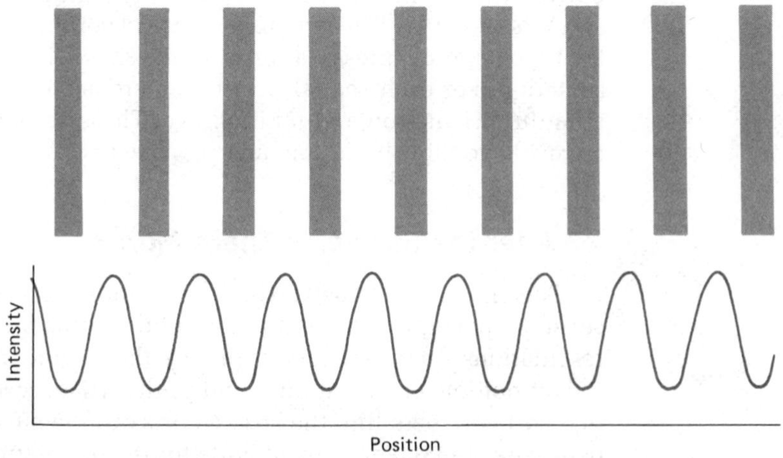

FIGURE 6.20 A spatial sine wave and how it looks in terms of varying degrees of brightness.

tive to detail at low frequencies than are humans, although humans have far better perception at higher spatial frequencies. Cats also demonstrate a more limited range of contrast detection than humans, having individual cells that are selectively responsive to only a small range of spatial frequencies. This difference in visual sensitivity is an example of adaptive evolution. Most of the action important to a cat takes place in the immediate surrounding area, and because of this more limited scope of activity, a cat can afford to see a "smaller world" than a human. Additionally, the cat's sensitivity to fine detail at lower frequencies enables it to survive in an environment where the slightest move by the prey can be detected.

Visual Images All of the foregoing experimental procedures on the visual system, as elegant as they are, have not shed light on how the brain creates visual images. That phenomenon which is in the border between sensation and perception is best illustrated by the case of Winny.

In spite of Winny's bad luck and ill health she remained bright and cheerful. Some said it was her faith in the church; others thought it was her devotion to her family. The reasons didn't matter, though, because this woman had a rare positive energy that was infectious. She worked in the daycare center—actually, she managed the formidable operation for the large neighborhood. The children love her, but Winny had not felt well for several weeks.

Many years before, she had contracted tuberculosis. This disease had spread to her spinal cord, leaving her paralyzed from the waist down. Frequent kidney infections had led to the removal of one kidney, and her most recent ill health was provoked by another plumbing failure. Her kidney had not been extracting and excreting enough poison from her blood and the poisons were at very high levels.

The operation to open the blocked channel from her kidney was difficult and complicated. At one point the surgeon worried that she had died, but she had suffered only a series of irregular heartbeats. Her blood pressure was very low, but her heart never stopped, and the operation continued over six hours.

Some two days later the anesthetic had worn off and she was still in coma from its effect. The operation had been a success. By the fourth day her kidney had begun to excrete more normally and Winny awoke. She awoke, however, with a pounding left-sided headache that no analgesic would relieve. It was the worst headache of her life.

Strangely, associated with this headache were recurrent images, first of her mother sitting on a chair knitting, then just of her mother's hands. These images were hallucinations. Her mother had not visited, and was certainly not present while Winny experienced this visual hallucination. On further description Winny noted that the images were only on the right side of her bed, and that they appeared suddenly. When they appeared they waxed and waned, becoming larger, then smaller than life. They were always accompanied by a headache, which usually occurred after the hallucinations disappeared. When examined, Winny had a slight paralysis affecting only her right side, with decreased sensation to touch, movement, heat, cold, and pain, and a right homonymous deficit in vision. The homonymous deficit in right-field vision indicated that the left temporal retinal half of the left eye and the left nasal retinal half of the right eye were not functioning. In the context of the mild right hemiparesis (slight paralysis) and sensory loss, this right-field deficit could only indicate a small stroke in the left parieto-occipital cortex.

The most fascinating aspect of her condition, the formed hallucinations, was supported by EEG evidence. During the time of the episode of hallucination the EEG recorded left parieto-occipital spike and wave pattern. Subsequent brain scan revealed a small stroke in the left parieto-occipital cortex. Winny was experiencing visual auras of a formed nature because of seizure activity in the parieto-occipital cortex caused by vascular accident, possibly due to her low blood pressure. Although there is no definite explanation for her mysterious hallucinations, speculation centers on the premise that some sort of abnormal neural transmission resulting from the stroke generates these striking visual images. Winny was promptly treated with Dilantin, and the EEG focus of seizure stopped, as did the hallucinations.

Several months later, a repeat exam revealed almost complete resolution of her hemiparesis and hemisensory defect. Her visual defect was resolved. She reported no more hallucinations, and for that she was happy. Researchers in vision, however, may not be happy until they discover just exactly how visual images are stored.

Summary

Where does analysis of the basic and primitive elements of a visual stimulus end, and subjective visual perception begin? The answer to this question is clearly years away from being obtained. Yet the ingenious investigations of neuroscientists throughout the past 20 years have revealed a number of phenomena about the visual process.

The visual process begins at the retina where the transduction of electromagnetic (light) energy to electrochemical energy occurs. Rods and cones, through changes in chemicals, transmit electrical impulses across a converging series of synapses to the brain. In humans, the peripheral field and detailed central vision form the visual world, but these aspects depend in the first instance on the photoreceptor. Laura's story illustrates the importance of the ganglion cells in the eye. Disruption of the neural message at this stage results in a constricted peripheral field, and loss of color vision and acuity. For humans the mere appreciation of light, or of movement, is simply inadequate.

The orderly flow of information must pass retinal cells first. Some fibers then go to the tectum. Most, however, are projected with great specificity and orderliness to the cortex via the lateral geniculate body. Thus messages from the temporal retina and nasal retina of the opposite eye are singularly represented by the cells in the lateral geniculate body, and just as singularly projected to the cortex. Here the cells are even more complex, with additional selective trigger features. For example, a ganglion cell may respond to an edge of light; in order for a cortical cell to respond, this edge must have a specific orientation, say 15° oblique to the horizontal. Light-message-sensitive cortical neurons may be more specific than those cells in lower centers, but their receptive fields are wider, complying with the convergence principle. Complex cells and simple cells, orientation and ocular dominance columns further define the specificity of the message.

Yet we still do not understand the total perceptual process involved in viewing, for example, a great work of art. In similar fashion, but focusing on the disrupted system, we do not understand migraine headaches which produce visual images of fortifications. Nor do we understand even more complex visual hallucinations that are complex formed mirages. Explanations of the stories of Carole and Winny are as elusive as the appreciation of beauty. Clearly the challenge remains to relate the anatomical findings to the psychological processes.

References

Benevento, L. A., and J. H. Pallon. 1975. The ascending projections of the superior colliculus in the Rhesus monkey *(Macaca mulatta). J. Comp. Neurol. 160*:339–362.

Berlucchi, G., M. S. Gazzaniga, and G. Rizzdatti. 1967. Microelectrode analysis of visual information by the corpus callosum. *Arch. Ital. Biol. 105*:583–596.

Bishop, P. O. 1965. The nature of the representation of the visual fields in the lateral geniculate nucleus. *Proc. Australian Assoc. Neurol. 3*:15–25.

Blakemore, C. 1975a. Development of cat's visual cortex following rotation of one eye. *Nature 257*:584.

Blakemore, C. 1975b. Central visual processing. In: M. S. Gazzaniga and C. Blakemore, eds. *Handbook of Psychobiology*. New York: Academic Press.

Brindley, G. S., P. C. Gautier-Smith, and W. Lewin. 1969. Cortical blindness and the functions of the non-geniculate fibres of the optic tracts. *J. Neurol. Neurosurg. Psychiat. 32*: 259–264.

Brown, P. K., and G. Wald. 1964. Visual pigments in single rods and cones of the human retina. *Science 144*:145–151.

Burkhardt, D. A. 1968. Cone action spectra: Evidence from the goldfish electroretinogram. *Vision Res. 8*:839, 853.

Butter, C. M. 1974. Visual discrimination impairment in Rhesus monkeys with combined lesions of superior colliculus and striate cortex. *J. Comp. Physiol. Psychol. 87*:918–929.

Campbell, F. W., L. Maffei, and M. Piccolino. 1973. The contrast sensitivity of the cat. *J. Physiol. 229*:719–731.

Cowey, A., and C. G. Gross. 1970. Effects of foveal prestriate and inferotemporal lesions on visual discrimination by Rhesus monkeys. *Exp. Brain Res. 11*:128–144.

Daniel, P. M., and D. Whitteridge. 1961. The representation of the visual field on the cerebral cortex in monkeys. *J. Physiol. 86*:353–380.

Dowling, J. E. 1967. The site of visual adaptation. *Science 155*:273–279.

Dowling, J. E., and B. B. Boycott. 1966. Organization of the primate retina: Electron Microscopy. *Proc. Roy. Soc. London 166*:80–111.

Dreher, B., and L. J. Cotter. 1974. Visual receptive field properties of cells in area 18 of the cat's cortex before and after acute lesions in area 17. *J. Neurophysiol. 3*:735–750.

Gross, C. G. 1973. Visual functions of inferotemporal cortex. In: R. Jung, ed. *Handbook of Sensory Physiology*. Berlin: Springer-Verlag, Vol. 7, pp. 431–482.

Haaxman, R., and H. G. J. M. Kuypers. 1975. Intrahemispheric cortical connexions and visual guidance of hand and finger movements in the Rhesus monkey. *Brain 98*:239–260.

Harting, J. K., K. K. Glendenning, I. T. Diamond, and W. C. Hall. 1973. Evolution of the primate visual system: Anterograde degeneration studies of the tecto-pulvinar system. *Amer. J. Phys. Anthropol. 38*:383–392.

Hartline, H. K. 1940. The receptive fields of optic nerve fibers. *Amer. J. Physiol. 130*: 690–699.

Hebb, D. O. 1949. *The Organization of Behavior*. New York: Wiley.

Hubel, D. H., and T. N. Wiesel. 1961. Integrative action in the cat's lateral geniculate body. *J. Physiol. 155*:385–398.

Hubel, D. H., and T. N. Wiesel. 1962. Receptive fields, binocular interaction, and functional architecture in the cat's visual cortex. *J. Physiol. 160*:106–154.

Hubel, D. H., and T. N. Wiesel. 1965. Receptive fields and functional architecture in two non-striate visual areas of the cat. *J. Neurophysiol. 28*:229–289.

Hubel, D. H., and T. N. Wiesel. 1967. Cortical and callosal connections concerned with the vertical meridian of visual fields in the cat. *J. Neurophysiol. 30*:1561–1573.

Hubel, D. H., and T. N. Wiesel. 1968. Receptive fields and functional architecture of monkey striate cortex. *J. Physiol. 195*:215–243.

Hubel, D. H., and T. N. Wiesel. 1974. Sequence regularity and geometry of orientation columns in the monkey striate cortex. *J. Comp. Neurol. 158*:267–294.

Hubel, D. H., and T. N. Wiesel. 1963. Shape and arrangement of columns in cat's striate cortex. *J. Physiol. 165*:559–568.

Hurwich, L. M., and D. Jameson. 1957. An opponent process theory of color vision. *Psychol. Rev. 64*:384–404.

Kluver, J., and P. C. Bucy. 1939. Preliminary analysis of functions of the temporal lobes in monkeys. *Arch. Neurol. Psychiat. 42*:979–1000.

Kuffler, S. W. 1960. Excitation, and inhibition in single nerve cells. *Harvey Lectures 54*: 176–218.

Kuffler, S. W. 1953. Discharge patterns and functional organization of mammalian retina. *J. Neurophysiol. 16*:37–68.

Kuypers, K. G. J. M., M. C. Szwarcbart, M. Mishkin, and J. E. Rosvold. 1965. Occipitotemporal cortico-cortical connections in the Rhesus monkey. *Exp. Neurol.* *11*:245–262.
LeDoux, J. E., and M. S. Gazzaniga. 1977. *The Integrated Mind.* New York: Plenum.
Marks, W. B. 1965. Visual pigments of single goldfish cones. *J. Physiol.* *178*:14–32.
Marks, W. B., W. H. Dobelle, and E. F. MacNichol. 1964. Visual pigments of single primate cones. *Science* *143*:1181–1183.
McIlwain, J. T., and H. L. Fields. 1971. Interactions of cortical and retinal projections on single neurons of cat's superior colliculus. *J. Neurophysiol.* *34*:763–772.
Mishkin, M. 1965. Visual mechanisms beyond the striate cortex. In: R. Russell, ed. *Frontiers of Physiological Psychology.* New York: Academic Press.
Norton, T. T. 1974. Receptive field properties of superior colliculus cells and development of visual behavior in kittens. *J. Neurophysiol.* *37*:674–690.
Rocha-Miranda, C. E., D. B. Bender, C. G. Gross, and M. Mishkin. 1975. Visual activation of neurons in inferotemporal cortex depends on striate cortex and forebrain commissures. *J. Neurophysiol.* *38*:475–491.
Rodieck, R. W. 1973. *The Vertebrate Retina, Principles of Structure and Function.* San Francisco: Freeman.
Rodieck, R. W., and J. Stone. 1965a. Response of cat retinal ganglion cells to moving visual patterns. *J. Neurophysiol.* *28*:819–832.
Rodieck, R. W., and J. Stone. 1965b. Analysis of receptive fields of cat ganglion cells. *J. Neurophysiol.* *28*:833–849.
Sachs, M. B., J. Nachmias, and J. G. Robson. 1971. Spatial-frequency channels in human vision. *J. Opt. Soc. Amer.* *61*:1176–1186.
Schneider, G. E. 1969. Two visual systems. *Science* *163*:895–902.
Sprague, J. M., G. Berlucchi, and A. DiBernardino. 1970. The superior colliculus and pretectum in visually guided behavior and visual discrimination in the cat. *Brain Behav. Evol.* *3*:285–294.
Stiles, W. S. 1949. Increment thresholds and the mechanisms of human color vision. *Docum. Ophthal.* *3*:138–163.
Stiles, W. S. 1959. Color vision: the approach through increment-threshold sensitivity. *Proc. Nat. Acad. Sci.* *45*:100–114.
Talbot, S. A., and W. H. Marshall. 1941. Physiological studies on neural mechanisms of visual localization and discrimination. *Amer. J. Ophthal.* *24*:1255–1264.
Tomita, T., A. Kancko, M. Murakami, and E. Pautler. 1967. Spectral response curves of single cones in carp. *Vision Res.* *7*:519–531.
Uttal, W. R. 1973. *The Psychobiology of Sensory Coding.* New York: Harper & Row.
Wald, G. 1959. The photoreceptor process in vision. In: J. Field, ed. *Handbook of Physiology.* Section I: Neurophysiology, Vol. 1. Washington, D.C.: American Physiological Society, pp. 671–692.
Wald, G. 1968. Molecular basis of visual excitation. *Science* *162*:230–239.
Wald, G. 1964. The receptors of human color vision. *Science* *145*:1007–1017.
Wald, G. 1966. Reflective color vision and its inheritance. *Proc. Nat. Acad. Sci.* *55*: 1347–1363.
Witkovsky, P. 1968. The effect of chromatic adaptation on color sensitivity of the carp electroretinogram. *Vision Res.* *8*:825–837.
Young, R. W. 1967. The renewal of photoreceptor cell outer segments. *J. Cell. Biol.* *33*: 61–72.
Young, R. W. 1969. A difference between rods and cones in the renewal of outer segment protein. *Invest. Opthal.* *8*:222–231.
Zeki, S. M. 1969. The secondary visual areas of the monkey. *Brain Res.* *13*:197–226.
Zeki, S. M. 1974. Comparison of the cortical degeneration in the visual regions of the temporal lobe of the monkey following the section of the anterior commissure and the splenium. *J. Comp. Neurol.* *143*:167–175.

CHAPTER 7

Hearing and Language Mechanisms

Although it is hard to impose a hierarchical ordering of the senses, most people would agree that audition is one of the most important senses. Life without sound is a lonely existence. Some might say that those who have never experienced the pleasures of a Beethoven symphony or a Bach fugue or even a song by Bob Dylan have never lived, and surely all would agree that being deprived of ever hearing laughter or conversation again would be a cruel and unusual punishment.

Since both vision and audition are sensory processes, they appear to function in similar ways. Receptor cells receive the stimulus and convert it into a neural impulse, which is then propagated along various neural pathways through the brain. We know more about the visual processes, however, than the auditory processes. One of the problems involved with researching the auditory system is that it is less accessible than is the eye, and there are technical problems involved in getting to the mechanisms of the hearing system. The inner ear is encased in a bony cavity of the skull, and the cortical areas (in humans) are buried in the depths of a fissure. Thus, the hearing process, from the first step of sound stimulus converted into a neural impulse, to the integration processes that go on at the highest level of the cortex, is difficult to understand. An additional problem with research in the field of audition is that one of the most important functions, language-processing, is, at least as we know it, unique to humans, and thus experimental observations of this process are not possible with animal subjects.

Despite these problems, a great deal is known about the nature of the sound wave, the anatomy of the ear, and the central pathways in the brain. Much, too, has been learned about how we locate a sound in space. In this chapter, we shall look at each of these topics, and shall also look at what is known about how we identify a sound. How is it that we decode spoken words? Are there specialized feature detectors as in the visual system? Some answers to these questions will be discussed as we examine audition in development and the role of audition in the production and perception of vocal sounds. First, though, from the medical clinics we have an example of how devastating yet subtle a hearing loss can be.

Karl had always been in the top tenth of his class. Both college and business school had been games for this budding financial wizard. Before graduation he was managing large sums of money. So it was no surprise that he quickly grew impatient working at Hornblower. The corporate presidents simply could not advance him fast enough, and to keep him Karl was promoted to an executive vice presidency. In the last six months, though, there had been a dramatic decrease in his extraordinarily productive efforts. Frankly, he became at once irascible and diffident. Some related it to the inevitable corruption of power. More sensitive thoughts prevailed though, and the president suggested he see a doctor.

The most remarkable part of the history taking was Karl's almost constant "I beg your pardon." He simply could not hear. In fact, when questioned about his hearing, he told of a ringing noise that recurred often throughout each day for the last year. Never before had he experienced this phenomenon. Minor head trauma occurred years ago, but there had been no loss of consciousness or hearing difficulty.

This ringing noise, called tinnitus, irritated him to a point where concentration was impossible. Headaches, occurring for the first time in the last two weeks, were an unwelcome additional symptom.

Examination was remarkable for a Weber test showed hearing only in the left ear. For this maneuver a tuning fork is placed on top of the skull. Vibrations of the tuning fork should be heard and felt in both ears. When the eighth cranial nerve is not functioning properly only the remaining healthy nerve senses the vibration. Simply quietly whispering into each ear often does not reveal the loss, although it was simple in Karl's case because he was deaf in his right ear.

Karl went into the hospital for this combination of hearing loss, tinnitus, headaches, and personality change. Early investigation included analysis of his cerebrospinal fluid. This waterlike material circulates within the ventricles of the brain, around and over the hemispheres and down the spinal column. It acts as a cushion for the central nervous structures, and certain products of brain metabolism are carried in this fluid. The analysis revealed a very high protein level, and this suggested inflammation, perhaps from a tumor. Further neurological x-rays confirmed the diagnosis of mass expanding against the eighth cranial or acoustic nerve. And at operation this mass was identified as an acoustic neuroma.

Sadly, Karl lost the hearing in that ear, but he could be sure that the maddening tinnitus would not recur. His headaches ceased, but the corporate presidents at Hornblower were still unsatisfied. This time the reason was different. Karl felt so good after the operation, he quit to manage his own firm.

The Anatomy of a Sound Wave

The auditory stimulus consists of a movement of molecules of air called a sound wave. One should not think of a sound wave as a traveling group of molecules, but instead as a pressure generated, in the case of a tuning fork, by the oscillations of the tongs, or in the case of a vocal sound, by the vibrations of the vocal cords (Figure 7.1).

The forward motion produces a compression of air, and the backward motion produces a slight vacuum, called a rarefaction. A mechanically generated tone produces a repetitive sound wave (called a pure sine wave), but as a tuning fork gradually stops its oscillating motion, the pressure gradually subsides, so the amplitude, or height, of the sound wave gradually diminishes. The regions of greatest compression (thus of maximum pressure) are called crests; the regions of greatest rarefaction

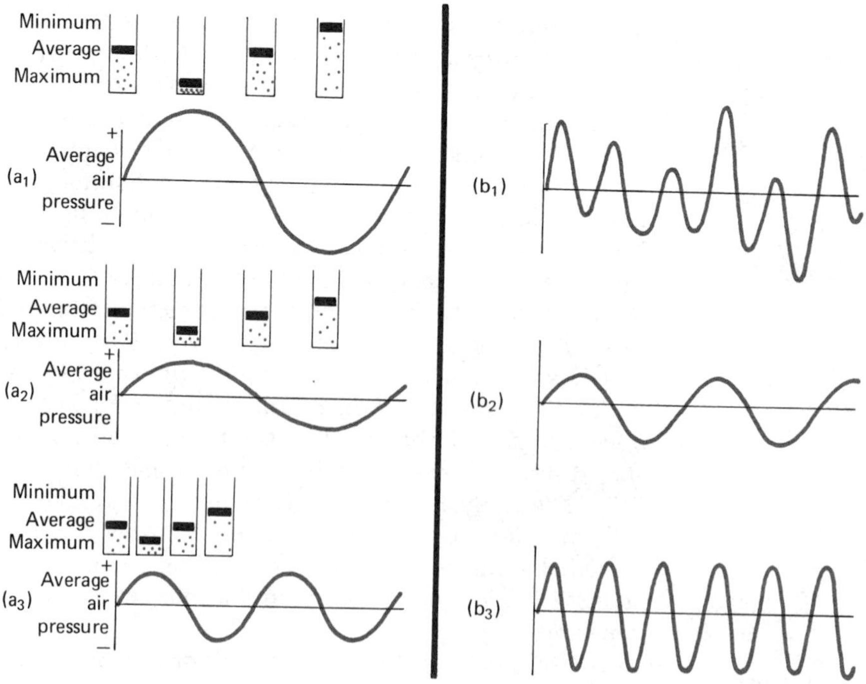

FIGURE 7.1 A sound wave. Sound production causes a movement of air molecules that may be regular, as in the case of a pure sine wave, or may, as is more common, vary irregularly. The sound waves, or vibrations of air, are received by the ear and transformed into neural impulses.

(thus of minimum pressure), troughs. The wavelength is the separation between the crest and the crest; the amplitude, which is one-half the wavelength, accounts for the loudness of a sound. Amplitude, sometimes called the intensity of a sound, is measured in decibels (dB). A decibel is not a unit, per se, but expresses a ratio, a logarithmic scale, each decibel being 10 times the physical energy of the preceding value.

A typical amplitude for, say, a quiet background noise level is about 20 dB. Most normal conversations are at 50 dB. Some rock concerts have been measured at 100 dB, coming dangerously close to the threshold of pain, 130 dB. Permanent damage can be inflicted by noise at 150 dB.

Frequency, or the number of times the pressure oscillates per unit of time, accounts for pitch, or the subjective impression of a tone. Frequency is measured in units called hertz, or cps, each hertz being one cycle per second. A stable, unmodulated frequency accounts for what is called a pure tone, but except for certain synthetic instruments, we rarely hear pure tones. Musical instruments produce a mixture or combination of pure tones, with the fundamental, or lowest tone, furnishing the overtones, or timbre, of the instrument. The difference between the sound of a clarinet and a violin, for example, is in the harmonics they generate.

If there are no regular, repetitive patterns of sound waves involved, and there are frequencies that are not in harmonic relation, then the sound is classified as noise. According to this definition, human speech is generally classified as noise, or dissonant sound, since the sound waves of our speech patterns mapped into waves rarely present a harmonic relationship, being instead an irregular pattern with many fluctuations of amplitude and frequency. We can hear sounds ranging from 20 to 20,000 cps, and our most sensitive range, that is, where we can hear close to 0 dB, is between 1000 and 3000 cps. Most music and speech fall within this range. As we get older, we become less sensitive to the higher frequencies.

Thus it is evident that everyday noises are not simple; our auditory system must be capable of decoding complex stimuli. Yet despite the complicated patterns of sound waves, humans and other animals are able to respond appropriately to a vast array of sounds, ranging from things that go bump in the night to the sweet words of love whispered in our ears.

The most popular hypothesis of how we hear assumes that we break down the stimuli into simple components. The simple components of the sound are encoded neurally and sent to the higher levels of the brain. To some extent we analyze the component frequencies, as when we hear a musical chord and can distinguish the different notes. The following examination of the neural processing system will present the various theories of hearing.

The Ear: Peripheral Receptor

The role of the ear, the receptor organ of the auditory system, is to take the sound waves, however complicated they might be, and transform them into coded neural impulses that can then be decoded and processed. There are three main divisions of the ear: outer, middle, and inner ear (Figure 7.2). Each part is important to the transduction process, but the functions of the outer ear and middle ear are purely mechanical; neural impulses are not generated until the sound wave reaches the organ of Corti in the inner ear. Nonetheless, these mechanical modifications are significant in reducing the size of the sound waves and generally increasing the intensity, thus expediting the transduction process executed in the small chambers of the inner ear.

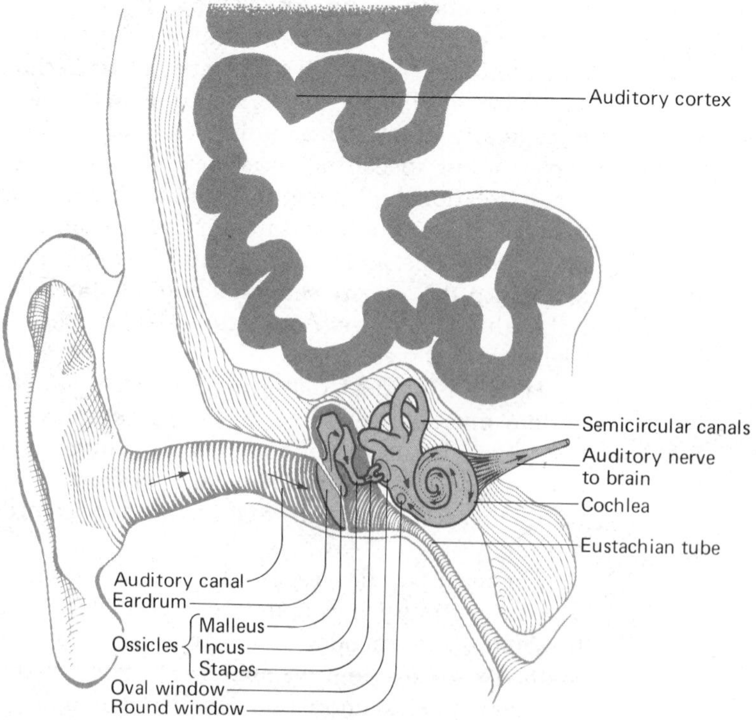

FIGURE 7.2 The ear. Shown here are the outer, middle, and inner portions of the ear, each of which plays an important role in the transduction process.

The Outer Ear and Middle Ear: Hearing Begins

The pinna, the fleshy, cartilaginous mass generally referred to as the ear, acts as a funnel or hearing horn to collect sound waves. Animals can tilt or move their ears to better hear sounds, but most humans have lost that ability. Consequently, the pinna can be considered a vestigial organ in humans, useful for displaying earrings, but not fulfilling the use suggested by its design. Nonetheless, all waves to be processed pass through the pinna and travel through the auditory canal (also called the external meatus), an opening about 6 mm in diameter and about 3 cm long. The outer ear terminates at the tympanic membrane, the conical-shaped membrane commonly called the eardrum. Vibrations of the eardrum caused by the sound waves are transmitted to the middle ear to a chain of three tiny bones called the ossicles.

These three bones, the malleus, the incus, and stapes (commonly called the hammer, anvil, and stirrups), perform the mechanical function of compressing the sound waves to a much smaller area, thus resulting in a more intense signal. That is, the amplitude of the wave is reduced, but the pressure is increased.

The middle ear not only is capable of essentially increasing the signal by reducing the amplitude and increasing the pressure; in the event of loud noises, the muscles of the inner ear can contract so that the signal transmitted by the ossicles is actually less intense than it might have been. This reflex cannot occur fast enough to lessen the intensity of a sudden sound, but it can protect us from the noise generated by an approaching airplane, a loud concert, etc. This mechanical modification of the auditory stimulus is similar to the action of the pupil in controlling the amount of light that enters the eye.

The middle ear, though separated from outside air by the tympanic membrane, is connected to outside air by a rather unusual passageway, the Eustachian tube, which connects the middle ear and the throat. That is why the pressure felt in your ear when riding in a very fast elevator or sometimes in airplanes can be relieved by opening your mouth to yawn. The temporary inner pressure caused by the rapid change in atmospheric pressure is dispelled through the Eustachian tube. If this passageway becomes clogged, as when you have a cold and mucus obstructs the tube, a buildup of pressure may be felt in the middle ear that cannot be released by yawning.

The Inner Ear: Site of (Neural) Transduction

The mechanical modifications by the outer and middle ear are important in transforming the sound stimulus to a form more readily processed by the inner ear. However, as mentioned before, the stimulus does not actually enter the nervous system until it reaches the inner ear, and specifically the organ of Corti.

The inner ear is composed of two main parts: the *cochlea,* which is the primary auditory mechanism, and the *semicircular canals,* or vestibular apparatus, which are concerned with balance, and will be discussed later in Chapter 9. The middle ear and the inner ear are separated by the oval window, a membrane-covered aperture at the large end of the cochlea (Figure 7.3). The cochlea itself, which houses the all-important *organ of Corti,* is a small, tapered tube coiled up like a snail shell, having in humans about 3½ windings, and in some animals, as many as 5 windings. The tube is divided into three parts by two membranes. One part, the *scala vestibuli,* is separated from a second part, the *scala media,* by Reissner's membrane, an ionic barrier that is only a single cell in thick-

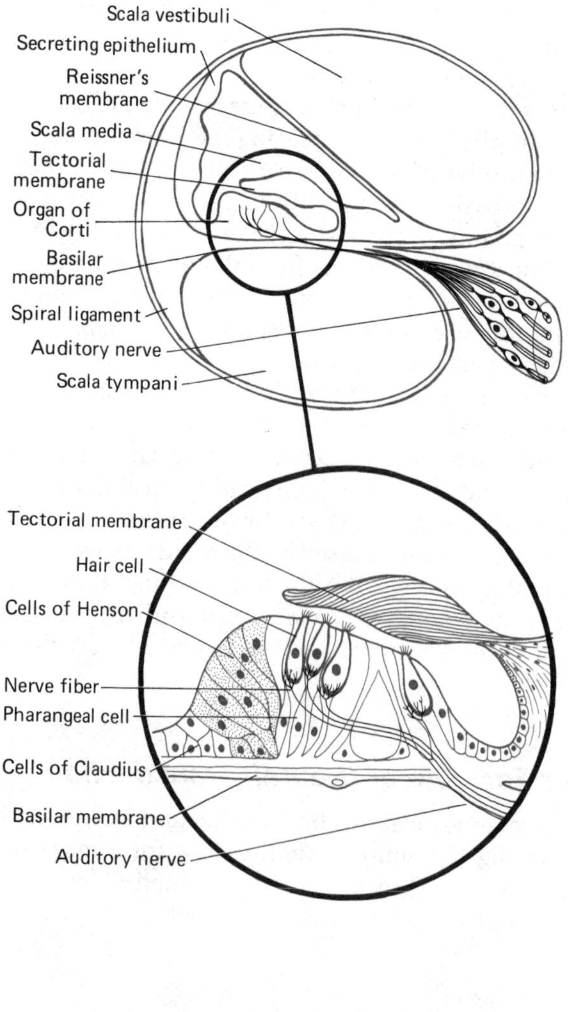

FIGURE 7.3 The cochlea. The organ of Corti is shown inside the cochlea. The shearing action of the tectorial membrane against the hair cells initiates the actual transduction process.

ness. The scala media is separated from the *scala tympani* by the basilar membrane. Actually, the scala vestibuli and the scala tympani are parts of a single surrounding cavity, being joined through a small hole called the helicotrema at the small end of the cochlea. All three cavities are fluid-filled, and since the scala vestibuli and scala tympani are connected, they have the same fluid, which is perilymph, a high-sodium-content fluid. The scala media, however, is filled with endolymph, a fluid dominated by potassium.

In the transduction process, the scala media is the most important part of the cochlea, for it is there that we find the receptor cells of the ear, the hair cells. Although how they function is not fully known, the hair cells are without a doubt the site of the neural transduction for sound. They are attached to the basilar membrane and covered by a loose flap of tissue called the tectorial membrane, which is connected to the wall of the scala media at only one end and supported separately from the basilar membrane. The hair cells, basilar membrane, and tectorial membrane collectively form what is called the organ of Corti.

The hair cells are arranged in four parallel rows. The three rows toward the outside of the spiral cochlea contain the outer or external hair cells, while the single row facing the inside of the spiral contains the inner hair cells (Figure 7.4).

A hair cell synapses almost immediately, having no elongated axonal processes, but instead having synaptic connections at the base of the cell, which is called a basal body (Engstrom et al., 1965). The basal body connects to the dendrites of the cells of the auditory nerve.

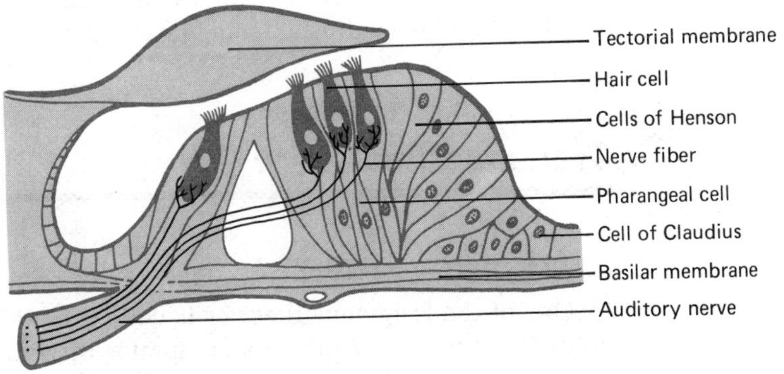

FIGURE 7.4 Hair cells. The receptor cells of the auditory system are difficult to study because of their inaccessibility. However, it is thought that there are inner and outer hair cells, and that the terminals may be either afferent or efferent.

The Transduction Process

The transduction process begins when the vibrations of the ossicles (the tiny bones in the middle ear stimulated by sound waves) are transferred to the oval window, which separates the middle ear from the scala vestibuli of the inner ear. These vibrations set the fluid of the scala vestibuli (the perilymph) in motion, and in turn transfer through Reissner's membrane and set the fluid of the scala media (the endolymph) in motion. Essentially, then, the sound wave creates a wave motion in the cochlea that causes all of the membranes (Reissner's, tectorial, and basilar) to move up and down.

Since the tectorial membrane is attached at only one end, it is free to move against the hair cells, resulting in a shearing or bending motion of the hair cells. It is this action that is believed to produce the receptor potential that is transmitted to the auditory nerve. Somehow, the hair cells are excited by the bending motion, undoubtedly through some kind of depolarization, and the impulse is transmitted through the basal body lying below each hair cell to the cochlear nerve fibers. Since Newton's law states that every action must have an equal reaction, vibrations of the scala media and the stretching down of the basilar membrane result in a corresponding movement of the perilymph of the scala tympani, the cavity below the scala media. This induced pressure is released through the round window, which bulges out into the middle ear. That pressure is then, as mentioned before, released via the throat through the Eustachian tube.

Such a simplistic description of the transduction process covers only the barest mechanical details. Trying to determine just how pitch and loudness are actually encoded by the auditory receptors is a complicated task, particularly since there are still gaps in what we know about the transduction process. At present, theories of hearing can largely be classified under two headings: frequency and place.

Transduction Theory

Frequency Theory

One of the frequency theories is called the telephone theory, which holds that the basilar membrane vibrates up and down at a rate that is the same as the frequency of the wave, and its amplitude, or height, corresponds in a ratio to the amplitude of a sound wave. Thus, because the hair cells are stimulated at the peak of each pulse, they transmit the correct frequency, and according to this theory, respond to the amplitude

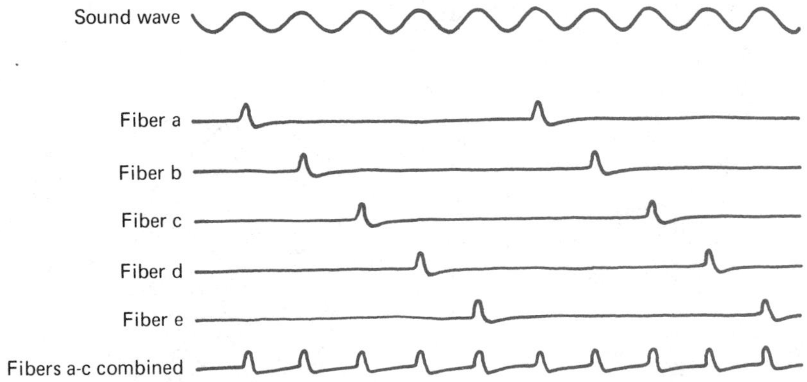

FIGURE 7.5 The volley theory. Individual fibers of the auditory nerve are assumed to respond as a group to a given frequency, with each axon being phase-locked to fire at a specific interval. Their combined output is interpreted by the brain to signify the particular frequency.

either by firing at a higher rate or having a higher percentage of axons fire at one time.

Although this theory sounds logical, it cannot account for all frequencies of audible sound simply because an axon is incapable of responding at a rate higher than about 1000 pulses per second. Thus, if this theory alone accounted for our hearing processes, any frequency higher than 1000 cps could not be transmitted, yet we know that it is possible to hear frequencies up to 20,000 cps. Also, given that increased output per pulse would signify increased intensity, it would be difficult to distinguish amplitude increases from frequency increases in the low range of the audible spectrum.

A modification of frequency theory that allows for some of the complications is the volley theory (Figure 7.5). This theory assumes that not all axons transmit a pulse at each peak of the sound wave. Rather, they are synchronized (phase-locked is the more appropriate term) to fire at intervals corresponding to time between peaks (Rose et al., 1969). That is, one axon may fire at every third peak, starting with the first. Another may fire at every third peak starting with the second, and so on. Thus, while it is true that no one neuron could fire faster than 1000 pulses per second, neurons firing sequentially as a group could accommodate higher frequencies. After all, there are thousands of nerve fibers forming the cochlear nerve. However, even the volley theory is not complete for it cannot explain how the high frequencies at the farthest range of the audible spectrum are transmitted.

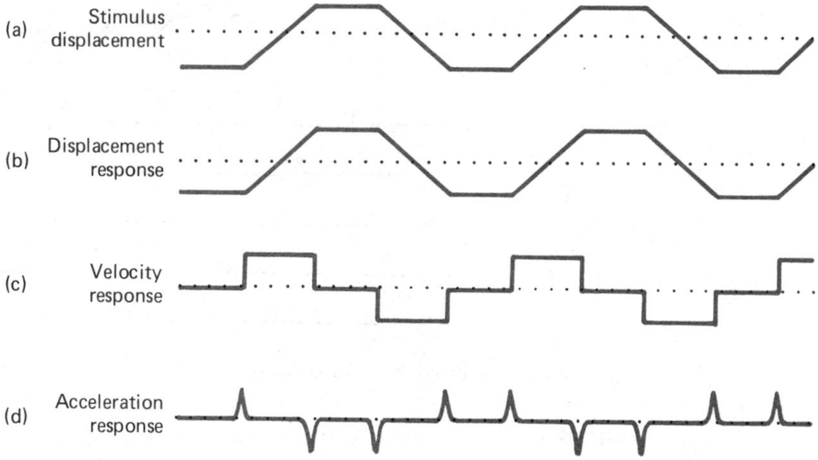

FIGURE 7.6 Place theory. These four drawings are rough examples of how a given sound wave looks when recorded (a), and then of how the response of the cochlea (called the cochlear microphonic) would be expected to look according to three different theories of the transduction process. Part (b) shows how it would look according to place theory, part (c), how it would look according to the velocity hypothesis, and part (d), how it would look if it were an acceleration sensitive response. The actual recording of the cochlear microphonic in response to the sound looks most like (b); thus von Bekesy's place theory of hearing is supported.

Place Theory

Naturally, like the frequency theories, place theory depends on the physical characteristics of the sound wave and the mechanical action induced by the wave, but as the name suggests, place theory holds that different sounds stimulate the basilar membrane in different places according to the frequency of the sound wave (Figure 7.6). Also called the traveling wave theory, this idea assumes that a high-frequency wave, being a relatively short wave, will travel only a short distance, while a low-frequency wave, being longer, will travel further. According to place theory, neurons firing from a specific place on the membrane signal a certain frequency to the brain; neurons firing from another place signal a different frequency.

Most of the research on place theory was done by Georg von Bekesy, who received the Nobel prize in 1962 for his work. Through experiments with many cochleas, he mapped the basilar membrane, finding relatively similar patterns of vibration from one cochlea to another in response to sound waves. Such regularity certainly lends support to von Bekesy's view that the basilar membrane vibrates selectively (von Bekesy, 1960). However, place theory, too, has its shortcomings. One of the problems associated with place theory is that the range of vibrations of the basilar membrane varies only from 1 to 100, whereas the average range of hearing varies from 1 to 10,000. In other words, place theory could not accommodate enough different specific frequencies to account for our wide range of hearing (20 to 20,000 cps). A second problem is that the basilar membrane does not seem to vibrate selectively for low frequencies.

Thus, it seems that both frequency and place theories have attendant problems. The frequency theory, as mentioned before, will not work for high frequencies. Conversely, the place idea does not seem to hold for low frequencies. Both theories, however, possess a certain validity, and ultimately it is probably some combination of the two that will explain the first step of how we hear.

Cochlear Microphonic

One interesting property of the cochlea is its ability to transmit sound. By attaching recording electrodes to the cochlea, one can hear exactly what input the cochlea is receiving. Because the electrical response of the cochlea is essentially merely a relay of the sound stimulus, it has been termed the cochlear microphonic. The function of this electric potential is not fully known, but it is believed to act as the generator or receptor potential, stimulating the auditory nerve cells, which then encode the sound according to whatever neural code is used to designate tone and amplitude.

The Central Auditory Pathways

However the receptor potentials are generated, they are transmitted from the receptor cells to the bipolar cells whose cell bodies collectively form the spiral ganglion, which is embedded in the bony structure of the skull. The axons of these cells form the cochlear nerve, the acoustic division of cranial nerve VIII.

The cochlear nerve is unique among the sensory nerves in the number of decussations, or crossing of fibers, it has between the receptor organ (the ear) and the cortex. There are at least four places where the nerve bifurcates; thus every structure along the pathway has bilateral input. This is in marked contrast to the visual system, which has only one decussation (the optic chiasm) and hence does not have bilateral innervation of structures until the collicular and thalamic levels and does not have binocularly driven cells until the cortex. This difference between the auditory and visual systems reflects the more difficult process of locating a sound in space compared with locating a visual stimulus. The numerous crossings of auditory input allow for comparison of the sound from each direction at each level of the pathway in the brain, thus facilitating the location of the sound source. The process of localization will be discussed in detail later.

The organizational pattern of the auditory system is tonotopical, an organizational principle similar to the retinotopic design found in the visual system (Figure 7.7). In the auditory system, that means that

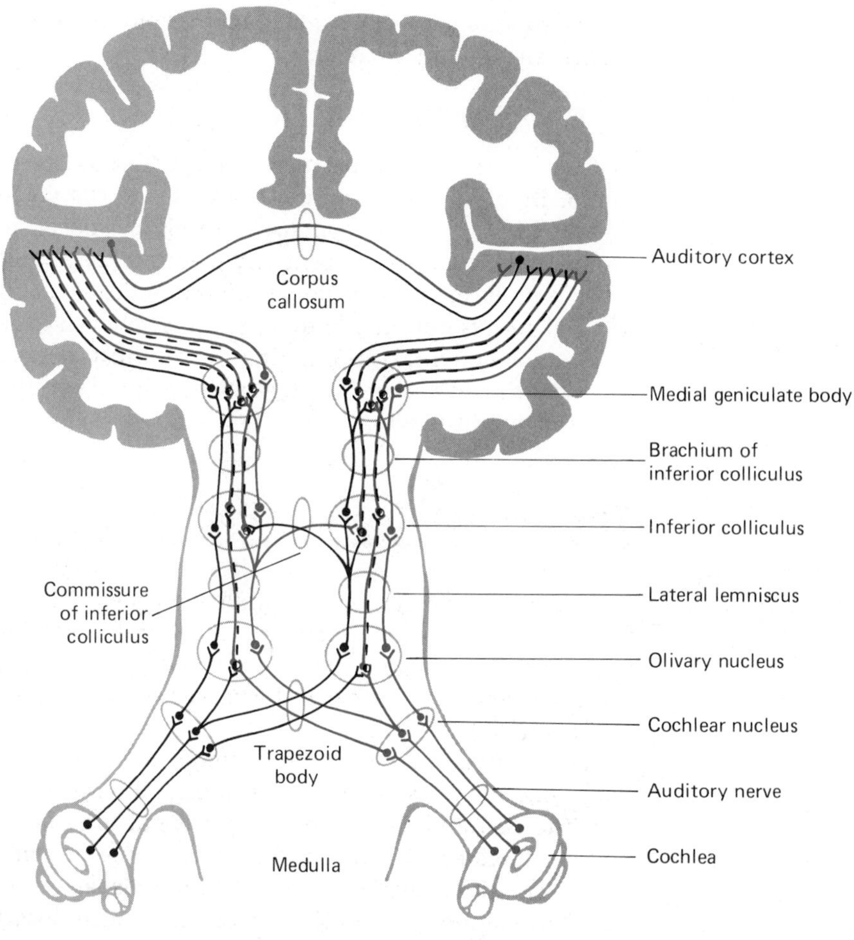

FIGURE 7.7 Auditory pathways. The auditory system pathways show a large number of decussations, or crossings, allowing for much comparison processing of input from the two ears.

notes of a musical scale stimulate adjacent neurons. The first note stimulates one neuron (or, more likely, group of neurons); the second note stimulates the neuron (or group of neurons) next to the first. The experimental procedure for finding this pattern of organization is relatively simple. A microelectrode is lowered into a particular neuron. Various tones are sounded until the neuron fires. Most neurons respond to a range of tones, but exhibit a stronger response to one particular tone. In other words, any one neuron in the auditory system is generally most sensitive to a small range of frequencies, called the "best" frequencies. Within any one structure the neurons are lined up according to their "best" frequencies, that is, from low to high, or vice versa (Evans and Whitfield, 1964). If an electrode is used to record from each neuron along its path of penetration, then one might find that the first neuron is most sensitive to a tone of, say, 100 cps, while the second yields a maximum response to a tone of 102 cps. If one assumes the place theory to be valid, an analogy can be made between the way the visual system preserves the retinal pattern of organization and the way the auditory system preserves the cochlear (basilar membrane) pattern of organization. In the auditory system, the arrangement of neurons is not necessarily a linear organization, but adjacent neurons will likely show a gradual increase in frequency (see Webster and Aitkin, 1975) (Figure 7.8).

The tonotopic principle of organization exists from the cochlear to the cortex, but not all auditory neurons respond simply to a tone within the range of best frequencies. Some cells fire only at the onset of a tone, while others may fire continuously for as long as the tone is held constant (see Webster and Aitkin, 1975). Other cells may decrease their firing when a tone is on, yet may be sensitive to fluctuations in frequency or amplitude. Single-cell recording has revealed many different response patterns. One factor that may affect the response pattern is whether the animal is awake or anesthetized. It seems that cells that may under normal conditions have a complex response pattern may present a rather simplified reaction if the animal is anesthetized, thus suggesting that an accurate picture of perceptual processes requires an alert animal with all its faculties intact.

Another problem experienced in single-cell recording in the auditory system is that irregular response patterns are often recorded. Since auditory research is done with clicks or pure tones, one explanation of why the patterns are irregular is that the cells are tuned for more complex stimuli, such as changes in amplitude or frequency (Evans, 1968). This argument is logical in the evolutionary sense in that clicks and tones are seldom encountered in natural settings, and it is improbable that our hearing mechanisms have evolved to detect such artificial sounds. Thus, it is not out of line to suggest that biologically significant sounds should be used as stimuli in hearing experiments, although ob-

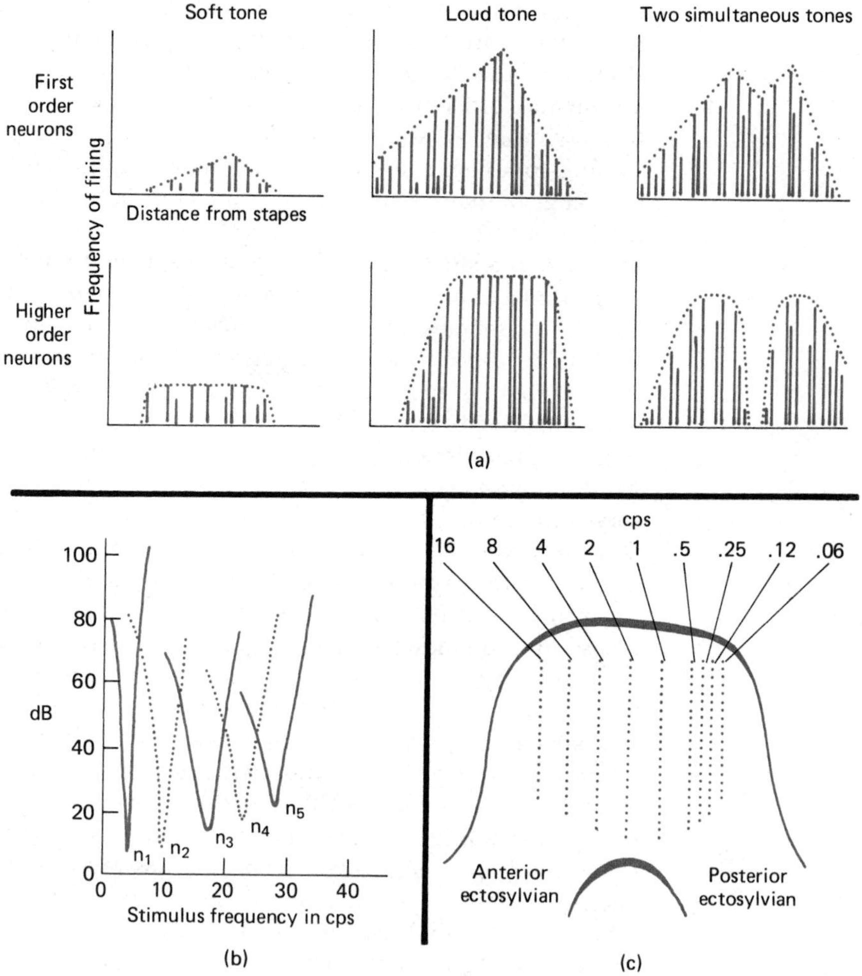

FIGURE 7.8 The tuning of auditory neurons. (a) Neurons at each level of the auditory pathway generally exhibit a definite sensitivity to a certain frequency. (b) Some neurons also show a preference for a certain range of intensity. (c) Adjacent neurons in cortex display a range of frequencies.

viously, more complex stimuli introduce the possibility of more complex experimental problems.

First Stop: Cochlear Nucleus

The cochlear nucleus is the first stop for auditory neurons (Figure 7.9). The cochlear nerve, formed by the axons of the bipolar cells of

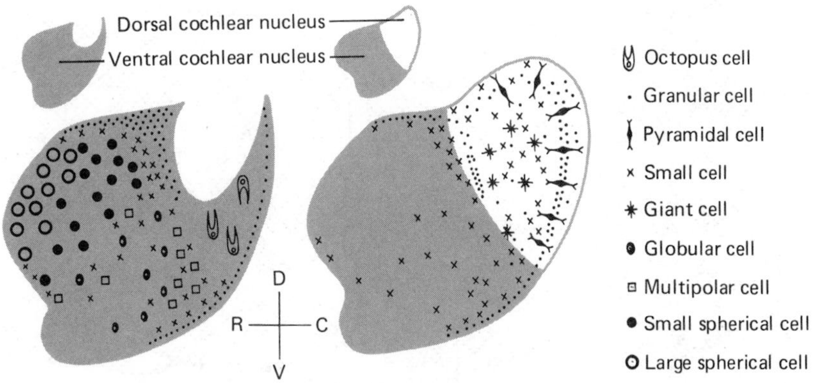

FIGURE 7.9 Cells of the cochlear nucleus. The complexity of the cochlear nucleus is evident from an examination of the various cells composing the nucleus. Although specific functions of the particular cell types are not fully known, it is believed that the cochlear nucleus is capable of considerably transforming the input from the cochlear nerve.

the spiral ganglion, enters the central nervous system at the level of the lower brain stem and synapses on the dorsal and ventral portions of the cochlear nuclei. The tonotopic organizational pattern of the auditory system is immediately evident in the cochlear membrane. A single tonotopic projection from the ipsilateral ear is found in the dorsal cochlear nucleus, and two tonotopic representations are found in the ventral cochlear nucleus (Mountcastle, 1968).

Projections from the dorsal and ventral cochlear nuclei follow two essentially different pathways. The ventral cochlear nucleus sends fibers to the dorsal cochlear nucleus and to both the ipsilateral and contralateral superior olivary nuclei, which are located in the medulla (Mountcastle, 1968). Thus, the superior olivary nucleus is significant in that it is the first site of bilateral innervations along the auditory pathway. Fibers going to the contralateral superior olivary nucleus form what is called the trapezoid body. The dorsal cochlear nucleus projection, on the other hand, goes to the contralateral lemniscal nucleus, which gives off fibers forming the lateral lemniscal tract, important as both a sensory and motor pathway. For example, axons from the superior olivary nuclei follow the lateral lemniscal tract, with the primary projection being to the inferior colliculus.

On to the Inferior Colliculus

The inferior colliculi, like the superior colliculi of the visual pathway, are two small "bumps" on the surface of the tectum in the midbrain. The colliculi are considered to be a major relay station for both the

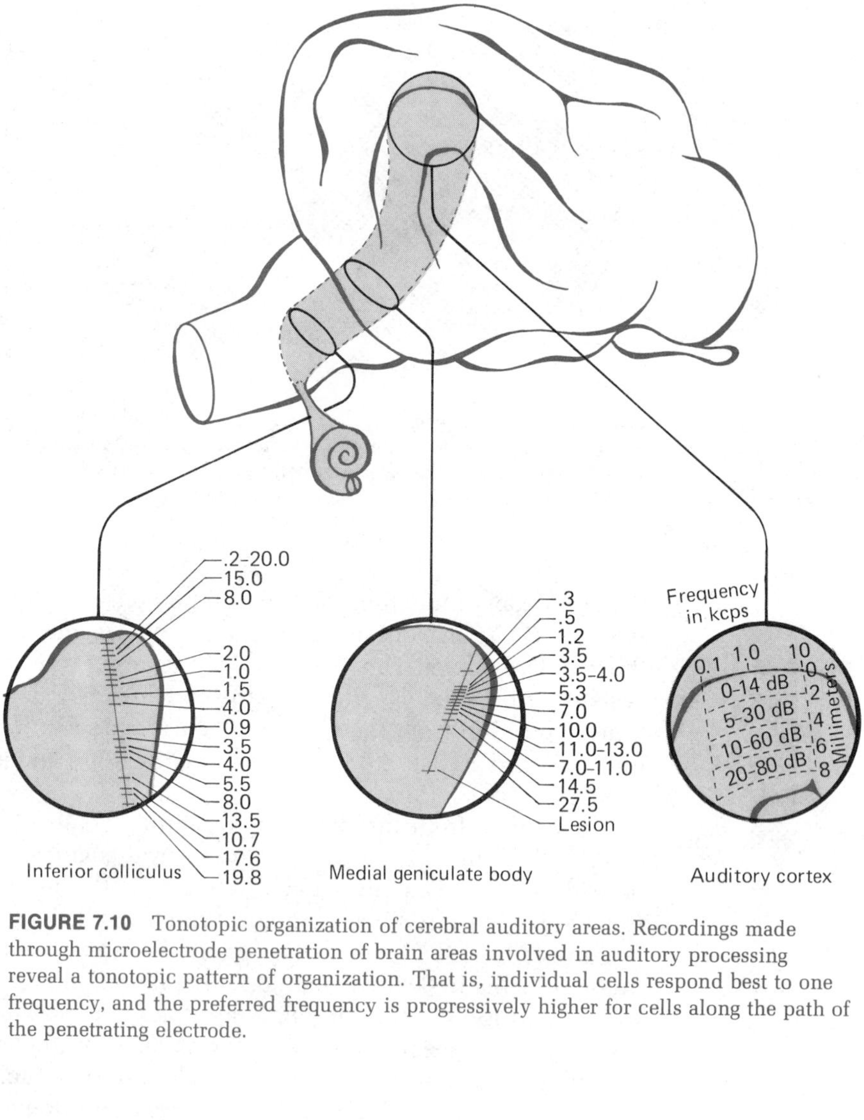

FIGURE 7.10 Tonotopic organization of cerebral auditory areas. Recordings made through microelectrode penetration of brain areas involved in auditory processing reveal a tonotopic pattern of organization. That is, individual cells respond best to one frequency, and the preferred frequency is progressively higher for cells along the path of the penetrating electrode.

afferent and efferent pathways. Although the colliculi maintain a tonotopic organizational pattern, over 50 percent of the cells tested in the inferior colliculus responded to stimulus intensity rather than to tone alone (Rose et al., 1963). Some neurons showed a decreased rate of firing as stimulus intensity increased, suggesting complex excitatory and inhibitory interactions in the inferior colliculus (Figure 7.10). The auditory tract bifurcates again at the level of the colliculus, with some fibers going to the contralateral inferior colliculus and some going to the medial geniculate body of the thalamus. Thus, both ears are represented in each colliculus, not once but twice, there being two bilateral representations in each colliculus.

Medial Geniculate Body

Like the inferior colliculus, the medial geniculate body (MGB) functions as a relay nucleus. The MGB, itself a division of the thalamus, is further subdivided into the dorsal, medial, and ventral divisions, and it is the ventral division that is most involved with relaying the auditory pathway. The ventral portion of the MGB contains a tonotopic representation of the auditory input, while the dorsal and medial portions are best described as having diffuse auditory projections.

Cortical Auditory Areas

The thalamic projection goes to the cortex, specifically to the primary auditory area, AI (Figure 7.11). The auditory areas of the cortex are located in the temporal lobe, and in the case of primates and humans, buried in the depths of the superior temporal convolution, called Heschl's gyrus. Again, area AI has a tonotopic representation of the auditory world through the thalamic projection. The other cortical auditory areas also have tonotopic fields (Merzenich and Brugge, 1973); in fact, the cat may have as many as six separate tonotopic projection fields in

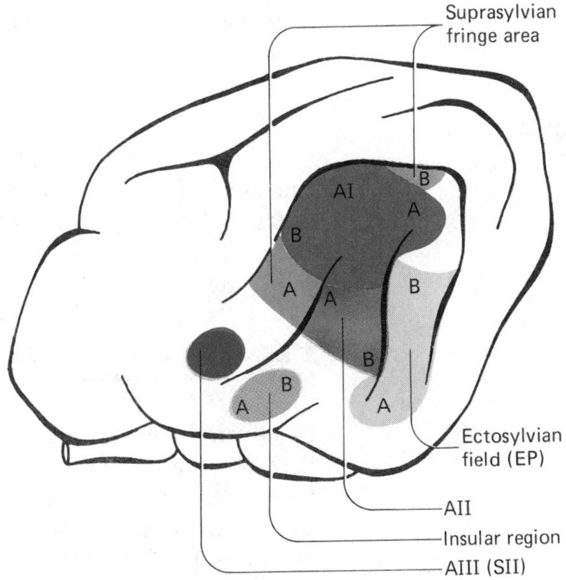

FIGURE 7.11 The auditory cortex of the cat. The feline auditory cortical areas are somewhat spread out over the lateral surface of the brain. AI is the primary auditory cortex, and it is surrounded by AII, the ectosylvian area (EP) and the suprasylvian fringe area. Separate from this main complex are two other auditory regions. AIII is located in what is properly called the second somatosensory area (SII). The last area is found buried in the insular region. Although it is on the external surface in the diagram, it is actually located inside one of the fissures.

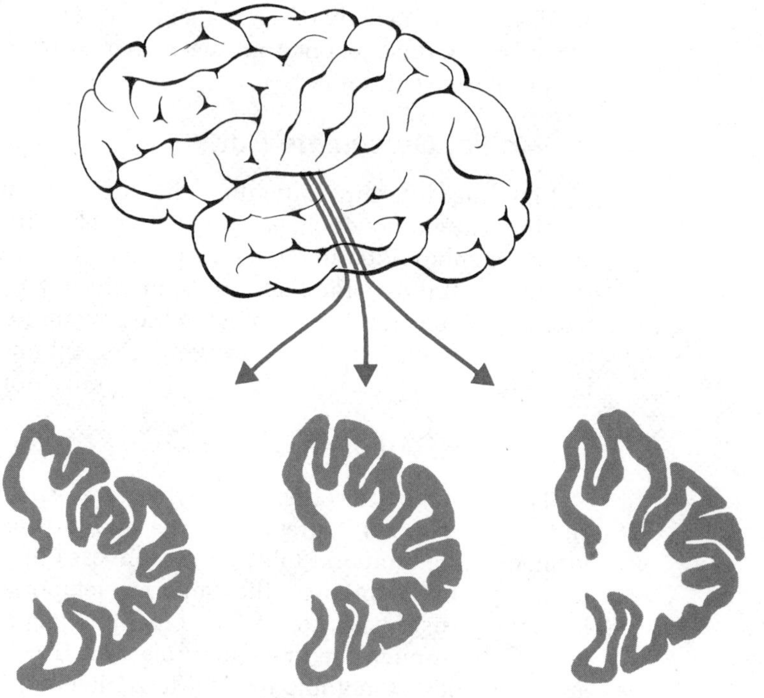

FIGURE 7.12 Auditory areas of the cerebral cortex of the primate. The auditory areas of the primate are, unlike the cat (see Figure 7.11), not exposed on the lateral surface of the cortex. Instead, they are largely buried in the sylvian fissure, though they also run along the outer surface of the superior temporal gyrus. Because these areas are less accessible than in the cat, much more work has been done on the cat.

the auditory cortex (Woolsey, 1961). Presumably, the tonotopically organized cortical areas outside the area AI derive this organization from cortical connections (Figure 7.12).

Perception of Sounds

Given the anatomy of the auditory system, it is still not clear how we decode sounds. The tonotopic organization of most of the auditory system is responsible for detecting the frequency (pitch) of a sound, but it cannot account for the way we differentiate between words such as "bad" and "dad." The perceptual processes involved in audition are complex, and although sometimes considered similar to the feature detection processes of vision, are not nearly so well understood. Complex language decoding mechanisms, in particular, are difficult to research because of their uniqueness to humans. Nonetheless, progress is being made in the area of speech perception, particularly since mechanisms analogous to our speech processors have been found in animals.

There are at least two steps involved in "decoding" any sound we hear. Generally, one of the first things we do when we hear a sound is figure out where it is located. Determining the location may give us clues to aid in the next step, which is deciding what the sound is. Of course, these two processes do not always occur in this order. Sometimes we may hear and recognize a sound but not immediately be able to pinpoint it. For example, if you are outside and hear the telephone ring, it is often hard to tell whether the sound is coming from your house or the one next door.

Sound Localization

An important step in the perception of a sound is to locate the source of the sound. This basic process, called localization, is greatly facilitated by the fact that we have two ears and thus get binaural input (Figure 7.13). As discussed earlier, there are many opportunities along the ascending auditory pathway for binaural interaction. Decussation occurs

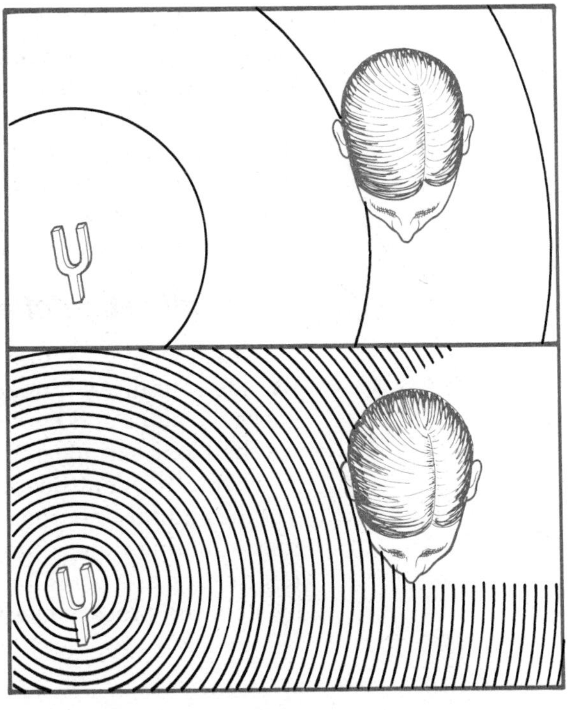

FIGURE 7.13 Localization of sounds. Because the sound waves of low-frequency sounds are relatively far apart, we locate low-frequency sounds by detecting differences in the phase of the sound arriving at each ear. High-frequency sounds, on the other hand, which generate more frequent sound waves, would not have a detectable difference in phase, but the difference in intensity or amplitude of the sound between the two ears helps us locate the sound.

first at the level of the lower brain stem in the superior olivary nucleus, and the auditory fibers may cross at least three more times before reaching the cortex, where the information of each hemisphere may travel to the other via the corpus callosum and the anterior commissure. The many points of binaural interaction allow for frequent comparisons of input from each ear, and thus help us locate a sound in space.

There are three characteristics of a sound that can give clues to the location. One is amplitude, or intensity; the other two are phase and time of arrival. The specialization of the auditory system for responding to these factors is evident through cellular recordings that show that some cells are sensitive to intensity differences, but not to phase differences, whereas other cells react to phase differences but not to differences in intensity (Rose et al., 1966). Neurons in the auditory system are known to preserve the phase dimension of the stimulus at least through second-order and third-order neurons (Eruklar et al., 1968), and this information is probably used in determining the direction the sound is coming from. However, some hold that it is not the phase difference that is used to locate the sound, but the delay of the sound getting to the second ear that is used to locate the sound.

Amplitude differences are most important at higher frequencies, since the waves over about 2000 cps are short enough to be obstructed even by an object as small as a human head (about 200mm). Consequently, the ear closest to the source will hear a louder sound than the other ear. Low frequencies, on the other hand, have longer wavelengths and thus an obstruction the size of the head has little effect on the number of waves reaching each ear. There is, however, a difference in the time of arrival of the sound at each of the two ears. Though the time varies with the angle from which the sound strikes the head, generally at least 2 msec elapses before a sound reaches the other ear. Whether it is the delay or the phase difference that is the clue to locating the sound is still debatable (Henning, 1974). In the case of a short click, delay, not phase difference, is believed to be the determining factor. In the case of a low frequency tone, however, it may be the phase difference.

Identification of a Sound

After locating a sound, the other half of perceiving a sound is to identify the sound. As humans, we are particularly interested in how language develops and how we decode language. In the following sections, we shall look at some of the language mechanisms.

Naturally, identification of a complex sound is not a simple process. Yet the auditory neurons can simplify the process by breaking the complex stimulus down into simple properties and using the elementary information as a basis for perception. Thus the stimulus is decoded step by step, the process facilitated by the intricate connections among the neurons of the auditory system. This mode of auditory processing is called feature extraction, and is believed to be somewhat similar to the feature detection processing observed in the visual system. Naturally, though, the specific characteristics vary from sensory system to sensory system. While visual feature detectors are attuned to such properties as edges, corners, and direction of movement, auditory feature detectors are attuned to simple properties of the auditory stimulus such as voice onset time (VOT), changes in tone, and changes in amplitude (Darwin, 1976).

Speech and Nonspeech Auditory processing has long been thought to differ for speech and nonspeech sounds. However, recent experiments have shown that the modes of processing appear to be quite similar. In fact, the distinction between the processing of speech and nonspeech sounds may be only that the language processing features act as a supplement, not a substitute, for the other auditory processing mechanisms. While it is true that speech is processed primarily by the left side of the brain, other sounds that are processed by both hemispheres are processed more efficiently by the right side of the brain (Kimura, 1961; 1964). It is only when a sound is perceived as a speech sound that it goes to the left hemisphere for processing. In other words, certain acoustic features may not be construed as speech sounds unless heard in a speech context. In fact, when there is a speech context, we tend to interpolate the sounds we hear to fit the auditory form we expect. Sounds that may only slightly resemble each other may be perceived as the same word if heard in the appropriate grammatical context. Consider the many different accents that can be heard when traveling through a country, yet because the basic clues are present, the language can be comprehended.

Selective Adaptation A good example of similar processing is seen in selective adaptation experiments involving either speech or nonspeech sounds. Just as visual cells can be selectively adapted, so, it seems, can auditory cells. The group of neurons that are selectively tuned to the particular characteristics associated with a specific sound can become fatigued or weakened with repeated exposure to a sound. As a result, the perception of sound may be distorted, particularly if the sound presented is ambiguous, that is, similar to the sound to which the group of neurons has been adapted.

Selective adaptation experiments use similar sounds such as "ba" and "pa," which differ only in the initial sound. It has been found that after repeated exposure to, say, "ba," the listener is less sensitive to that sound and may confuse "ba" with "pa" in borderline cases (Eimas and Corbit, 1973). Thus, it is as if the neurons (feature detectors) that are most sensitive to the "b" sound become exhausted just as visual feature detectors can become exhausted with repeated exposure to the same visual stimulus.

A similar experiment using nonspeech sounds has demonstrated that nonspeech feature detectors shift boundaries after selective adaptation in a manner resembling the speech syllable adaptation process (Figure 7.14). For example, a listener can at first clearly differentiate between the sound of a stringed instrument that is plucked, and that of a stringed instrument that is bowed, but after prolonged exposure to one of the sounds, the listener is apt to incorrectly identify the sounds that are borderline cases (Cutting et al., 1976). That is, if the sound is similar to both a "pluck" and a "bow," a person who has been repeatedly exposed to a pluck will be likely to classify the ambiguous sound as a bow, since presumably the neurons that respond to a pluck have been fatigued and thus require a stronger (less ambiguous) stimulus to respond.

Adaptation, then, is a phenomenon occurring at the simple acoustic feature level (nonspeech) and the single-syllable (speech) level. For some reason, however, adaptation occurs more readily with a sound perceived as a speech sound than with an acoustic feature alone (Warren, 1968). In addition, adaptation may occur at levels above these simple features. For example, if one listens to a word repeated over and over, the word may begin to sound like another word. This adaptation may likely be attributed to the adaptation of several units of neurons that combine to respond to a particular word (Lackner and Goldstein, 1974).

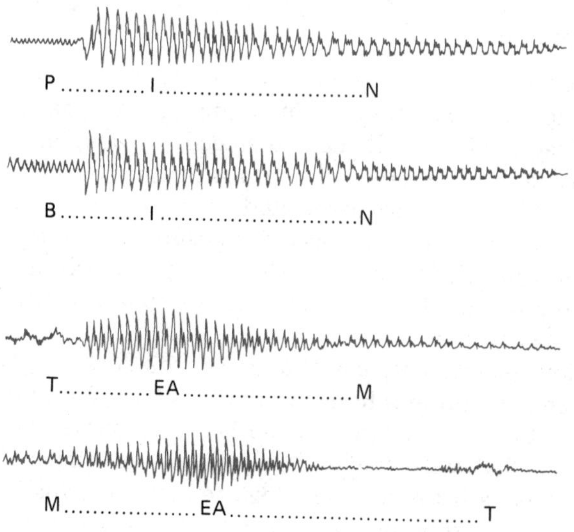

FIGURE 7.14 Sound waves generated by speech. Differences in voiced and voiceless stop consonants, such as "B" and "P," are evident in the patterns generated by recording the sounds. Presumably, our feature detectors are responsible for differentiating between the sounds.

Animals, too, demonstrate selective responding. Chincillas, for example, can discriminate between "ba" and "pa" (Kuhl and Miller, 1975). Even more effective in evoking a selective response, however, are sounds that are biologically significant to the animal. A frog, for instance, will show a greater response to the sound of a cricket than to a click or a tone.

Consequently, there is interest in designing auditory experiments that utilize biologically significant sounds rather than artificial sounds. Biologically significant sounds may be divided into two groups: those that are environmentally significant (such as the sounds a laboratory animal associates with feeding time) and those that seem to be natively or genetically significant (such as the mating call of the species). However, classifying sounds as genetically significant is a controversial issue. Are animals actually born with programmed auditory neurons that respond to species-specific calls, or are the neurons programmed after birth when the animals are exposed to the sounds of the other animals around them—that is, are they environmentally conditioned? In other words, the issue is once again "nature or nurture."

Hearing and Voice . . . Song There are many approaches to this problem, but one of the most interesting combines the study of auditory perception and vocal production. Naturally, the processes of perception and production of vocal sounds are similar, so they are bound to have some kind of integral relationship. Genetic factors dictate the major characteristics of the sounds produced by an animal (obviously, a bird will not "meow"), but auditory experience also plays a part in vocal learning. What an animal hears—whether it be a self-produced sound or an external sound—influences the direction of vocal development.

Developmental studies examining these two processes in birds have revealed that aberrant speech patterns often develop when there is no auditory feedback, and that exposure to abnormal or cross-specific calls can also affect the song produced by a bird.

Clearly, vocal learning is a complex process. One theory proposes two stages of learning a complex sensory-guided motor skill (such as vocal production) (see Worden and Galambos, 1972). The first stage requires constant integration of motor commands and sensory feedback. The second stage, however, is more stable—the efferent or motor programs become fixed and are carried out independently of direct feedback or with only a slight dependence on feedback. One idea associated with this theory of vocal production is the concept of an auditory template, which is a pattern-detecting mechanism within the auditory processing system that lets the organism know whether or not a stimulus of a particular class has occurred (Worden and Galambos, 1972). Although there are some who hold that the auditory template is genetically prescribed, others hold that it is a *memory* of a sound formed through experience, though acknowledging at least some genetic input. Once the template is formed, birds such as the white-crowned sparrow may be reared in auditory isolation, yet develop normal song. However, if the bird is deafened before forming the auditory template, the song produced will be as abnormal as the song of a bird that was never exposed to an auditory model.

Evidence of the complexity of the relationship between auditory perception and vocal production is that it varies for different kinds of birds (see Nottebohm, 1975). Chicks, doves, and turkeys are all in the group that does not require either a model (for imitation in vocal learning) or auditory feedback. A second group, including canaries (*Serinus canaria*), requires no model, but without auditory feedback does have some discordant screeches and hisses in the vocal repertoire. A third group, which includes song sparrows (*Melospiza melodia*), has a more stringent need for auditory feedback and some need also for an auditory model. Without an auditory model, the birds develop at least some songs of fairly normal wild-type quality, though they may develop other songs that are quite abnormal. A fourth group, including some meadowlarks, chaffinches, white-crowned sparrows, cardinals, and zebra finches, requires both an auditory model and auditory feedback. Without a model, these birds develop abnormal song patterns. If the bird is deafened before the onset of song, the song patterns produced by the bird are even more aberrant than those of birds reared without a model.

The aberrant songs produced by deafened birds are often attributed simply to the lack of access to essential auditory feedback. But deafened birds may have abnormal endocrine levels and a different motivational system. Thus, it is sometimes hypothesized that the hormonal differences (specifically, a depressed testosterone level) cause the abnormal song, since deafened chaffinches with added testosterone produce more song than deafened chaffinches without added testosterone. However, a castrated canary that is subsequently implanted with extra testosterone and exposed to an auditory model develops normal song, whereas a castrated and deafened canary also implanted with extra testosterone develops abnormal song (see Worden and Galambos, 1972). Thus, the logical conclusion is that auditory feedback is essential for normal vocal development.

In addition to the auditory requirements, vocal learning is also dependent on timing. There is a certain critical period when vocal learning is possible. It is during this critical period that the bird must have exposure to auditory models and learn the song. If the bird learns the "wrong" song (aberrant singing) and produces the final adult pattern, a process called crystallization, no amount of tutoring can correct the bird's song.

Here again, though, manipulation of hormonal levels can change the normal expected pattern. If a male canary is castrated, the critical period for vocal learning is extended from one to two years (Nottebohm, 1970).

Thus, it is clear that vocal learning is a complex process, and is interdependent upon a number of factors, including auditory experience and feedback, timing, and hormone levels.

In the following sections we shall examine some of the problems that can develop in language mechanisms.

Audition and Language: Study of Dysfunction

The term aphasia refers to the inability to understand or use both the written and spoken symbols of language. Incomplete loss of these language capacities is often referred to as dysphasia. Another class of aphasia, known as expressive or motor aphasia, specifically involves the loss of the ability to speak and write. The person is unable to carry out the specific motor skills required for language, although there is an absence of paralysis or rigidity. In these cases, the lesion occurs in the frontal lobes, specifically in the posterior portion of the inferior frontal gyrus and the lowest part of the precentral gyrus (Figure 7.15).

The speech disturbances vary with the severity of the lesion. An expressive or motor aphasic will often mispronounce words but may be able to produce several words correctly, if the damage is not very severe. Assuming there is no damage to the region of the temporal lobe concerned with auditory-verbal memories, the expressive aphasic is able to recognize the mistakes but is often unable to correct them. In the mildest

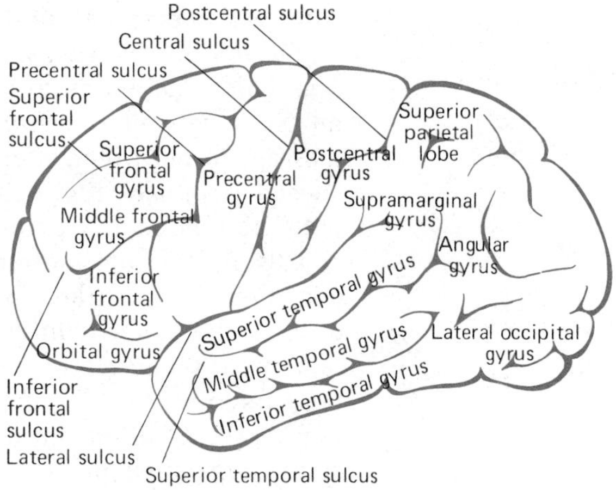

FIGURE 7.15 Lateral view of the left cerebral hemisphere, indicating the major gyri and sulci.

forms of this disorder, only occasional words create difficulty, and the patient might learn to compensate for this by using synonyms for the problematic words.

The loss of the ability to understand the meaning of spoken or written language is called receptive aphasia. It occurs in spite of the fact that the person has normal hearing and vision. In cases of receptive aphasia, it seems that the storage site for the auditory memories of words has been damaged. Most of the clinical and pathological evidence points to the involvement of the posterior portions of the temporoparietal region (usually in the dominant hemisphere) (Geschwind, 1965). This deficit may also be called auditory agnosia because the patient cannot recognize the auditory symbols of speech.

Expressive aphasia is not only a disturbance of language but also a disturbance of motor behavior. Expressive aphasia is also considered a specific case of a whole class of motor disorders known as the apraxias, which are described in Appendix II. Most aphasic patients tend to exhibit both receptive and expressive impairments in varying degrees.

Helen had more and more difficulties after the operation. She had had rheumatic heart disease as a child, and now in her late sixties, the damaged heart valves caused such instability in her blood circulation that she could not negotiate one flight of stairs without extreme breathlessness. So two years ago the cardiac surgeons replaced one of the valves in her heart. For many months she experienced improved exercise tolerance, and easily walked up the steps to her apartment. Over the subsequent months, though, she needed progressively increased doses of medicine to maintain this improved state. Another complicating factor was that she would not stop eating ham hocks, pork, and other salty meats. Her cardiologist warned her against increased salt consumption because of her inability to rid herself of the extra water that inevitably came with increased salt intake.

One morning she was to have her hair fixed at the local beauty shop. She dialed the phone to confirm the appointment but could not make any sense when her friend answered. Finally, she was able to relay the message to her friend that she had a headache and felt confused. Her speech was fluent; that is, she produced runs of well-articulated speech, with grammatical structure and the rhythm of normal speech, but it conveyed little information. In fact, the beautician reported Helen kept describing the weather in response to each question. The beautician asked Helen if she would be late. Helen responded, "I was going off to that and if I made it then all would be all right. Wait, wait . . . the sign appears to be a . . . something's wrong . . . wait . . . wait. . . ." Sensing her frustruation through the cryptic language Helen produced, the beautician called for an ambulance and had Helen taken to the hospital. There she had no change in her cardiopulmonary status, and her vital signs were normal. Further, the staff thought she was demented, as she seemed to understand their questions but her verbal responses bore no relation. Later on, with careful testing, it was clear she had a conduction aphasia. Her disorder represented a fluent aphasia, in that the flow of speech appeared normal. She made some naming mistakes, often literal paraphasias. For example, she called a tie a "neck . . . neck . . . f . . . f . . ."; a pen became a "poof"; a belt buckle became a "bettle." When asked to perform motor tasks, even in a four-step command, she easily complied. Her comprehension was intact. Writing was disordered in a similar manner to her speech disorder.

Helen suffered a stroke, and in this case the localized destruction of brain tissue was probably caused by a small clot of blood from her heart that traveled into the brain and blocked a nutrient vessel. With the vessel blocked, no further blood could supply glucose and oxygen to the brain downstream from the clot, so an area of brain in the left parietal lobe died.

Helen was treated with anticoagulant so no further clots could form and travel to distant sites. Anticoagulation is the process of interfering with the normal process of hemostasis (blood coagulation). Drugs can diminish the clotting process in such a way to decrease the incidence of another stroke episode, yet not cause overwhelming hemorrhage.

Three months later her other defects were gone completely. Helen's aphasia had also markedly improved. Her speech regained meaning, and the dense circumlocution receded. She still made naming errors of the literal paraphasic kind; in fact, she still called a belt buckle a "bettle buck."

As in many cases of clinical neuropathology, the effects of damage to a specific area of the cortex can often result in widespread neurophysiological deficits. Since the capacity for verbal memory underlies many other linguistic and cognitive functions, disruption of these verbal memory abilities will cause disruptions in the functions that build upon these abilities. For example, the loss of verbal memories will produce losses in the patient's vocabulary and syntactical knowledge. This may show up as an expressive language difficulty. The patient may use incorrect or nonsense words and will be unable to recognize the mistakes if the verbal memory capacity is not functioning properly. If the lesion includes some parieto-occipital damage, then the patient will exhibit some difficulty in reading. Parts of the parieto-occipital region are concerned with the visual symbols of speech. Lesions spreading into this area will not only produce reading difficulties (dyslexia), but the patient will often exhibit dysgraphia (interference with writing abilities) as well. This may stem from the patient's inability to comprehend the meaning of the symbols the patient has written down.

Another and perhaps more important impairment that may result from a disturbance of auditory-verbal memories is an interference with the patient's thinking processes. It is generally believed that a great deal of thinking is done in words, and therefore a disturbance in auditory-verbal memory will necessarily have some deleterious effects on these thinking capacities.

Researchers have encountered many problems in trying to localize specific areas of the brain associated with the different types of aphasia. A large part of the problem is the fact that the two most common causes of aphasia are vascular disorders, such as strokes, and tumors. In the case of vascular disorders, the disturbance often occurs in the middle cerebral artery, which supplies blood to the entire area of the brain associated with the expression and comprehension of language. In a similar manner, brain tumors that cause aphasia are often not so well circumscribed, or they can cause swelling or vascular problems at considerable distances from the main body of the tumor.

Whereas research with animals allows for more controlled experiments and often yields fruitful insights into issues of importance for humans, in this particular case, the relevance of animal research is lost since animals do not have a capacity for auditory verbal processes as we know it.

Summary

Listening to the subtleties of a Bach fugue, the critical shouts of buying and selling, or even the singsong tedium of the beautician's recounting of the weather, all turn out to involve a highly accessible sensory receptor. This reception system begins with the great collectors of sound—the ears. Delicate mechanisms of juxtaposed bones and membranes continue the transduction process. To the cells of the cochlea is left the task of finally transducing the mechanical pulse of sound waves and fluid movement into a neural message.

Just as the visual system began with the peripheral receptor, so is the cochlear microphonic the beginning of the ascending pathway. Encoded messages are transferred to the cochlear nucleus in the brain stem. Here there is a definite division of neurons into groups that will respond to various acoustic stimuli with different response patterns. Multiple representation and tonotopic arrangement are the keys to the organization of the system. From the cochlear nucleus the message is projected to the olivary complex, and binaural convergence into single neurons takes place here. Proceeding via the lateral lemniscus to the inferior colliculus, and then to the medial geniculate nucleus complex, mixed but tonotopically organized messages are transferred to cortical processing areas. Identification and localization of sound are crucial to the human process of communication. This is a complex process, however, in which the auditory neurons divide the signal stimulus into simple properties, in order to extract specific features. In the auditory system, feature detection depends on qualities such as voice onset time, tone change, and amplitude change.

Auditory information is organized tonotopically at each level of the pathway. And this basic feature of specifically tuned neurons, coupled with sound localization, allows humans to understand the spoken language. Once decoded, the message must be sent to still another cortical area to obtain the appropriate semantic referents. For the function of the system is the organization and interpretation of sound.

References

Bekesy, G. von. 1960. *Experiments in Hearing.* Trans. and edited by E. G. Wever. New York: McGraw-Hill.

Cutting, J. E., B. S. Rosner, and C. F. Foard. 1976. Perceptual categories for musiclike sounds: implication for theories of speech perception. *Quart. J. Exp. Psychol. 28*: 361–378.

Darwin, C. J. 1976. The perception of speech. In: E. C. Carterette and M. P. Friedman, eds. *Handbook of Perception.* Vol. II. New York: Academic Press.

Eimas, P. D., and J. D. Corbit. 1973. Selective adaptation of linguistic feature detectors. *Cog. Psychol.* 4:99–109.

Engstrom, H., H. W. Ades, and J. E. Hawkins. 1965. Cellular pattern, nerve structures, and fluid spaces of the organ of Corti. In: W. D. Neff, ed. *Contributions to Sensory Physiology.* New York: Academic Press.

Eruklar, S. D., P. G. Nelson, and J. S. Bryan. 1968. Experimental and theoretical approaches to neural processing in the central auditory pathway. In: W. D. Neff, ed. *Contributions to Sensory Physiology.* New York: Academic Press.

Evans, E. F. 1968. Upper and lower levels of auditory system: a contrast of structure and function. In: E. R. Caianello, ed. *Neural Networks* (Proceedings of the School) New York: Springer-Verlag.

Evans, E. F., and I. C. Whitfield. 1964. Classification of unit responses in the auditory cortex of the unanesthetized and unrestrained cat. *J. Physiol. 171*:476–493.

Geschwind, N. 1965. Disconnection syndrome in animals and man. *Brain 88*:237–294.

Harrison, J. M., and M. E. Howe. 1974. Anatomy of the descending auditory system (mammalian). In: W. D. Keidel and W. D. Neff, eds. *Handbook of Sensory Physiology.* Vol. V/1. New York: Springer-Verlag, pp. 363–388.

Henning, F. B. 1974. Auditory localization. In: M. S. Gazzaniga and C. Blakemore, eds. *Handbook of Psychobiology.* New York: Academic Press.

Kimura, D. 1961. Cerebral dominance and the perception of verbal stimuli. *Can. J. Psychol. 15*:166–171.

Kimura, D. 1964. Left-right differences in the perception of melodies. *Quart. J. Exp. Psychol. 16*:355–358.

Kuhl, P. K., and J. D. Miller. 1975. Speech perception by the chinchilla: Voiced-voiceless distinction alveolar plosive consonants. *Science 190*:69–72.

Lackner, J. R., and L. M. Goldstein. 1974. The psychological representation of speech sounds. *Cognition* 2:279–298.

Leiberman, P. 1965. On the acoustic basis of the perception of intonation by linguists. *Word* 21:40–54.

Merzenich, M. M., and J. F. Brugge. 1973. Representation of the cochlear partition on the superior temporal plane of the macaque monkey. *Brain Res.* 50:275–296.

Mountcastle, V. B. 1968. Central neural mechanisms in hearing. In: V. B. Mountcastle, ed. *Medical Physiology.* St. Louis: Mosby.

Nottebohm, F. 1970. Ontongeny of bird song. *Science* 167:950–956.

Nottebohm, F. 1975. A zoologist's view of some language phenomena with particular emphasis on vocal learning. In: E. H. Lenneberg and E. Lenneberg, eds. *Foundations of Language Development.* New York: Academic Press.

Osen, K. K. 1969. The intrinsic organization of the cochlear nuclei in the cat. *Acta Oto-Laryngol.* 67:352–359.

Rose, J. E., J. F. Brugge, D. J. Anderson, and J. E. Hind. 1969. Some possible neural correlates to combination tones. *J. Neurophysiol.* 32:402–423.

Rose, J. E., D. D. Greenwood, J. M. Godlberg, and J. E. Hind. 1963. Some discharge characteristics of single neurons in the inferior colliculus of the cat. *J. Neurophysiol.* 26: 294–320.

Rose, J. E., N. B. Gross, C. D. Geisler, and J. E. Hind. 1966. Some neural mechanisms in the inferior colliculus of the cat which may be relevant to localization of a second source. *J. Neurophysiol.* 29:288–314.

Warren, R. M. 1968. Verbal transformation effect and auditory perceptual mechanisms. *Psychol. Bull.* 70:261–270.

Webster, W. R., and L. M. Aitkin. 1975. Central auditory processing. In: M. S. Gazzaniga and C. Blakemoje, eds. *Handbook of Psychobiology.* New York: Academic Press.

Woolsey, C. N. 1961. Organization of cortical auditory system. In: W. A. Rosenblith, ed. *Sensory Communication.* New York: Wiley.

Worden, F. G., and R. Galambos. 1972. Auditory processing of biologically significant sounds. *Neurosci. Res. Program Bull.* 10 (1).

CHAPTER 8

Body Sense, Body Schema

The somatosensory system is considered the gateway to the tactile, sensual world of feeling. The receptors of the somatosensory system enable us to feel everything from the gentle caress of a spring breeze to the biting cold of a winter storm. This system is responsible, on one hand, for our ability to enjoy the physical aspects of a sexual experience, and on the other hand, for the capacity to experience pain. Whether relaxing in a whirlpool bath or doubled over with stomach cramps, we owe our experiencing of these sensations to the action of the somatosensory system.

Somatosensory literally translated means "body sense," *soma* being the Greek word for "body." This translation describes well the physical sense of self, the body awareness derived from the somatosensory system. The body, inside and out, is constantly subjected to a barrage of sensory information, and a majority of this information must be processed by the somatosensory system. In short, everything we feel in the realm of touch, temperature, pain, or body position is transmitted through the pathways of the somatosensory system. Moreover, it is on these sensations that we base most of our motor movements, and losing this sense is thus tantamount to losing the capability for movement.

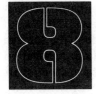

Given the wide variety of sensations experienced through the somatosensory system, its action is somewhat more complex and less well understood than that of other sensory systems, which deal with only one stimulus modality. *Modality* is a word that means "pertaining to structure as opposed to substance." While the visual system deals with several aspects of vision, for example, color, intensity, and brightness, these characteristics are all part of the modality of light. Likewise, the auditory system handles both the pitch and loudness of a sound, but both characteristics are obviously of the same modality. The somatosensory system, on the other hand, receives and processes several different classes of stimuli, or modalities. In this regard, the workings of the somatosensory system are necessarily somewhat more complicated than those of the visual or auditory systems. Further, add the confounding factor of the infinite possibilities for receiving a sensation through the somatosensory system; virtually every area of the body, inside and out, with the possible exception of the brain and a few internal organs, is supplied with sensory receptors of the somatosensory system. The result is that the somatosensory system is necessarily more complex than a system in which the stimulus reception process is limited to one organ, say either the eye or the ear.

In this chapter, then, we shall deal with four modalities: touch, temperature, pain, and body position. In the first section we shall describe the several classes of sensation, including how they are classified, generated, and measured. Next we shall discuss the receptors, including the various types and where they are located. Here, too, will be examined the question of whether the receptors are modality specific, which is one of the important issues in studying the somatosensory system. The third section will cover the transduction process: how the somatosensory stimulus, whether it be mechanical (touch), thermal, or painful, is converted into a neural impulse. Next we shall trace the pathways of the somatosensory system, from the receptors of the peripheral nerves to the spinal cord and brain trajectories. Finally, we shall explore some facets of the somatosensory self, looking at mechanisms of pain perception and attempts to control it, including the recently discovered enkephalins, the brain's own natural painkillers.

Somatosensory Modalities

The various sensory modalities labeled somatosensory are generally divided into four categories on the basis of the nature of the stimulus involved. Mechanoreceptive stimuli are defined as those that produce a mechanical deformation of tissue, with examples being touch, pressure, and vibratory stimuli. Proprioceptive stimuli are similar to mechanoreceptive stimuli but occur inside the joints and ligaments of the skeletal part of the body. Thermoreceptive stimuli are those that produce noticeable changes in temperature, either hot or cold. Nociceptive stimuli are painful, defined as those that actually damage tissue.

TABLE 8.1 Classification of Somatosensations

Contact Group
Touch, pressure, vibration, tickle, tactile paresthesia
Pain Group
Superficial "pricking," deep "aching," discomfort, itch, painful paresthesia
Thermal Group
Cold, warm
Sensory Blends
Cold, pain, wetness, smoothness, heat, etc.
Position
Sense of position in space, kinesthesia

(Adapted from Sinclair, 1967.)

Discriminating between the different modalities of somatosensory sensations is not easy (see Table 8.1), and placing a stimulus in one of the modal categories may be difficult because of the overlapping characteristics of the stimulus. For instance, should a piece of very cold metal applied to the skin be classified as a mechanoreceptive, thermoreceptive, or nociceptive stimulus? Experiments measuring sensitivity to touch may be compounded by such variables as the temperature of the stimulus used. A piece of metal chilled by normal room air conditioning, for example, may elicit a different reaction than one that is warmed to body temperature. Consequently, in this first section we shall look at a few of the means of generating somatosensory stimuli and of controlling and measuring stimulus intensity.

Mechanoreception Mechanoreceptive sensations are of three types. The sensation of touch results from stimulation of tactile receptors in the skin or just below it. The sensation of pressure is experienced when touch extends to deeper tissues, and the sensation of vibration occurs when rapidly repetitive stimuli touch the skin (Guyton, 1976).

Mechanoreception can also be experienced inside the body, since there are mechanoreceptors in the muscles, lungs, and intestines, for example. However, these receptors operate mainly at unconscious levels and thus do not produce noticeable sensations.

Proprioception Proprioception can be considered the inner counterpart to mechanoreception. Through receptors located in the joints and ligaments, we are able to sense the position of the limbs and body. Some of these receptors are constantly firing, whereas others transmit signals only if the position changes. Thus we are peripherally conscious of body position at all times, but may become more aware of various body parts if they are moved. The body schema section later in the chapter will cover this in more detail.

Experiments involving proprioception have mainly been limited to animals, for the deep-lying proprioceptive receptors are not easily accessible.

Thermoreception The sensation of thermoreception is experienced when a stimulus generates a noticeable difference in temperature. Such a sensation is generally experienced on the outer surface of the body, but some inner organs, such as the stomach, also possess receptors capable of transmitting thermoreceptive sensations.

Early researchers in the area of thermoreception no doubt utilized crude methods for generating stimuli, but today's work is based on sophisticated techniques. The most precise method for heat stimuli is radiant heat. An incandescent light that approaches the infrared portion of the light energy spectrum is aimed at a spot on the skin darkened to at-

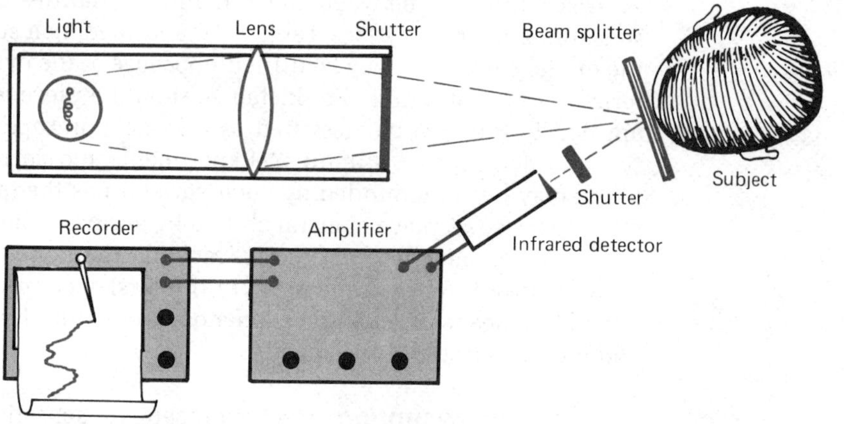

FIGURE 8.1 A typical apparatus for generating thermal stimuli is this one using an incandescent light as the source of heat. Included in the apparatus is a radiant energy skin thermometer, which measures the temperature of the forehead without touching the skin.

tract heat (see Figure 8.1). Radiant energy generated by the bulb causes the skin to feel heat. If the wavelength is varied, the amount of heat transmitted can be precisely measured.

Nociception Stimuli classified as painful are those that actually damage the tissue (Guyton, 1976). Three commonly accepted categories of pain, which are by no means inclusive of all the kinds of pain a person can feel, are pricking, burning, and aching (Mountcastle, 1974). Pricking pain, also called fast pain, can be accurately pinpointed. When the noxious stimuli are removed, the sensation of pricking pain is almost completely relieved. Burning pain is a slower, longer-lasting pain, and is more diffuse than pricking pain. That is, the affected area may not be limited to simply one small area, and pain may persist even after removal of the noxious stimulus. Aching pain is even harder to localize, for it occurs inside the body, either in the viscera or deep in the somatic tissues. The most common form of aching pain is the headache.

Although there are many ways of inflicting pain, one painful stimulus that is efficiently measured is a nociceptive thermal stimulus. The number of degrees that a person is able to withstand before labeling the sensation "pain" is more easily measured objectively than, say, when a pinch becomes painful. Thus many experiments studying pain involve thermal stimuli also.

Receptors of the Somatosensory System

The somatosensory system is different from the sensory systems discussed in previous chapters because there are no specific receptor cells. Instead, sensory impulses are received by receptor terminals—structures that are at the distal ends of the fibers of the parent cell bodies. The dorsal root ganglia lying just outside the spinal cord contain the parent cells (see Figure 8.2). The receptor-transduction process is not that different, however, for these receptor terminals seem to function in approximately the same manner as receptor cells in other sensory systems. They receive the stimulus and convert it into a neural impulse, a process that will be discussed in the transduction section of this chapter.

Receptor terminals of the somatosensory system may be divided into two general classes: free nerve endings and encapsulated nerve terminals. It is generally agreed today that free nerve endings serve as the pain receptors, and that the encapsulated nerve terminals receive mechanical and thermal stimuli. However, there are exceptions to this generalization, for the free endings in the cornea are receptive to touch as well as to pain (Lele and Weddell, 1959).

Free nerve endings, which branch out from either myelinated or unmyelinated nerve fibers, show little variation. In contrast, encapsulated nerve terminals are of many shapes and sizes (at least 100), but their shape has little to do with how they respond. All varieties consist of nerve terminals surrounded by tissue, and the shape of the various encapsulated receptors has nothing to do with the neural impulse generated. The size or number of nerve fibers inside the capsule may vary, and thus the rate of adaptation of the different types of receptors may be dif-

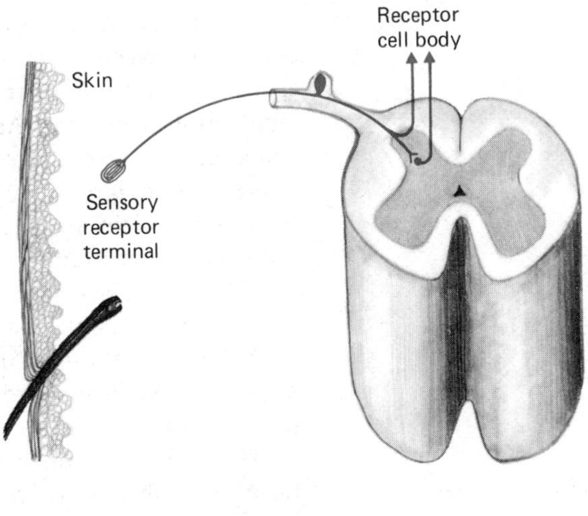

FIGURE 8.2 Peripheral portion of the somatosensory system. The stimulus is received by receptor terminals at the end of the neural fiber from the cell body in the dorsal root ganglion. Some of the somatosensory fibers (those of the spinothalamic tract) synapse in the dorsal horn; others go all the way up the spinal column before synapsing in the medulla.

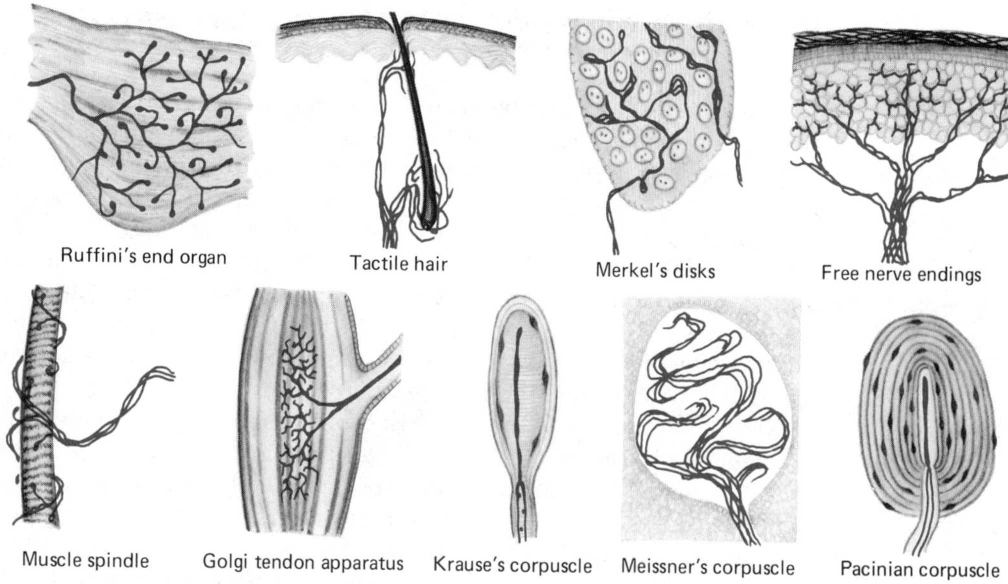

FIGURE 8.3 Examples of some of the receptor terminals of the somatosensory system. (Adaped from Guyton, 1976.)

ferent, but the tissue capsule itself serves only a nonneural function. As you will see in the discussion of transduction, stimulation of the fiber nerve terminal leads to production of the generator potential. Figure 8.3 shows only a few of the many varieties of encapsulated receptors and compares them to free endings.

Distribution of Receptors

The most common receptor terminals of the somatosensory system are free nerve endings, which are sensitive to pain and mechanical stimuli. They are found throughout the skin and in many other tissues, particularly the viscera. As a rule, they are not concentrated in any one place in the viscera, but are diffusely scattered, so visceral pain is most severe when large areas are stimulated. With regard to encapsulated terminals, Pacinian corpuscles, which are especially sensitive to rapid stimulation by touch (vibration), are found both in the skin and in the deep tissues (viscera) of the body; Meissner's corpuscles are found in the fingertips, the back, the bottom of the foot, and other areas of the body with low thresholds. Merkel's disks are also abundant in these same areas; and Ruffini's endings are commonly found throughout the skin (see Figure 8.3).

Hairy skin and nonhairy (smooth) skin differ in the kinds of receptor terminals. The hair follicles themselves have receptor terminals (see

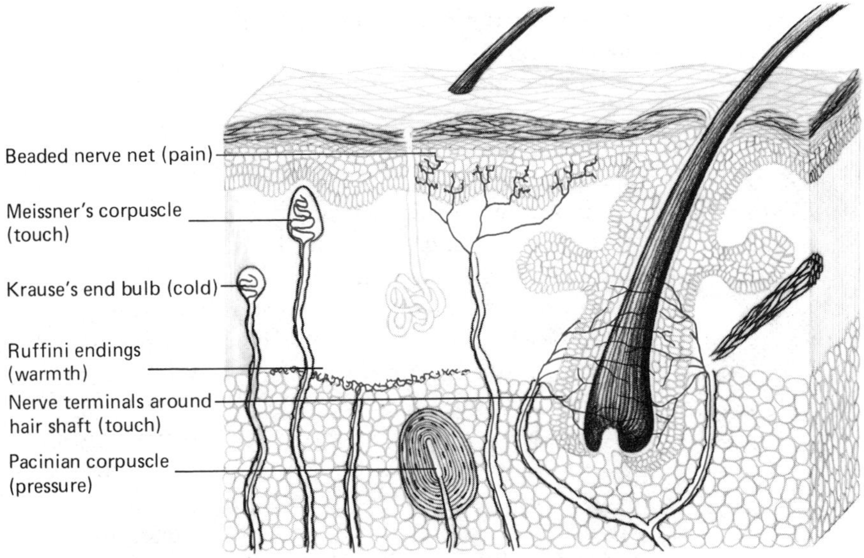

FIGURE 8.4 Receptor terminals of the somatosensory system. Shown here is a section of skin with different types of receptor terminals occurring at various levels. (Adapted from Peele, 1961.)

Figure 8.4), which are simply unmyelinated fibers terminating within the follicles. Incidentally, the sexual organs are not blessed with special sensory receptors (Quilliam, 1966). Their extreme sensitivity is due to both the concentration of receptors found there and the mental processing that accompanies sexual arousal.

Encoding Information Impulse: Labeled Line or Pattern

Like other aspects of the somatosensory system, the coding of neural impulses is more complicated than in other sensory systems because of the diversity of stimuli presented. Not only must the coding signify the location, frequency, and intensity of the stimulus; it must also specify the modality.

One controversial issue in studying the somatosensory system is in deciding just how specifically tuned any particular receptor is. Proponents of the "labeled line" theory hold that each receptor is narrowly attuned to one kind of stimulus, so a terminal that is sensitive to cold will not register a response to touch. Pattern theorists, on the other hand, maintain that receptors are broadly tuned. A number of receptor terminals will be excited in the vicinity of the stimulus, no matter what modality it is. However, of that large group of receptors, a few are more directly tuned to, say, touch, so the pattern, or the relative amounts of activity of the excited cells, will determine what sensation is received by the brain.

Both of these theories are based on the concept of receptive fields. A receptive field in the somatosensory system encompasses the area of skin or tissue in which a particular neuron or group of neurons can receive sensations. As in other sensory systems, the receptive fields get larger as the sensory pathway progresses to the higher levels of nervous system processing. For example, the receptive field of one neuron in the spinal cord may include only a small area of the hand. In the thalamus, however, sensory input has been condensed so that input from several areas on the hand are reflected by the information carried in a single neuron. Thus the receptive field of that neuron encompasses a larger area of the hand.

Both theories have supporting evidence. One study of receptor distribution held that sensitivity of the skin to different modalities was arranged in a punctate manner, with spots on the skin sensitive to cold, spots sensitive to warmth, spots for touch, and spots sensitive to pain. However, the existence of specific sensory spots came to be doubted when it was discovered that the location of the spots shifts during the course of the day. Such shifting obviously could not be caused by the receptors actually moving. An interpretation of this shifting indicates that the specific sensitivity of receptors may change during the day, thus supporting the pattern theory with its broadly tuned receptors and challenging the notion of labeled lines or very narrowly tuned receptors. Still, an experiment involving the sensory receptor located in a hair follicle revealed that bending a hair even 5° will evoke an action potential in the nerve fiber, and that even this one stimulated fiber can produce the sensation of being touched. Such information supports the labeled line theory. Since one fiber can elicit the sensation of touch, that fiber must be "labeled" touch.

As happens so much of the time with conflicting theories in science, each with some supporting evidence, both the labeled line and the pattern theory seem to be at least in part correct. The emerging theory, which is a synthesis of both, holds that receptors are indeed receptive to more than one kind of stimulus, but are not so broadly tuned as the pattern theorists would have us believe. In other words, each receptor terminal is thought to have a definite lowest threshold for one particular kind of stimulus, and thus, according to this modified pattern theory, the pattern of responding forms a sort of neural code for informing higher brain areas of the identity of the stimulus.

One undisputed fact of receptor distribution is that the density of innervation varies from one part of the body to another. For example, the fingertips and lips have far more receptors and thus are more sensitive than areas such as the back. This is easily demonstrated by giving the "two-point test" to a friend. Chances are that a person will quickly distinguish two points when applied 5 mm apart on the hand, but will find it hard to distinguish between two close points applied to the back (see Figure 8.5).

Even in regions of the body that do not have heavy concentrations of somatosensory receptors, there are overlapping receptive fields supplied by two or more sets of nerves. Thus the neural representation of things touched stimulates two sets of fibers, generating a two-point pattern of responses. This two-point system yields greater acuity in determining the fine details of the object touched.

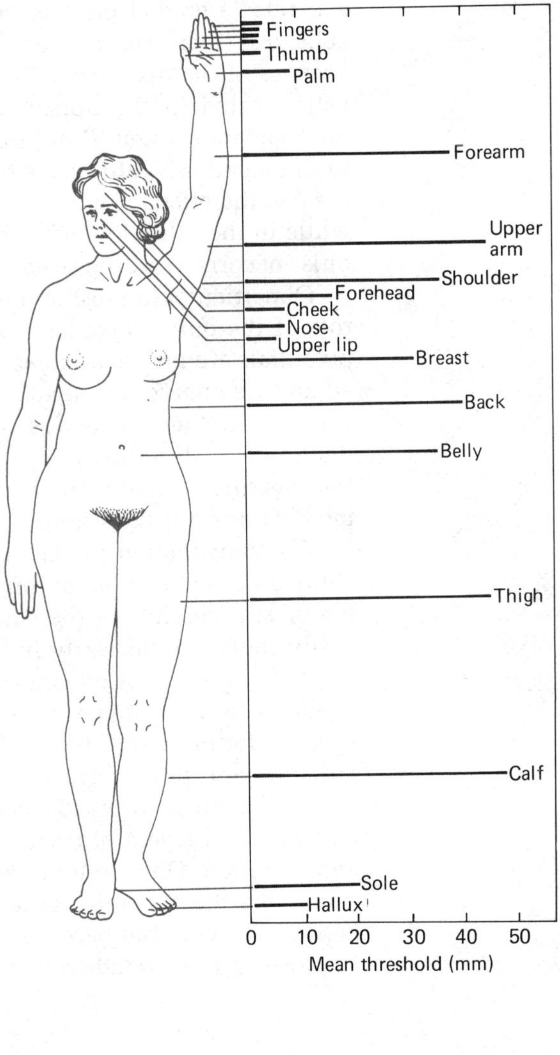

FIGURE 8.5 Two-point discrimination values for different parts of the body. One can distinguish between two points less than 5 mm apart on the hands, but two points on the calf must be more than 45 mm apart in order for a person to distinguish between them. (Adapted from Weinstein, 1968.)

The Transduction Process

Because the somatosensory system has receptor terminals rather than receptor cells, the transduction process is a bit different from the sensory systems discussed prior to this. The receptor terminal must perform the function of receiving the mechanical impulse, converting it into a neural impulse (here called a generator potential rather than a receptor potential as in receptor cells) and then initiating a spike, or action, potential in the nerve fiber. Aside from the terminology, this process, as far as we know, is basically the same whether the stimulus is received by a cell or nerve terminal.

In other sensory modalities, such as vision or audition, the stimulus generates a graded electric potential that goes directly to the receptor cells less than 1mm away. However, in the somatosensory system, because of the distance between the receptor terminal and the receptor cell (located in the dorsal column of the spinal cord), the stimulus must generate a neural impulse at the receptor terminal to travel to the receptor cell. The difference between the two processes is simply that in the one the effect of the stimulus is passed directly to the receptor cell, while in the other the effect of the stimulus is to generate a neural impulse of corresponding strength to be relayed to the receptor cell.

Of particular interest in the case of the somatosensory receptors is the role of the outer capsules surrounding the nerve terminals. Generator potentials are produced in essentially the same way in both encapsulated and free nerve terminals. The capsule covering the nerve ending of encapsulated terminals does not play a role in the actual neural transduction of a stimulus. In some instances, as in the Pacinian corpuscle, the covering mechanically modifies the stimulus, while in other cases it merely transmits the stimulus to the nerve terminal.

The transduction process of the somatosensory system is most often studied in the Pacinian corpuscles. These receptor terminals are among the most accessible of the somatosensory system, being large and thus easily found, particularly in the mesentery (tissue supporting the viscera). An additional advantage to researchers is that the Pacinian corpuscles can be removed from the body, and if placed in an appropriate saline solution, will function for several hours, a feature that greatly facilitates neurophysiological research.

The Pacinian corpuscle, consisting of a central nerve fiber surrounded by several layers of tissue, is particularly responsive to quick touch and vibration. One method used to determine the role of the capsule in producing the generator potential is to carefully strip away the outer capsule, leaving the bare nerve exposed (see Figure 8.6). Then, neural impulses are recorded from the stripped corpuscle and from an intact

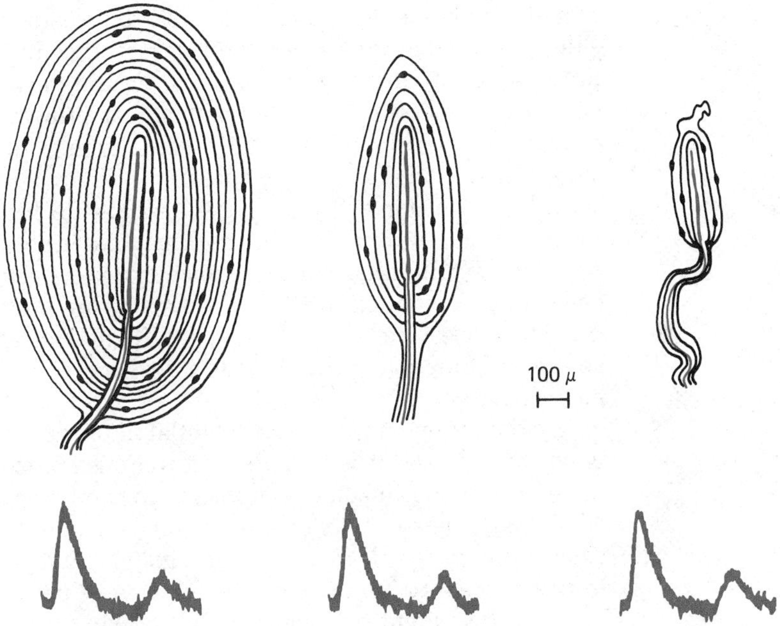

FIGURE 8.6 Intact and stripped Pacinian corpuscle. Layers of tissue can be peeled from the capsule surrounding the nerve ending, but spike potentials from the denuded nerve ending are virtually identical to those from an intact Pacinian cell. (Adapted from Lowenstein and Rathcamp, 1958.)

Pacinian corpuscle, using a stimulus of constant pressure. The generator potentials from the two cells differ, but the spike potentials are the same. In the intact corpuscle, there is one generator potential response at the onset of the stimulus and another when the stimulus is finished, whereas the bare capsule emits one continuous generator potential, beginning with the onset of the stimulus and lasting until the end of the stimulus. However, the important fact is that both cells display the same spike potential pattern: One spike is recorded at the onset of the stimulus, and another is recorded at the end of the stimulus. In other words, given that the actual neural response is the same, it appears that the effect of the outer covering of the Pacinian corpuscle is mainly a mechanical modification of the stimulus that does not affect the neural impulse (Lowenstein and Rathkamp, 1958).

The mechanical action of the Pacinian corpuscle is not complex. As mentioned earlier, this receptor terminal is one that is particularly sensitive to touch. Accordingly, pressure on a Pacinian corpuscle produces a slight deformation of the layers of tissue surrounding the nerve ending, which stimulates the nerve. However, the elastic properties of the capsule are such that the tissues in effect rearrange themselves to absorb the pressure, thus releasing the pressure on the nerve. (An analogy might be poking your finger into a foam rubber pillow.) When the stimulus or pressure is removed from the outside of the capsule, the layers again shift to regain their normal shape, and this movement of the layers again stimulates the nerve. Apparently, the capsule functions as an energy-saving efficiency device, peaking the generator potential at the onset and offset of the stimulus. Without the capsule, the generator potential fires continuously, though with no corresponding continuous spike potential. The nerve terminal is obviously designed to register the presence or absence of touch, and the capsule serves merely to modify the stimulus mechanically.

Exactly how the generator potential is produced in the nerve ending is not known, but it is thought that the mechanical deformation of the inner membrane in some way results in the firing of the cell. Undoubtedly, the permeability of the membrane is changed, perhaps by a chemical reaction caused by pressure, or it may be that the pores change shape in response to pressure. That this change in permeability is caused by pressure is evident from recordings showing the relationship between

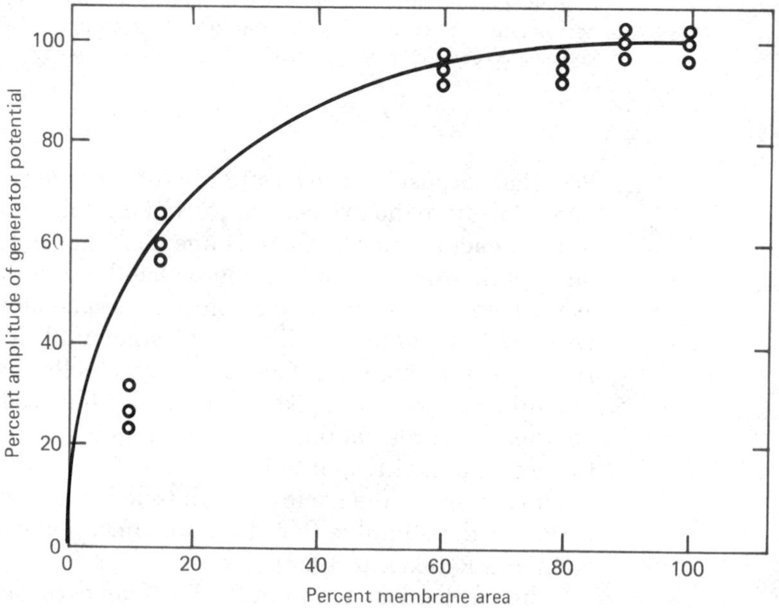

FIGURE 8.7 Relationship between the generator potential and the amount of the nerve terminal stimulated. As the percentage of the membrane area stimulated increases, so does the generator potential. (Adapted from Lowenstein, 1961.)

the size of the generator potential and the extent of the nerve terminal that is stimulated (Lowenstein and Rathkamp, 1958) (see Figure 8.7). At any rate, the change in permeability allows an ion redistribution that results in the production of the generator potential. The generator potential, in turn, must produce the "all or none" spike potential (see Chapter 2). This task is accomplished at the first node of Ranvier, which is the only node specialized for converting generator potentials into spike potentials.

Not much is known about the transduction process in thermal receptors or in pain receptors. One theory holds that thermal reactions are, like the touch reactions, caused by a mechanical deformation of the nerve membrane, but with temperature the surrounding tissues expand or contract in response to heat or cool. As in the Pacinian corpuscle, this deformation could cause the release of a chemical or could change the shape of the pores. The generator potential in pain receptors, which are free nerve endings, is believed to be triggered by the release of certain chemicals from the injured tissues, and the nociceptive nerve terminals are believed to be chemoreceptors (Mountcastle, 1974) that respond actively when the chemical is released.

Adaptation of Receptors

One distinguishing feature of somatosensory cells is that the various types adapt to stimuli at different rates. That is, some cells, such as the *Pacinian* corpuscles, adapt very rapidly to a prolonged stimulus. The elasticity of the Pacinian corpuscle is mainly responsible for the cell responding just at the onset and offset of a stimulus. Other rapidly adapting receptor terminals are *Meissner's* corpuscles, which are particularly sensitive to light touch, and the hair follicle receptors.

Both of these terminals are important for signaling even small movements on the surface of the skin. Since the surface of the skin is constantly under stimulation, it is probably fortunate for us that these cells do adapt rapidly. Otherwise the central nervous system would be cluttered with unimportant sensations such as one's shirt touching the skin of the back.

On the other hand, having some receptor terminals that adapt slowly, especially those located in the deeper layers of the skin, is fortunate, since prolonged pressure to the skin can be damaging. *Merkel's* disks adapt slowly, thus balancing the rapidly adapting Meissner's corpuscles with which they are generally found. *Ruffini's* endings, also located in the deeper tissues of the body, do not adapt rapidly. Some of the proprioceptive receptors are slow to adapt, maintaining a continuous firing pattern even in response to an invariant stimulus. Such receptors enable one to know at all times the position of one's body and limbs.

Proprioception is perhaps more properly conceived as the realm of sensory-motor function, for this modality, more than any of the others in the somatosensory system, involves the most intimate interaction between the sensory receptors and motor efferents.

As mentioned earlier, proprioception is rather difficult to study since the receptor cells are located deep inside the joints. The most common type of receptor terminal in the proprioceptive system is the Pacinian corpuscle, which, as described earlier, is sensitive to deformations or pressure on the outer capsule. Other sensory receptors found at joints are the muscle spindles and tendon organs. These will be discussed in connection with the motor system (see Chapter 9).

Pathways of the Somatosensory System

Although some of the peripheral pathways of the somatosensory system are as long as 4 feet, they are quite simple. Essentially, the somatosensory system may be thought of as having many separate pathways, for the receptor nerve terminals are at the end of peripheral nerves, which go all the way back to the dorsal root ganglia of the spinal cord without synapsing. These nerves band together in groups or bundles to travel back to the spinal cord, but they remain functionally discrete all the way. The vast network of afferent and efferent fibers innervating virtually every part of the body form what is called a nerve net, or plexus (see Figure 8.8).

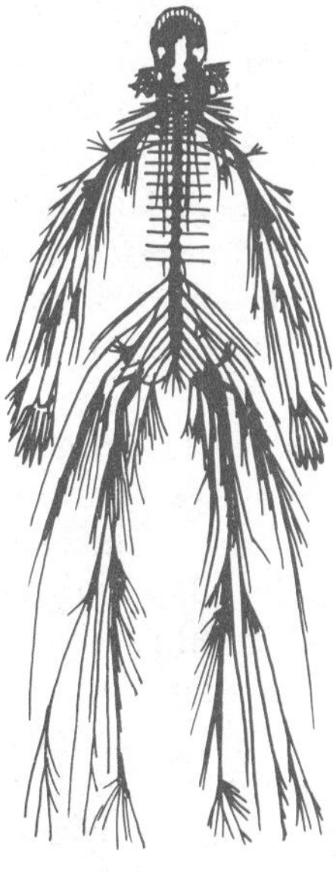

FIGURE 8.8 The fibers of the peripheral nervous system form a very efficient network for sensing and responding to incoming stimuli. The more heavily innervated areas of the body can be pointed out in this figure of a human body with all nerves outstretched. (Adapted from Time-Life, Inc. photo.)

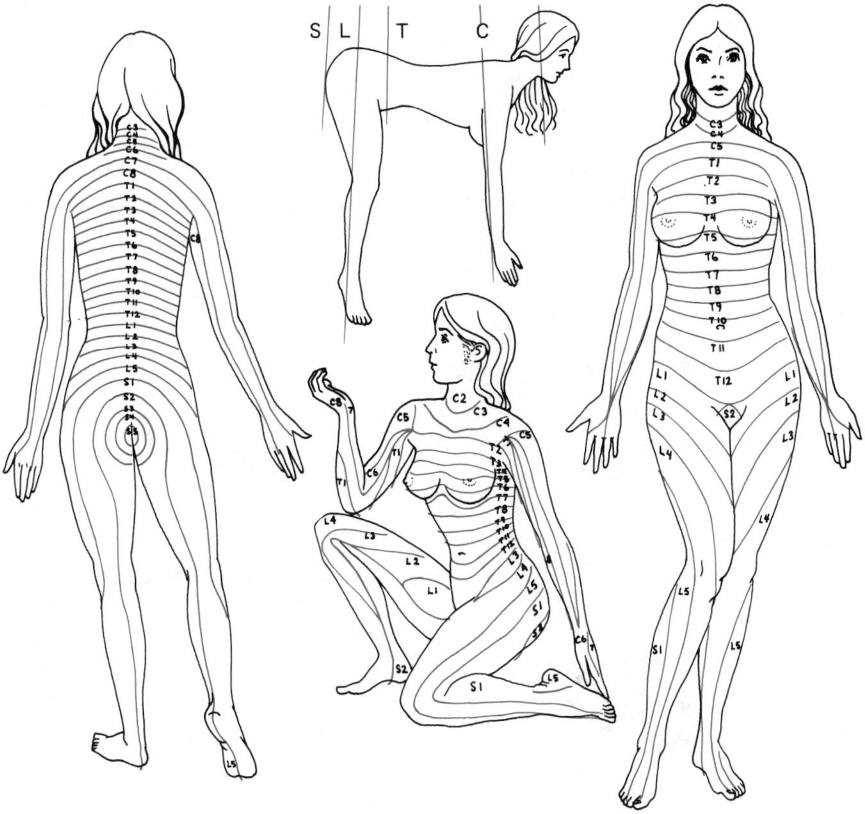

FIGURE 8.9 Dermatomes of the body. It is important to remember that the dermatomes overlap to some extent, thus aiding in two-point discrimination. Additionally, because of this overlap, injury to one spinal cord segment may not result in loss of sensation to the area of the body innervated by that segment since the surrounding segments also contribute to the innervation of that area.

Organization of the peripheral nerves is not random. Issued from each spinal cord segment is a group of fibers supplying one particular area of the skin, called a dermatome (see Figure 8.9). The dermatomes constitute the receptive fields of the group of nerves supplying the area. The arrangement of dermatomes associated with a particular spinal cord segment is best remembered if one thinks of man as walking on four legs. If that were the case, the hind region would be the origin of the tail, or the most distal part of the body. Consequently, the nerves serving it issue from the lowest spinal cord segment. The pattern continues up to the head, which is supplied by the nerves issuing from the uppermost segments of the spinal cord. The facial area is innervated by cranial nerve V, the trigeminal nerve, a mixed nerve, serving both sensory and motor functions. Fortunately, dermatomes overlap, so even if one group of nerves is completely destroyed, the area of skin innervated by that group of nerves will still have feeling, as it is innervated by a second group of nerves.

The peripheral fibers carrying somatosensory impulses vary in size and consequently in speed of conduction (see Figure 8.10). The system of classification for nerve fibers is given in Table 8.2. In this system, fibers are rated A, B, and C, according to size, with A being the largest. Type A fibers are broken down into four divisions: alpha (α), beta (β), gamma (γ), and delta (δ). By far the largest number of fibers are type C, the very small unmyelinated fibers. While their rates of conduction are relatively slow, they are sufficiently fast for carrying messages of a nonemergency nature. Note that although slow pain is carried by type C fibers, fast pain, that which is relieved by quick removal of the noxious stimulus, is carried by the considerably faster type A(α) fibers.

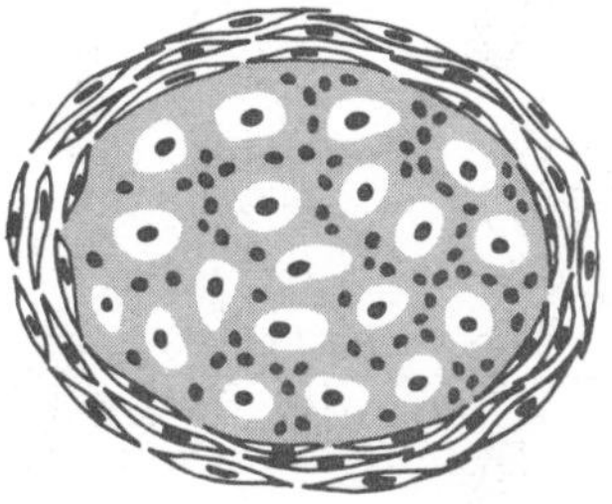

FIGURE 8.10 Within each nerve trunk are fibers of many different sizes, and this cross section shows both myelinated and unmyelinated fibers. The larger the nerve fiber, the faster it conducts impulses, with speed of conduction increasing in approximate proportion to the diameter of myelinated nerve fibers and in proportion to the square root of the diameter of unmyelinated fibers. In the somatosensory system, different sized fibers generally serve different functions (see Table 8.2). (From Guyton, 1976.)

TABLE 8.2 Properties of Different Nerve Fibers

Type of Fiber	Diameter of Fiber	Velocity of Conduction (m/sec)	Duration of Spike (msec)	Function
A(α)	13–22	70–120	0.4–0.5	Motor, muscle proprioceptors
A(β)	8–13	40–70	0.4–0.6	Touch, kinesthesia
A(γ)	4–8	15–40	0.5–0.7	Touch, excitation of muscle spindles, pressure
A(δ)	1–4	5–15	0.6–1.0	Pain, heat, cold, pressure
B	1–3	3–14	1.2	Preganglionic autonomic
C	0.2–1.0	0.2–2	2.0	Pain, postganglionic autonomic, smell

(Adapted from Guyton, 1976.)

Because of the length of the peripheral pathways of the somatosensory system, a disorder affecting one of the nerves can affect points distant from the site of the disorder. For example, pressure on a peripheral nerve as it enters the spinal cord can cause excruciating pain. Not only may the muscles of the lower back be affected; the entire pathway along which the nerve runs may register some form of painful reaction. A case in point is Barbara.

Barbara had been a floor nurse for 10 years, and had run the hemodialysis (kidney machine) unit for another 10 years. She enjoyed the daily contact with patients, especially the long individual relationships that were inevitable in a chronic-care facility like the dialysis unit. But not all memories of the dialysis unit were pleasant, for six years ago, while off balance leaning over the machine to change the coil, she had strained her back. That moment marked the beginning of a painful lumbar backache that would episodically leave her prostrate with pain and paresthesia (loss of sensation).

The first episode was by no means the most severe, but the characteristic pattern established a precedent. She fell helplessly after the strain, her lower back muscles tight in spasm. She was carried home by her colleagues. There she lay in bed with severe lumbar back pain, which by the third day radiated down the right side of her buttock into her posterior thigh and along the course of the nerve innervating the thigh and leg, called the sciatic nerve. When she rose to go to the bathroom she kept herself bent forward and leaned her back to the left. This posture took pressure off the right lumbar roots descending in the lower tip of the spinal cord (cauda equina) and exiting between the vertebrae. This extreme pain lasted a week, and she finally sought attention.

On examination she had numbness and decreased sensation to all modalities over her great toe on the right, up her foot, and on the lateral aspect of her calf. Testing for muscle strength was uninterpretable because of the pain. Muscle reflexes on her right side were depressed. Elongation of the nerve by passive straight leg raise, or extending the knee with the leg flexed at the hip, consistently provoked pain, and increased the feeling of numbness over the great toe. Finally, she displayed weakness of the muscles in her buttocks. Reluctantly she consented to admission, whereupon she was treated with further bed rest, sedation, and analgesics. Over a two-week period the spasm relented and she was able to walk in the exercise room. The numbness and decreased sensation remained.

These attacks occurred about twice a year, and as the last attack did not respond to bed rest, she underwent myelography. This is an x-ray study where radioactive opaque dye is injected into the spinal subarachnoid space, and the patient, on a tilt table, is positioned at various angles so that the dye can outline the entire space. Barbara had a large herniated disk, as expected. That is, one of the cushioning disks between the spinal vertebrae had ruptured, thus placing pressure on a nerve. Because her disk had not responded to conservative management (i.e., bed rest and avoiding back strain), Barbara went to surgery. It was uncomplicated; the disk was removed and the lumbar-sacral root freed. Her pain was relieved; only the numbness persisted. She returned with new vigor to her nursing responsibilities.

Pressure on the sciatic nerve had caused Barbara pain all along the course of the nerve, but in particular had caused numbness and tingling in her foot and lower leg. Obviously, the affected area reflected the dermatome of the damaged nerve.

The Spinal Cord: Pathways to the Brain

The peripheral pathways terminate just outside the spinal cord in the dorsal root ganglia. From that point on, central pathways take over the function of transmission of somatosensory impulses. Two pathways carry the bulk of the somatosensory information: the dorsal column-medial lemniscal system and the spinothalamic system. For quite some time the dorsal column-medial lemniscal system was thought to be the pathway for discrete touch, that is, sensations of touch that deal with specific features of an object, such as its edges, shape, and texture. The spinothalamic pathway was thought to be involved with more diffuse forms of touch sensitivity, as well as with pain and temperature. In recent years, however, a new view of somatosensory organization regarding the pathways for touch has emerged. The distinction between the two pathways seems to be based more on active vs. passive touch than on discrete vs. diffuse touch, per se (Semmes and Mishkin, 1965; Wall, 1975). Support of this conslusion is found in cases in which the dorsal column is severed (Wall, 1970). In such cases, the person or animal loses the capacity for learning tactual discriminations that require active exploration of the stimulus features. However, the subject is still capable of making passive tactual discriminations, that is, those that have only one dimension upon which the correct performance is dependent (i.e., Which object is rough? Which is round?) (Wall, 1970). On the basis of this information, along with the existing notion concerning pain, temperature, and proprioception, the distinction between the two pathways now rests on active vs. passive touch. The dorsal column-medial lemniscal system is thought to be the pathway for active touch and proprioception, and the spinothalamic system is thought to handle passive touch, pain, and temperature sensation.

Dorsal Column-Medial Lemniscal System Fibers in this system leave the dorsal root ganglion and travel straight up through the spinal

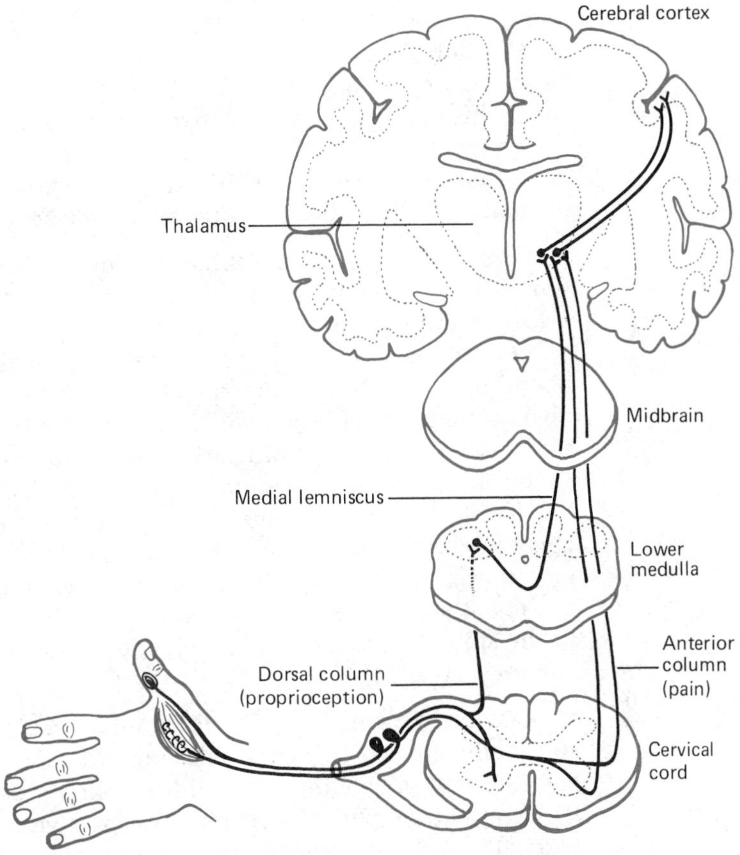

FIGURE 8.11 The dorsal column-medial lemniscal system, subserving active touch and proprioception. This pathway begins with neural fibers from the dorsal root ganglion, which enter the spinal cord and ascend without synapsing through the dorsal column. The first synapse is in the dorsal column nucleus in the medulla, where the tract then crosses over the midline to the contralateral half of the brain. Ascending through the medial lemniscal tract, the fibers synapse in the ventroposterolateral nucleus of the thalamus and then make their way to the somatosensory cortex.

cord, forming what are known as the dorsal columns (see Figure 8.11). These columns are, as the name suggests, in the dorsal region of the spinal cord, and are also known as the funiculus gracilis (containing fibers from the legs) and the funiculus cuneatus (containing fibers from the arms and head). Fibers ascending through these columns neither cross to the contralateral side of the cord nor synapse until they get to the level of the medulla in the lower brain stem. Here they synapse at the dorsal column nuclei (the nucleus gracilis and nucleus cuneatus) and then cross over to the other side of the brain, making this system totally contralateral.

In the brain these fibers form what is called the medial lemniscal tract. This tract makes its way to the ventrobasal portion of the thalamus, where the neurons of this pathway synapse for the second time in the ventroposterolateral nucleus (VPL) (Mountcastle et al., 1963). From the thalamus, the fibers head for the somatosensory areas of the cortex.

The Spinothalamic Pathway The spinothalamic pathway has proved to be somewhat more difficult to study than the dorsal column-medial lemniscal system, for the organization of the receptive fields differs. In the dorsal column-medial lemniscal system, the cells and fibers maintain an accurate somatotopic map, and adjacent cells and fibers innervate adjacent fields. In the spinothalamic system, the somatosensory map is not nearly as accurate (Poggio and Mountcastle, 1960). An added complication of the spinothalamic system is that receptive fields are not discrete. Receptive fields in the dorsal column-medial lemniscal system are small and generally surrounded by inhibitory zones; receptive fields of the spinothalamic system are larger and not completely surrounded by inhibitory regions. Additionally, cells in the spinothalamic system receive input from many types of specific afferents. (Wall, 1975).

Clinical Examples of Anatomic Principles Studies involving split-brain subjects (patients whose interhemispheric connections have been severed in an attempt to control epileptic seizures—see Appendix II) have lent support to the active vs. passive distinction between the two pathways, and illustrate some of the complicated anatomical points just discussed.

Given this anatomical organization of pathways, with the dorsal column-medial lemniscal system being completely contralateral and the spinothalamic system being both homolateral and contralateral, in split-brain subjects one would expect crisp lateralization of information transmitted by the dorsal column (active touch, proprioception), but various degrees of lateralization for information transmitted by way of the spinothalamic system. Indeed, many studies have confirmed this expectation.

Split-brain patients are able to report verbally the temperature or painful sensation when either hand is stimulated. In contrast, such patients are able to describe verbally the position of the limbs (proprioceptive sensory information) for only the right side of the body, and are unable to do so concerning the left side of the body. Since the language mechanisms are only in the left hemisphere, and this hemisphere receives proprioceptive information only from the limbs on the right side of the body, this demonstrates the anatomic principle of crisp lateralization of dorsal column information, and bilateral representation of spinothalamic information.

In studies of split-brain animals, it has been observed that when passive touch stimuli are used in discrimination training, and presumably this information is conveyed to the brain both homolaterally and contralaterally by the spinothalamic pathways, the untrained hand performs above chance on posttraining tests. However, if more complex stimuli are used, thus requiring active manipulation of the objects in order to ascertain the critical cue, and presumably reflecting information conveyed to the brain contralaterally only by dorsal column-medial lemniscal pathways, the untrained hand generally shows no signs of having benefited from the training of the other hand. These observations support the notion that dorsal column information (active touch and proprioception) is projected mainly to the contralateral hemisphere, whereas spinothalamic information from one side of the body is available, at least in part, to each half-brain (Gazzaniga and LeDoux, 1978).

The Proprioceptive Pathway

Aside from the two main pathways in the somatosensory system, another important one is the proprioceptive pathway. Afferent fibers from the muscle, tendon, and joint receptors travel to the parent cell bodies in the dorsal root ganglia. Fibers from these cells then enter the dorsal column and ascend through an undefined dorsolateral column, synapsing on cells of the dorsal column nuclei and then merging with the medial lemniscal pathway. However, the proprioceptive cells remain functionally discrete, projecting on cells with similar properties in the thalamus, and then continuing to the cortex, specifically to SI, the postcentral gyrus. An important offshoot of this pathway, however, projects not to the cortex, but to the cerebellum, where muscle tone, body postion, and motor control are unconsciously mediated.

In the next section, we proceed even further along the central pathways to examine cortical processing of somatosensory information.

Cortical Processing of Somatosensory Information

The somatosensory cortex has three principal subdivisions: SI, SII, and the association area, composed of areas 5 and 7. The SI and SII areas make up the primary somatosensory cortex since they are the only cortical areas that receive somatosensory input directly from the thalamus. Areas 5 and 7 are called association areas since they receive and process "secondhand" information from the primary somatosensory cortex. These areas all occupy the parietal lobes.

Most of the cortical processing is done in SI, which occupies the postcentral gyrus, and is composed of cortical areas 1, 2, and 3, according to the Brodmann map. Each of these areas contains a modality-specific topographical representation of the opposite side of the body (Mountcastle, 1957). Area 3 contains the representation of the tactile

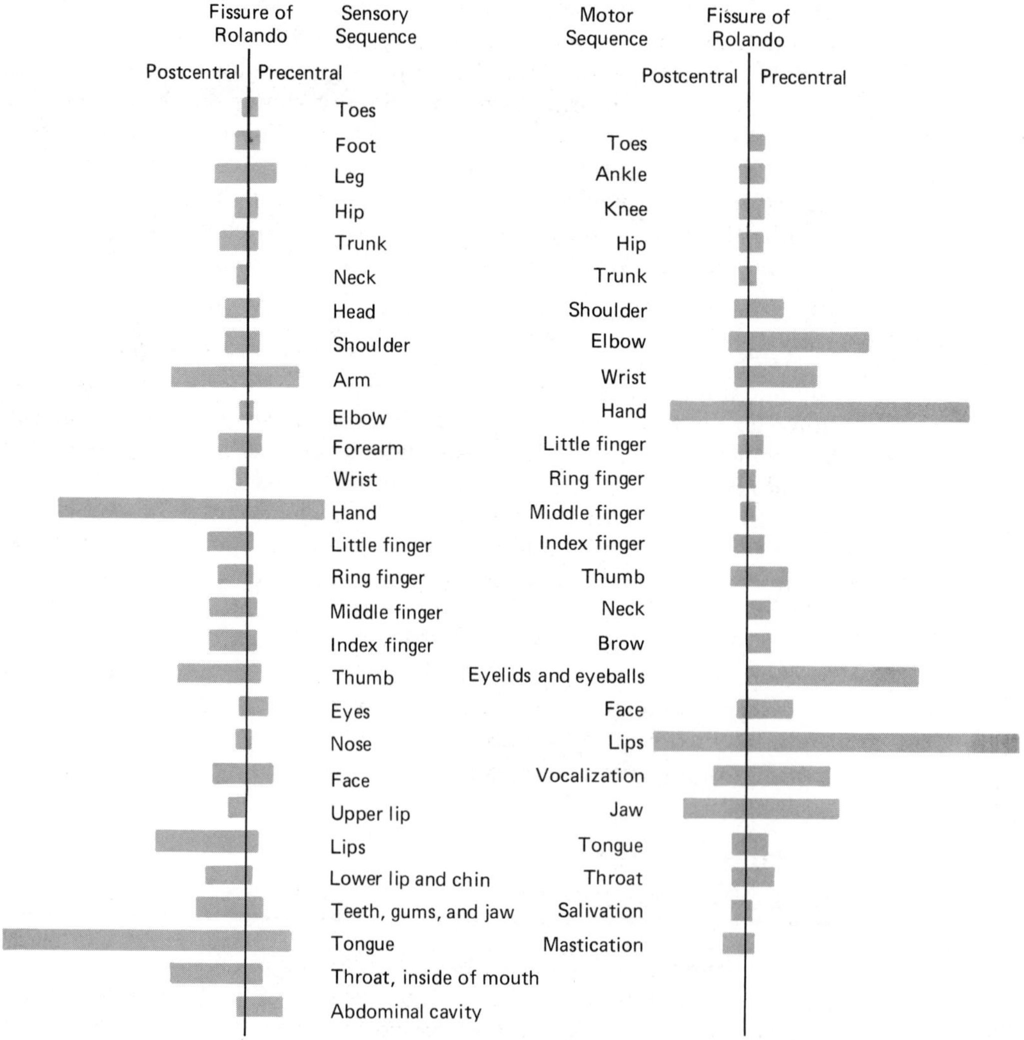

FIGURE 8.12 This distorted view of human body parts illustrates the percentage of sensory cortex and motor cortex serving each particular area. The face, and particularly the mouth, is heavily innervated. The hands also claim a fairly large share of the sensory motor cortex. (Adapted from Penfield and Rasmussen, 1950.)

(light-touch) modality, while areas 1 and 2 contain the representations of the deep senses (pressure and joint rotation). The tactile map of area 3 maintains a somatotopic organization. That is, stimulation of adjacent areas of the body produces excitation of adjacent areas of the cortex. Cortical organization also reflects the density of innervation by the peripheral nerves. For example, the lips and thumbs, which contain many somatosensory afferents, claim a proportionately large part of the cortex (see Figure 8.12).

The SII area occupies the parietal cortex of the superior bank of the sylvian fissure. Within SII, there is a somatotopic representation of the contralateral body, though it is less precise than the representations found in SI. In addition, there is a poorly localized representation of the ipsilateral body in SII, which receives input directly from the thalamus, but the input is from collaterals of the fibers going to SI (Jones, 1976).

Cortical association areas 5 and 7 receive no primary input. Area 5 depends on input from SI, and in turn supplies area 7. Area 5 contains a somatotopic representation of the body, but area 7 seems to lack topographic organization (Jones and Powell, 1970).

Studies of the Vertical Column Concept

The physiological studies of the somatosensory cortex by Mountcastle and his associates show that the basic functional units of SI are vertically oriented columns of cells, each column sensitive to a single modality of somatosensory input. Thalamic input to SI terminates in layers III and IV, and is processed vertically in the surrounding layers, with very little lateral spread. As a microelectrode vertically penetrates the cortex, all cells respond to the same modality and have nearly identical contralateral peripheral receptive fields. Columns in area 3 represent the tactile sense, while columns in areas 1 and 2 represent the deep senses.

The basic experimental setup used to determine this information requires an animal with recording microelectrodes implanted in the brain. This animal is then placed in a chair or on a table, and various stimuli are applied to the area of the body from which the particular cortical cell receives input. Say the electrode is in the area of the brain that processes information from the left paw. The paw is stimulated in some way, whether it be touched, tickled, pressed, warmed, or cooled. The cells in the particular cortical column will fire only when the stimulus is in one particular modality, say touch. If the electrode is moved either up or down in one vertical column, the cells in that column will respond only to touch. However, if the electrode is moved over to another column, the cells in that column may respond not to touch, but to a thermal stimulus.

Intrahemispheric connections of the somatosensory cortex seem to integrate information concerning different somatic modalities affecting the same body part. For example, the primary cellular connections in SI are between cells that have the same peripheral receptive fields, though the cells mediate different response properties for the same part of the body (Jones and Powell, 1970). Thus, the cells of the columns representing the deep senses (areas 1 and 2) of the forefinger are connected to the cortical cells registering light tactile stimulation of the forefinger.

The somatosensory cortex is unique, for it is the only primary sensory area that projects directly to the motor areas of the cortex. This is not too surprising since the interplay between the somesthetic system, which is responsible for the bodily sensations, and the motor system, which is responsible for motor control, is essential for smooth, coordinated movement.

Damage to SI, as you might expect, produces a loss of conscious sensations in the body areas corresponding to the lesion locus. If the damage is restricted to one hemisphere, the sensory loss is greatest on the opposite side of the body, though the ipsilateral side may also be affected. However, the ipsilateral side usually recovers rapidly (its innervation from the undamaged hemisphere being intact), and the contralateral side also generally recovers to some extent. The distal extremities, being innervated mainly by crossed pathways, are the least likely to regain sensation. Little is known concerning the consequences of damage to SII. Lesions of the parietal association areas produce a number of striking behavioral deficits, including the inability to perform complex tactual discriminations (probably of the active-touch type) in the absence of sensory loss (Corkin et al., 1970; Ettlinger et al., 1966), spatial disorientation (Semmes et al., 1960), and difficulties in manipulating items to construct spatial patterns. These observations, in conjunction with recent studies of the physiological response properties of single cells in areas 5 and 7, suggest that the somatic association areas play a major role in providing the organism with an appreciation of the relation between its bodily parts and the immediately surrounding spatial environment (Mountcastle et al., 1975).

Hence we have traced the anatomical basis of somesthetic sensations from the receptor level to cortical processing. In the next section we shall look at a few specific examples of the functioning of the somatosensory system.

The Experience of Pain

Aside from the pleasurable sensations we enjoy by way of somatosensory receptors, it is regrettably true that we are also subject to the experience of pain through somatosensory receptors. Pain may be brief, as in a stubbed toe or pinched finger, or it may be lasting, as in migraine headaches and back injuries. Fortunately, progress is being made in the area of controlling the perception of pain, and longtime sufferers are now finding some relief from their ordeal of enduring a life marred by incapacitating pain. Many of the new methods for controlling pain base their effectiveness on the principles of the gate control theory of pain, a theory proposed during the 1950s. Although the theory is not without its problems, it remains the most salient theory of how pain is perceived.

The Gate Control Theory of Pain

Painful stimuli differ from other stimuli in that they are carried by smaller, slower neural fibers. Like all other neural impulses, painful impulses are electrical, and a currently accepted theory of pain perception is based on the electrical activity in the spinal cord (Melzack and Wall, 1962). According to this theory, certain cells in the spinal cord, called T-cells, are responsible for transmitting impulses from the periph-

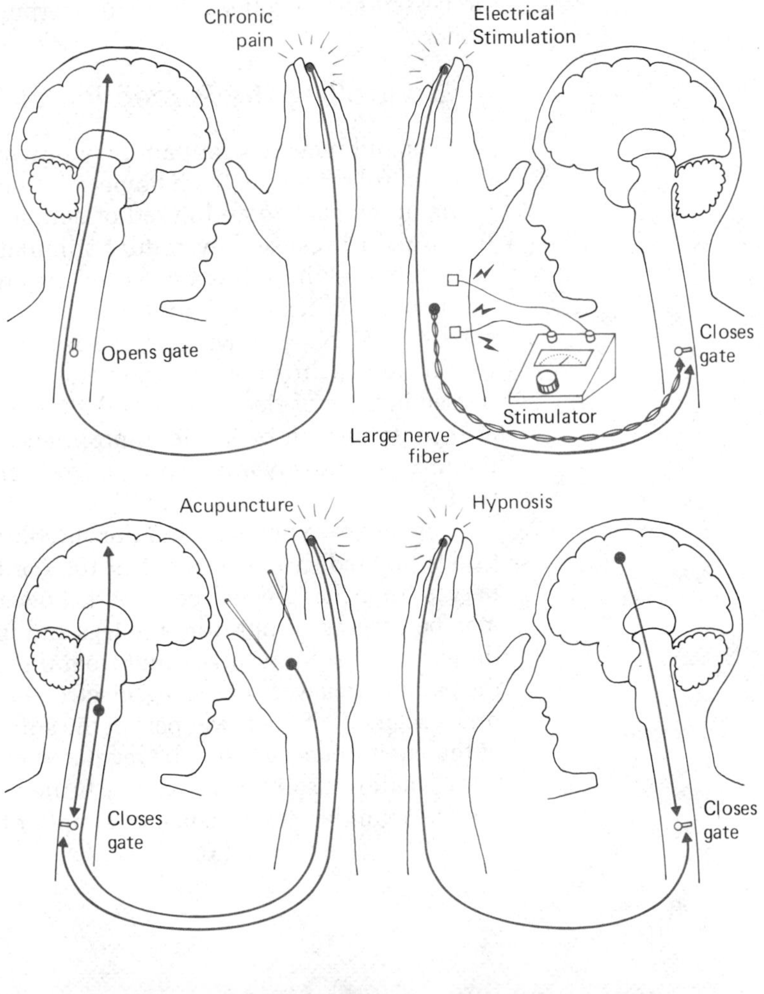

FIGURE 8.13 Input from large fibers can effectively "close the gate" to input from small fibers (which carry pain). Obviously, if the impulses do not get beyond the dorsal horn of the spinal cord, they will not reach the cortex for processing by the conscious part of the central nervous system.

eral nervous system to the brain. Input to these T-cells is controlled by a group of intrinsic neurons in the substantia gelatinosa area of the spinal cord (see Figure 8.13). Afferent input from large fibers to these interneurons results in presynaptic inhibition of cutaneous input (nociceptive, small fibers), while sufficient input from small fibers will reduce or stop the presynaptic inhibition. Up to a certain point, however, input from large afferent fibers can prohibit the impulses from small fibers (nociceptive) from ever being processed in the CNS. It is as if the neurons of the substantia gelatinosa act as a gate, metaphorically speaking, allowing input from large fibers to proceed, and prohibiting the input from smaller fibers that are excited by painful stimuli. Of course, it is important to remember that there is no actual gate mechanism, for the control is exerted electrically, but the effect is analogous to a gate.

The presynaptic inhibition imposed by the cells of the substantia gelatinosa is believed to occur only when the ratio between input from large and small fibers is at a certain level or below. When the painful stimuli outnumber other somatosensory stimuli, the painful input is processed and its effects tend to overpower any sensations from large fibers.

Controlling the Perception of Pain

Even old remedies for pain may unwittingly have been based on the gate control principle. Such home solutions as application of a hot water bottle or ice pack to an injured or aching part of the body no doubt relieved pain because they mildly stimulated certain somatosensory receptors (whose impulses are carried by large fibers), thus blocking transmission of the stronger impulses from nociceptive receptors (carried by small fibers). Now, however, there is a more direct and convenient way of blocking pain impulses. Somatosensory stimulation per se is bypassed in favor of electrical stimulation of the large afferent fibers, either at the site of pain or in the appropriate segment of the spinal cord or brain. By selectively innervating large fibers, pain can be effectively controlled.

One device, known as the dorsal column stimulator, involves electrodes planted in the segment of the cord that receives the peripheral nerves from the affected body part. Lower cord segments, you will remember, receive input from the legs and lower body, while segments of the cord higher up receive input from the arms and upper body. Thus, if the painful area were in the leg, electrodes would be placed in the appropriate segment of the lower part of the spinal cord. Electrical stimulation of the large fibers can then be regulated at will by the patient, who carries a small transmitter that can be turned on as the need to control pain arises. A similar device consists simply of a hand-held transmitter that can be rubbed gently over the painful area, electrically arousing the large fibers. A similar method, which is a bit more complicated, involves planting electrodes directly in the brain centers that control the perception of pain.

The Complexity of the Problem

Attitudes and Pain

In some instances, control of pain can become a case of mind over matter, and a person's attitude can have a large effect on the amount of pain perceived. Examples of this attitude effect are seen frequently in daily life. A person who is accidentally shoved is far more likely to feel hurt if the shove appears intentional. The sting of a facial slap inflicted in a lover's quarrel is likely to persist longer than a similar nociceptive stimulus such as, say, the pain from a volleyball hitting the face during the routine course of a game.

The physiological explanation for how attitude can reduce the perception of pain is based on descending impulses from the brain. Conscious manipulation of attitudes through counseling, then, can effectively alter people's attitudes and teach them to control pain. Individuals sometimes unconsciously thrive on the attention and rewards they get when they are suffering. In clinics set up for the sole purpose of treating pain, patients are forbidden to discuss their pain or dwell on it. Keeping their minds and hands busy with other projects, whether they be knitting or conscious relaxation procedures, has significantly helped many patients who formerly thought of almost nothing but their pain.

Some attitudes toward pain are fostered by the culture one lives in. An example of how culturally influenced attitudes affect perception of pain is in the act of childbirth. In many cultures, childbirth is regarded as an excruciatingly painful experience, but in others, it is seen as a joyous, life-giving occasion. Given the effects of attitude on the perception of pain, is it any wonder that in the latter case far less pain is felt by the mother? In some cultures, the event has perhaps of necessity been treated as a routine experience. The expectant mother stops working just long enough to give birth, then quickly returns to work without allowing herself the luxury of a recuperation period. Probably as an effect of the mother's attitude, the pain experienced is less than in other cultures. Current trends in western society are promoting methods of natural childbirth that emphasize the positive aspects of giving birth, stressing that much of the pain can indeed be controlled by a positive attitude toward the experience.

Pain Killers and the Brain

One of the more exciting discoveries in recent years has been an exploration of the biochemical mechanisms working in the perception of pain. It has long been known that the family of opiate drugs blocks the perception of pain. These drugs apparently act on specific receptor sites in the brain, and most of them are found in the limbic system. As a result, the euphoric effect these drugs have on patients, in addition to their analgesic effect, is thought to be caused by their acting directly on the "emotional" brain (Snyder, 1978) (see Chapter 11).

At this point the question might be asked, why does the brain have opiate receptors? At first glance the brain seems set up for drug abuse. The answer lies in the fact that the brain can generate its own opiates, which most likely are small peptides called enkephalins. While the exact site of a mechanism of synthesis is not known, it has been shown that these small peptides bind to the opiate receptors and allow for the analgesic effects that externally administered morphine produces. The mechanism of action is not completely understood, but Snyder (1975) believes the enkephalins act by inhibiting the amount of neurotransmitter secreted on excitation.

It may be that some persons are seemingly able to tolerate more severe pain than others because their body naturally produces more of these morphinelike substances. Likewise, some of the theories of pain control may in fact be based on somehow increasing the body's supply of enkephalins.

Still, there is much to be learned about pain. The following case tells of a person whose life was ruined by pain. Her perception of pain was seemingly unresponsive to her body's own supply of enkephalins, to externally administered painkillers, or to peripheral stimulation based on the gate control theory of pain.

Thelma spent most of her time doing research for her encyclopedia articles. She had been a journalist in a competitive city news department early in her career and had risen quickly to assistant city editor. But love of travel and faraway places had made the foreign office even more inviting, so she had seized the opportunity for change. In the foreign office her reporting had won her and the paper many prizes, but that is a long chronicle and another story. She stayed in that vigorous position for 45 years, and her retirement last year was a great commemorative event. She planned to continue writing—there was no way she could stop—but now at a more leisurely pace, with time to explore the magnetic byroads that always seemed to flash past too quickly.

Healthy and addicted to a vigorous physical fitness regimen of an early morning swim, she was nonplussed by the sudden severe headache she experienced. It passed by lunchtime, but she became suddenly aware of the loss of tactile sensibility on her right side. Her arm and face were more surely involved with this unusual sensation or lack of sensation. Everything she touched felt as though she were touching it through a glove; even the teacup did not seem hot. She was also suffering from proprioception loss, that is, loss of the sense of limb position. This part of her disorder was difficult to explain or gauge, and she described it as clumsiness.

Soon after this sudden onset of anesthesia to pain and temperature, along with the less profound loss of proprioception, she suffered a mild but definite hemiparesis (slight paralysis on one side). This weakness of her arm and face caused her to seek medical attention.

By the time she arrived at the hospital, her hemiparesis on the right hand had cleared. The sensory loss on objective testing was more profound for proprioception and vibration in the right hand than for pain or temperature, although the latter two modalities were also affected. She had no visual loss. Although she had no risk factors for atherosclerotic disease (lipid deposits in blood vessels) or cerebrovascular disease, it seemed her story represented the thalamic syndrome of Dejerine-Roussy. This rare stroke was due to occlusion of the thalamogeniculate artery and destruction of the ventrolateral thalamic nuclei.

Over the next two weeks of hospitalization Thelma was encouraged by the return of strength in her right hand, and she returned home relieved. In the next year, however, the anesthesia, less noticeable except on her face, underwent a distinct change. In fact, she now felt dyesthesias (burning pains) that grew to crescendo pitch until she would scream that it "felt like the flesh was being torn away" from her face and arm. These unfamiliar and bizarre sensory experiences replaced the anesthesia.

The mechanism of such central pain is unknown. Speculations include loss of afferent thalamocortical pathway with subsequent diminished cortical stimulation. It is also possible that reduction in cortical stimulation may lead to similar reduction in descending inhibitory impulses to the dorsal horn gate control of pain in the spinal cord.

Virtually any sensation could precipitate the sudden paroxysmal onset of Thelma's pain. Any event from change in temperature, to music in the room, to an argument, aggravated Thelma's condition. The inevitable personality change took place. She became continually aware of her affected arm; she shielded it, even cajoled it, as her arm had become a separate entity. She became quite depressed. No medicine or combination of medicines would help. Electrical stimulation, peripheral stimulation were also failures. After two years of almost constant agony, Thelma committed suicide, a tragic end for such a vibrant intellectual.

It is hoped that learning more about the central processing of somatosensory information will someday lead to help for individuals like Thelma.

In the next section, we proceed even further along the central pathways to examine cortical processing of somatosensory information.

The Body Schema

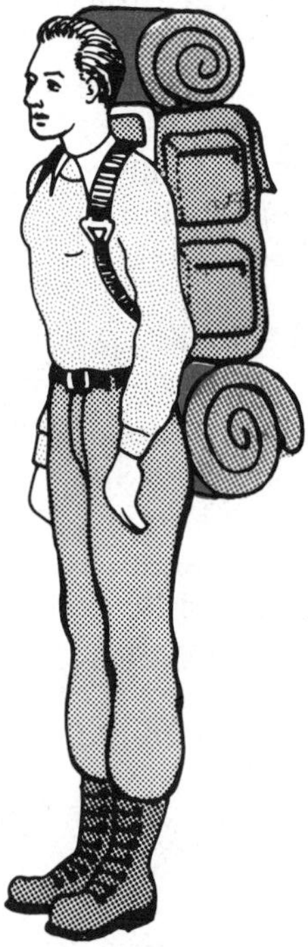

FIGURE 8.14 The body schema is extended to include projections that are not actually part of the body but become part of the body space. The hiker quickly learns to extend the sense of personal space to include the backpack.

Another example of a function of the somatosensory system is found in people's perception of their own bodies, that is, their mental representation of the spatial and physiological extent of their bodies. This representation is called the body schema. Naturally, the receptors of the somatosensory system provide most of the information on which the body schema is based. The proprioceptive sense, derived from receptors in the joints, muscles, and tendons, supplies information necessary for formulating an idea of the posture of the body, while the sensory impulses derived from receptors in the skin and subcutaneous tissues also contribute to a person's sense of body outline. A third element contributing to the body schema is visual input, but it is not essential, since even a congenitally blind person may have an accurate body schema.

Normally, the body schema is not considered part of the conscious experience; rather consciousness of the body is only peripheral. It is not until one's attention is specifically directed to a part of one's body that the body schema is consciously considered.

The body schema is a plastic concept. That is, the body schema can be extended to include tools one is using (such as a pen when writing) or projection (such as skis or a backpack) (see Figure 8.14). When maneuvering through a crowd, for example, a man wearing a backpack is aware that he must find room for himself and the backpack.

The neurologic site for construction of the body schema is most probably the parietal lobe, for disorders of the body schema are generally associated with lesions of the parietal lobe, which is the location of most of the cortical processing of somatosensory input.

The Phantom Limb

One common disorder of the body schema is its persistence even after amputation of a limb. Although the limb is gone, the person still seems to experience the spatial characteristics of the missing limb. The existence of the "phantom limb" is based on the body schema, which was firmly ingrained in the person's mind before the part was amputated. Generally, a person perceives the phantom limb almost immediately after surgery. The phenomenon does not disappear quickly; in some cases, phantom limbs have persisted for many years.

Perception of the phantom limb is based mainly on somesthetic characteristics. The position of the limb is at first constant, often assuming the position of the limb immediately prior to surgery (Frederiks, 1969). Eventually, a person can "move" the phantom limb, and this control over the limb can make it easier for the person to cope with the phantom limb phenomenon. Consider the case of a man whose phantom limb was awkwardly positioned on his back (Bornstein, 1949). He was forced always to sleep on his stomach.Had he been able to move the imaginary hand, it would have presented a far less substantial problem.

Strangely enough, another manifestation of the phantom limb phenomenon occurs in patients whose limbs are intact, but who at times experience a third limb (Critchley, 1965). This type of phantom limb is due to a lesion in the nervous system. The other type of phantom limb is much more difficult to explain. Any theory that attempts to explain it must deal with several aspects of the syndrome (Frederiks, 1969). Explanation can be based on a peripheral point of view, holding that severed nerves in the stump itself produce or contribute to the phantom limb. Another aspect of explaining the phantom limb lies in examining the role of central nervous system mechanisms, such as the integrating process of the somesthetic system in the cortex of the parietal lobe. However, because much cortical processing remains unexplained, particularly with respect to the normal body schema, discovery of a central mechanism that accounts for the phantom limb will undoubtedly come only after further successful research on cortical processing. Clearly an important aspect of the syndrome must be psychological processes. For example, a phantom limb may disappear once a person has clearly accepted the loss of the limb and no longer imagines the presence of the missing part. However, psychological explanations alone are insufficient.

Summary

Thus we see that a study of the somatosensory system—the sensory innervation of the entire body—and the disorders of this system covers a wide range of topics. As should be obvious by now, however, all sensory systems operate on the same basic principles. A stimulus is received when an adequate stimulus excites a receptor. By now it should be clear that the receptor may be regarded as a transducer capable of responding to a specific form of energy (light, sound, touch, pain). The neural impulse follows its particular pathway to the brain for processing.

The somatosensory system is no different. Whether the impulse is tactile, thermal, painful, or important information about joint position in space, the message is transduced at the receptor terminal. For this large nonhomogeneous system the modes of peripheral reception have unique receptors. Somewhat unlike seeing and hearing, where the most specific cell receptors are in the cortex, the somatosensory system viewed in toto begins with a complex peripheral organization.

But on closer study of this peripheral specificity and distribution of receptors, each subsystem more closely approximates the paradigm of the visual and auditory systems. For example, humans' appreciation of pain usually begins at the nerve ending far from the spinal cord. Traveling in the dorsal column the message is routed upwards toward the brain in the spinothalamic pathway to the thalamus. If this painful stimulus is induced by accidentally pressing on a hot iron, then heat is part of the neural message. As such, the perception of heat begins at specific thermal receptors. Temperature messages also travel through the dorsal roots and up to the brain in the spinothalamic tracts. In the hypothetical circumstance of a person leaning accidentally on an iron, proprioception, that is, the immediate position of one's limbs in space, is crucial too. Proprioception messages are also relayed through the dorsal horn but travel to the brain in the dorsal columns and medial lemniscus. The messages are projected to the thalamus and then to the cortex for the important integration with motor activity.

Naturally in the above case there is a reflex, (to be discussed later) which insistently pulls the wayward hand away from the iron much faster than waiting for this multifactorial sensory message to track all the way to the brain and back. Just as naturally this raises the question as to the anatomic level of certain behaviors. Obviously for some messages the spinal cord is enough. The relay between the access pathways in the dorsal root with intimate functional and anatomic coupling to the outflow motor pathways in the anterior horn allows an accurate perception of circumstances. And although other aspects of sensation probably enter consciousness at the thalamic level, it is the primary sensory areas of the cortex that are specially concerned with the integration of sensory experience and with the multifaceted discriminative qualities of sensation. In the next chapter we shall look at the essential integration of the somatosensory and motor systems.

References

Bornstein, B. 1949. Sur le phénomène du membre phantom. *Encephale* 38:32–46.

Cajal, Ramony, 1933. *Histology*. Baltimore: Wood.

Cavna, N. 1965. The effects of aging of the receptor organs of the human dermis. In: *Advances in Biology of Skin*. Vol. VI, *Aging. Proceedings of the Symposium held at the University of Oregon Medical School*, 1964. New York: Pergamon Press, pp. 63–96.

Chapman, L. F., A. O. Ramos, H. Goodall, and H. G. Wolff. 1961. Neurochemical features of afferent fibers in man: Their role in vasodilation, inflammation and pain. *Arch. Neurol.* 4:617–650.

Corkin, S., B. Miller, and T. Rasmussen. 1970. Somatosensory thresholds: Contrasting of postcentral gyrus and posterior parietal lobe excisions. *Arch. Neurol.* 23:41–58.

Critchey, M. 1965. Disorders of corporeal awareness in parietal disease. In: S. Wapner and H. Werner, eds. *The Body Percept.* New York: Random House.

Ettlinger, G., H. B. Morton, and M. Muffett. 1966. Tactile discrimination performance in the monkey: The effect of bilateral posterior parietal and lateral frontal ablations and of callosal section. *Cortex* 2:5–29.

Frederiks, J. A. M. Disorders of the body schema. 1969. In: P. J. Vinken and G. W. Bruyn, eds. *Handbook of Clinical Neurology.* Vol. 4. New York: Elsevier, pp. 207–240.

Gazzaniga, M. S., and J. G. LeDoux. 1978. *The Integrated Mind.* New York: Plenum.

Guyton, A. C. 1976. *Textbook of Medical Physiology.* Philadelphia: Saunders.

Hardy, J. D. 1956. The nature of pain. *J. Chronic Dis.* 4:22.

Hensel, H., and K. K. A. Boman. 1960. Afferent impulses in cutaneous sensory nerves in human subjects. *J. Neurophysiol.* 23:564–578.

Iggo, A. 1968. Electrophysiological and histological studies of cutaneous mechanoreceptors. In: D. R. Kenshalo, ed. *The Skin Senses. Proceddings of the First International Symposium,* 1966. Springfield, Ill.: Thomas, pp. 84–111.

Jones, E. G. 1976. Pattern of cortical and thalamic connexions of the somatic sensory cortex. *Nature* 216:704–705.

Jones, E. G., and T. P. S. Powell. 1970. An anatomical study of converging sensory pathways within the cerebral cortex of the monkey. *Brain* 93:793–820.

Kerr, F. W. L. 1975. The central spinothalamic tract and other ascending systems of the ventral funiculus of the spinal cord. *J. Comp. Neurol.* 159:335–356.

Lele, P. P., and G. Weddell. 1959. Sensory nerves of the cornea and cutaneous sensibility. *Exp. Neurol.* 1:334–359.

Lowenstein, W. R. 1961. Excitation and inactivation in a receptor membrane. *Ann. N.Y. Acad. Sci.* 94:510–534.

Lowenstein, W. R., and R. Rathkamp. 1958. The sites for mechano-electric conversion in a Pacinian corpuscle. *J. Gen. Physiol.* 41:1245–1265.

Melzack, R., and P. D. Wall. 1962. On the nature of cutaneous sensory mechanisms. *Brain* 85:331–352.

Mountcastle, V. B. 1957. Modality and topographic properties of single neurons of cat's somatic sensory cortex. *J. Neurophysiol.* 20:508–534.

Mountcastle, V. B. 1974. Pain and temperature sensibilities. In: V. B. Mountcastle, ed. *Medical Physiology.* Vol. I. St. Louis: Mosby, pp. 348–381.

Mountcastle, V. B., J. C. Lynch, A. Georgopoulos, H. Sakata, and C. Acvna. 1975. Posterior parietal association cortex of the monkey: Command functions for operations within extrapersonal space. *J. Neurophysiol.* 38:871–908.

Mountcastle, V. B., G. F. Poggio, and G. Werner. 1963. The relation of thalamic cell response to peripheral stimuli varied over an intensive continuum. *J. Neurophysiol.* 26: 807–834.

Nafe, J. P., and D. R. Kenshalo. 1962. Somesthetic senses. *Ann. Rev. Psychol.* 13:201–224.

Nathan, P. W. 1976. The gate-control theory of pain. *Brain* 99:123–158.

Peele, T. L. 1961. *The Neuroanatomical Basis for Clinical Neurology.* New York: McGraw-Hill.

Penfield, W., and T. Rasmussen. 1950. *The Cerbral Cortex of Man.* New York: Macmillan.

Poggio, G. F., and V. B. Mountcastle. 1960. A study of the functional contributions of the limniscal and spinothalamic systems to somatic sensibility. *Bull. Johns Hopkins Hosp.* 106:266–316.

Quilliam, T. A. 1966. Unit design and array patterns in receptor organs. In: A. V. S. De-Revack and J. Knight, eds. *Touch, Heat and Pain* (Ciba Foundation Symposium). Boston: Little, Brown, pp. 86–112.

Riddich, G. 1941. Phantom limbs and body shape. *Brain* 64:197–222.

Semmes, J., and M. Mishkin. 1965. Somatosensory loss in monkeys after ipsilateral cortical ablation. *J. Neurophysiol.* 28:473–486.

Semmes, J., S. Weinstein, L. Ghent, and H. L. Teuber. 1960. *Somatosensory Changes after Penetrating Brain Wounds in Man.* Cambridge, Mass.: Harvard University Press.

Snyder, S. H. 1975. Opiate receptor mechanisms. *Neurosci. Res. Program Bull.* 13 (1).

Snyder, S. H. 1978. *The Opiates.* The Harvey Lectures (in press).

Wall, P. D. 1970. The sensory and motor role of impulses traveling in the dorsal columns. *Brain* 93:505–524.

Wall, P. D. 1975. The somatosensory system. In: M. S. Gazzaniga and C. Blakemore, eds. *Handbook of Psychobiology.* New York: Academic Press, pp. 373–393.

Weinstein, S. 1968. Intensive and extensive aspects of tactile sensibility as a function of body part, sex, and laterality. In: D. R. Kenshalo, ed. *The Skin Senses.* Springfield, Ill.: Thomas, pp. 195–222.

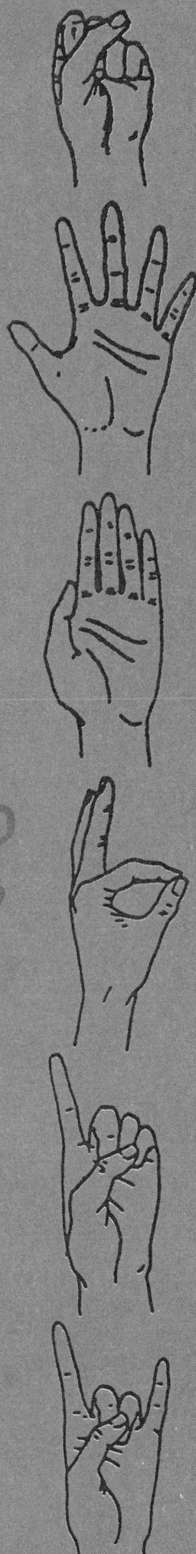

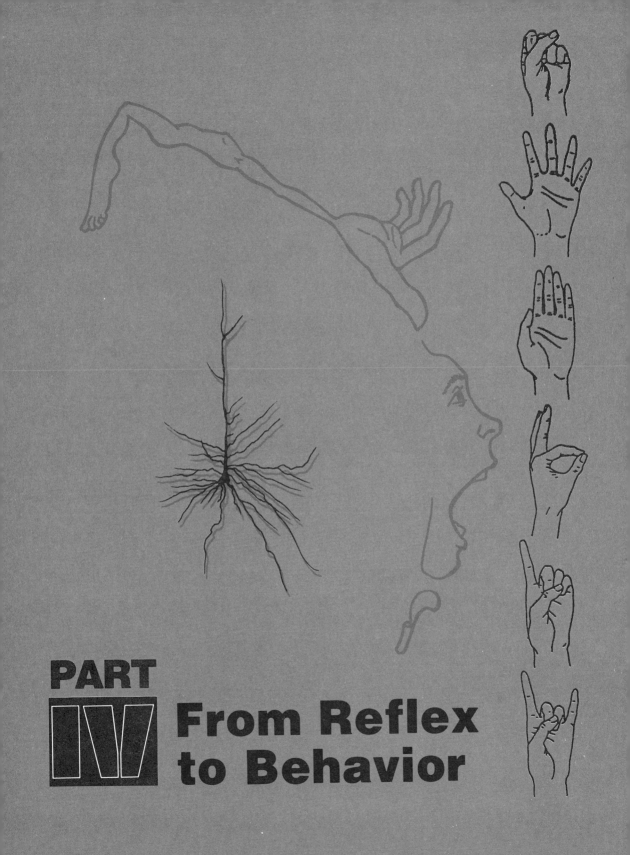

PART IV From Reflex to Behavior

CHAPTER 9

The Response System

The function of the CNS is to organize a response. Certainly man's abstract thought is a more complex brain function, but the ability to move at will is the extraordinary result of billions of neurons functioning together. Obviously, without the actions initiated by the motor areas of the brain and spinal cord, the body would no longer function. But at no time should the importance of the sensory input, with which we have been concerned in the last three chapters, be underestimated. Neither system should be thought of as a separate, autonomous entity; in fact, a more descriptive term emphasizing the coordination of the two systems is the sensory-motor system. However, because a discussion of either system alone constitutes a staggering amount of information, sensory-motor coordination forms another separate chapter.

Though the mechanisms involved in movement are numerous, each is relatively simple. In this chapter we shall explore the basic mechanisms that operate together to produce movement. We shall begin our discussion of the motor system with a description of the basic anatomy of the muscles themselves. Next, we shall discuss the innervation of those muscles, beginning with the spinal cord reflexes and moving up to those originating in the brain stem and in higher parts of the brain. The final section will cover the cerebral motor mechanisms and their descending pathways.

Muscles

Muscle Types

In our quest to understand muscular action, we begin with a discussion of muscle types. We shall also consider muscular innervation, sensory feedback in muscle action, and the neuromuscular junction. At least one-half of the body tissue is composed of muscle, either striated,

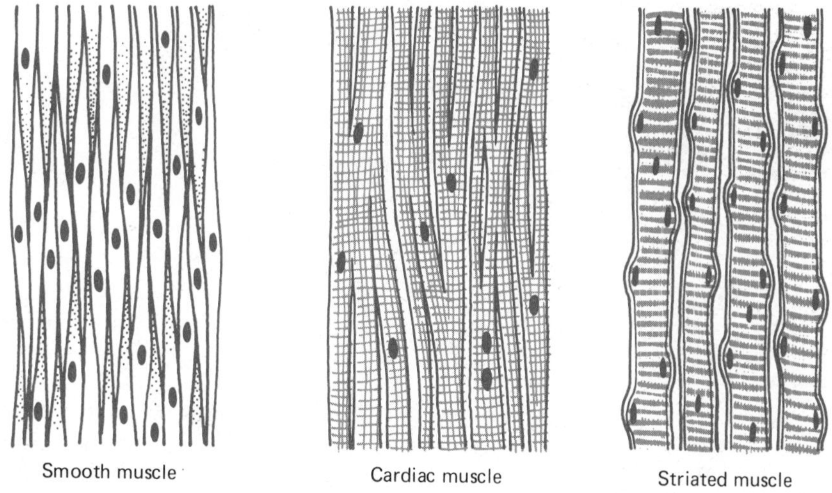

FIGURE 9.1 Muscle types. *Striated muscles,* so named because of their striped appearance, comprise the bulk of the bodily muscles. When we think or speak of muscles, we are usually referring to striated muscles. *Smooth muscles* are found in the internal organs. One organ, the heart, has its own special type of muscles, *cardiac muscles.* Cardiac muscles are a blend of smooth and striated, possessing some properties of both. (Adapted from Griffin, 1962.)

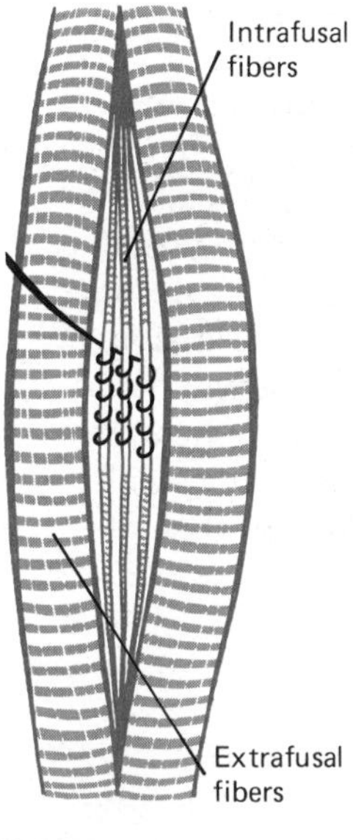

FIGURE 9.2 The juxtaposition of intrafusal and extrafusal fibers in a striated muscle fasciculus (Adapted from Barker, 1948).

smooth, or cardiac (see Figure 9.1). *Striated muscles* are by far the most common, being the muscles that move the skeleton. When the layman speaks of muscles, he is usually referring to striated muscles. *Smooth muscles* are found in the viscera, the internal organs. But one organ, the heart, has its own special type of musculature, the *cardiac muscles.* The smooth and cardiac muscles, while of course critical for maintaining life, are secondary to the striated muscles when it comes to behavior, as behavior usually involves movement of the skeleton. Consequently, we shall focus on the nature and function of the striated musculature.

Muscle Fibers The striated muscles, as their name implies, have a striped appearance. The striations are due to the way the strands of muscle fibers are grouped as they course from one end of the muscle to the other. Anatomically, three types of striated muscle fibers can be identified. Type A fibers are large, pale fibers, the color being light because the fibers contain only a few mitochondria (which among other things supply the cellular sources of energy). Type B fibers are smaller and darker than type A, and contain more mitochondria. Type C fibers, as you might guess, are the smallest and darkest of the three types of fibers, and contain the most mitochondria. Each muscle consists of many muscle fibers, and most muscles consist of a mixture of the three fiber types.

Another way of looking at striated muscle fibers involves the classification of such fibers as either intrafusal or extrafusal (see Figure 9.2). The *extrafusal fibers* are the main fibers, which actually do the work of the muscle, that is, they contract. *Intrafusal fibers*, scattered throughout the muscle, contain the sensory receptors (muscle spindles) of the muscles. These play an important part in controlling contraction by providing sensory feedback, as will be described.

The Mechanical Principles of Muscle Action

Since muscle fibers are capable of only one active movement, which is contraction, muscles are arranged in pairs, one on either side of the limb. Thus, extending one's arm is accomplished by contraction of muscles (extensors) on the underside of the arm. Flexing it requires contraction by muscles (flexors) on the top side of the arm (see Figure 9.3). Even though a muscle can be stretched, the stretching effect is not an active movement, but is the result of the contraction of another muscle. Consequently, the terms "agonist" and "antagonist" are used to indicate the muscles contracting and being stretched, respectively. The descriptive terms agonist and antagonist are applied interchangeably within a pair of muscles, depending on whether a limb is being extended or flexed.

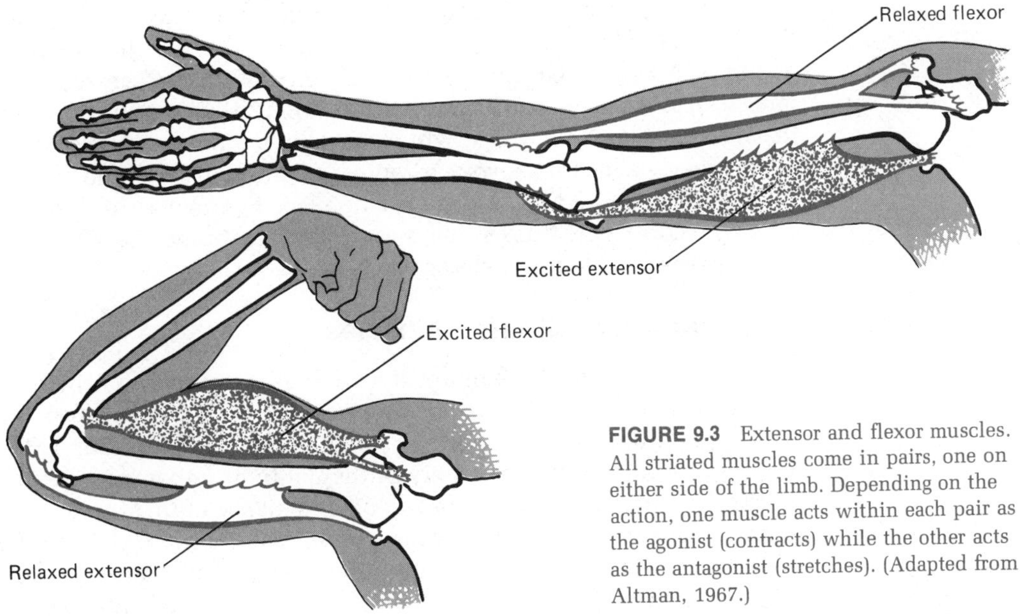

FIGURE 9.3 Extensor and flexor muscles. All striated muscles come in pairs, one on either side of the limb. Depending on the action, one muscle acts within each pair as the agonist (contracts) while the other acts as the antagonist (stretches). (Adapted from Altman, 1967.)

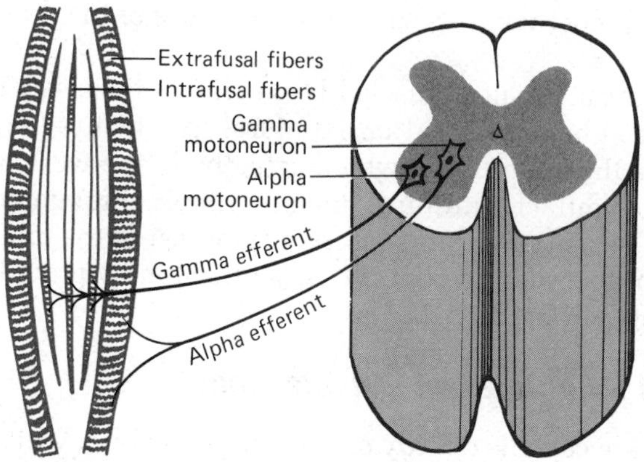

FIGURE 9.4 Alpha and gamma efferent systems. The alpha nerve fibers (as distinct from muscle fibers are the large alpha motoneurons of the spinal cord. These nerve fibers terminate on the extrafusal muscles. The muscles that contract the intrafusal system are composed of small gamma efferents. These gamma efferents terminate on the intrafusal fibers at the polar (end) region of the muscle fiber.

Peripheral Nerve-Muscle Interaction

Innervation of muscles is provided by two groups of nerve fibers: those arising from large motoneurons called *alpha cells*, and those arising from smaller motoneurons called *gamma cells*. The alpha and gamma systems together provide different types of muscular innervation. Alpha neurons provide direct control over the muscles by terminating for the most part on the extrafusal fibers, the fibers that initiate contraction. The gamma neurons, which make up one-third of the fibers in the ventral roots (the fiber bundles leaving the spinal cord en route to the muscles), control muscles indirectly. Gamma fibers mainly innervate the intrafusal muscle fibers, which contain the nuclear bag fibers and chain fibers, and are sensory receptors of the muscles. The extrafusal fibers do the work of muscle contraction (see Figure 9.4), and through a sensory feedback arc, the gamma system can cause muscles to contract to a predetermined length, as described shortly.

Excitation of Striated Muscles

The point where the efferent fiber actually synapses on the muscle fiber is called the *neuromuscular junction* (see Figure 9.5). Each muscle fiber is innervated by only one junction, and that junction is in the middle of the fiber. The anatomy of the neuromuscular junction is not drastically different from that of any other synapse in that there is a near junction between the neural ending and the muscle fiber, separated by a microscopic space called a synaptic cleft. The entire neural ending is called an *end plate*, and its many small protrusions are called *sole feet*.

As in other synapses, the synaptic action is effected by release of a neural transmitter, stored in vesicles in the neural ending. When a spinal motor neuron is stimulated, it sends a neural impulse, or action potential, along its axon. The arrival of the action potential changes the membrane potential and allows the transmitter *acetylcholine* to flow out. The transmitter immediately floods the *synaptic gutter*, a convoluted indentation in the muscle fiber, the folds of which greatly increase the amount of muscle exposed to the chemical action of the neurotransmitter. The released acetylcholine acts on the membrane of the muscle fibers, causing an *end-plate potential*, which is entirely analogous to an EPSP (excitatory postsynaptic potential). If the end-plate potential is sufficiently large, it causes an action potential in the muscle fiber, the fiber contracts, and the basic process of neuromuscular control is complete. Further excitation of the muscle membrane is prohibited by a "clean-up chemical," which destroys the ACh. *Cholinesterase*, the chemical that breaks down ACh, is normally accumulated around the edge of the synaptic gutter, and immediately breaks down the transmitter before it can act on the membrane a second time.

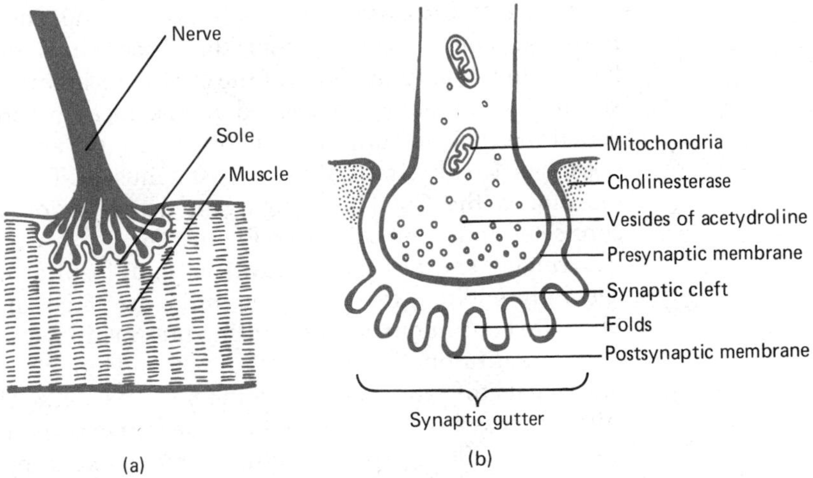

FIGURE 9.5 The neuromuscular junction. The neural innervation of the muscle fibers is similar to the neural-neural connections examined in Chapter 2. Part (a) shows the nerve arriving at the muscle fiber, and the sole foot of the nerve, which spreads over the muscle fiber. Part (b) shows the presynaptic-postsynaptic relations of the neuromuscular junction. Presynaptically, the sole foot of the nerve contains mitochondria and vesicles of ACh. Postsynaptically the motor end plate, the place of near contact with the sole foot, is folded over. The folds increase the surface area available for transmitter action. The depressed area of the muscle in which the sole foot terminates is called the synaptic gutter. The top edge of the gutter contains pockets of cholinesterase, the enzyme that breaks down ACh. (Adapted from Guyton, 1976.)

Excitation of Smooth Muscle

The neuromuscular junction of smooth muscles is different from the skeletal muscle junction because the nerve is not invaginated into the muscle membrane. Rather, axons of the nerve make contact with the muscle fibers by actually touching them. Two transmitters are known to be secreted by nerves innervating organs: acetylcholine (ACh) and noradrenaline (NA). ACh acts as an excitatory transmitter, but in some organs it has an inhibiting effect. In organs where ACh has an inhibitory effect, NA and ACh reverse roles, with NA serving as an excitatory transmitter, and ACh being inhibitory.

Neuromuscular Control

Alpha and gamma efferent systems, together with the afferent mechanisms of the muscle spindle organ, constitute a closed-loop feedback system. These feedback loops are especially important for highly skilled movements that require a high degree of control, because the feedback mechanism allows for the modulation of the necessary extent of muscle contraction.

Afferent Information The sensory input necessary for neuromuscular control comes from the three kinds of stretch receptors located in the muscles. Two of the stretch receptors, called primary and secondary afferents, are located in the receptor organ of the muscle called the muscle spindle. This organ is built around a small number (less than 10) of intrafusal fibers in the muscle. The third kind of stretch receptor is the Golgi tendon organ, which is located in the tendons connected to the muscles (see Figure 9.6).

Primary endings, also known as annulospiral endings since they generally encircle the muscle spindle, are large and highly sensitive. They fire continuously, transmitting information about the length of the muscle. Additionally, because they respond quickly, the change in firing rate signals the rate of change in the muscle length. The primary spindle afferent gives a dynamic, or velocity-sensitive response. *Secondary endings,* called "flower spray" endings, branch out to the muscle fibers, and register the length of the muscle. These secondary spindle afferents have little or no dynamic-response component.

The muscle spindle, which contains the primary and secondary afferents, and the tendon organ measure different aspects of the muscle stretch, and this is, at least in part, a result of their position relative to the fibers of the muscle. The muscle spindle is located parallel to the muscle fibers. When the extrafusal fibers contract, the ends of the intrafusal fibers around which the muscle spindle is built contract, and the pri-

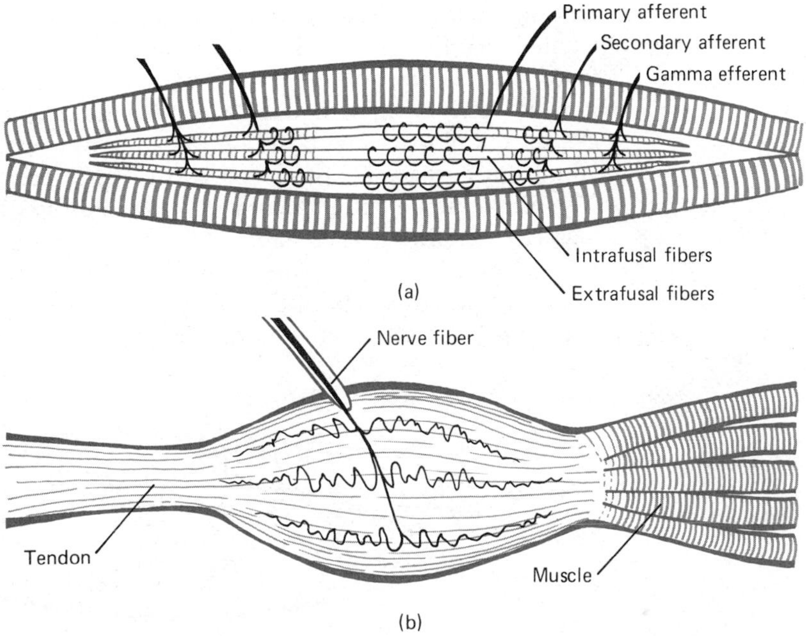

FIGURE 9.6 Sensory receptors of the muscles.(a) Primary afferent fibers are relatively large nerve fibers. Their terminals encircle the encapsulated central portion of intrafusal fibers (usually not more than 10). Primary receptor terminals are also known as annulospiral receptors. The smaller, secondary afferent fibers give rise to "flower spray" or sensory receptors. The primary and secondary afferents and receptors make up the muscle spindle. (b) The Golgi tendon organ has its terminals in the tendon.

mary and secondary endings can measure the change in the muscle length and the velocity of the change. In contrast, the Golgi tendon organ is located in series with the contractile elements, and is receptive to the force, or tension, of the stretch.

Efferent Program The efferent system originating in the small gamma motoneurons of the ventral horn of the spinal cord acts by stimulating the muscle spindle organ. When the gamma fibers excite the polar (end) regions of the muscle spindle, the intrafusal muscle fibers contract in such a way as to stretch their central portion (see Figure 9.7). This action stimulates the primary and secondary afferent receptors of the muscle spindle organ. The afferents then send impulses through the dorsal root back to the spinal cord, where either alpha motoneurons or interneurons connected to alpha motoneurons are excited (see Figure 9.8). The motoneurons, in turn, stimulate the extrafusal muscle fibers so that their degree of stretch matches that of the muscle spindle. In this way, the muscle spindle organ, through the gamma efferent system, provides the afferent feedback needed to modulate major movements produced by the alpha efferent system.

This fundamental anatomical relationship is like a piece of well-integrated machinery; each element by itself performs one basic function. For example, one set of muscular fibers (the intrafusal) performs only a sensory function within the muscle. Another set of muscle fibers (the extrafusal) actually contracts to achieve the movement. Likewise, one

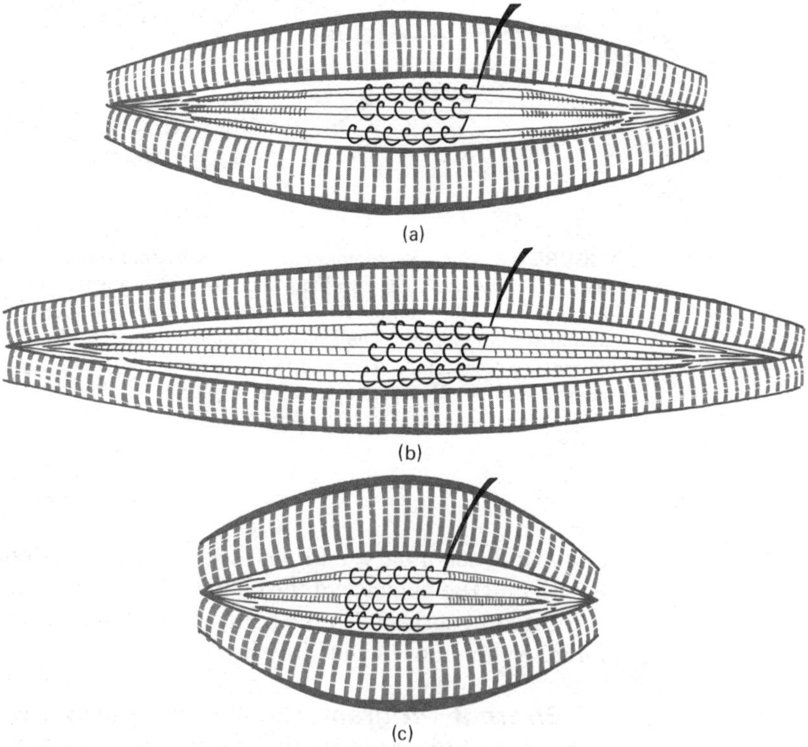

FIGURE 9.7 The muscle spindle consisting of intrafusal fibers is shown at rest in part (a). The intrafusal fibers contract only at the polar regions (due to interaction between sensory afferents and gamma efferent messages). The sensory receptors are stretched as a result (b) and this action excites the alpha motoneurons, which in turn cause the extrafusal muscle to contract (c). Later the spindle returns to its normal length. This is called the stretch reflex, and is described in the next section. (Adapted from Guyton, 1976.)

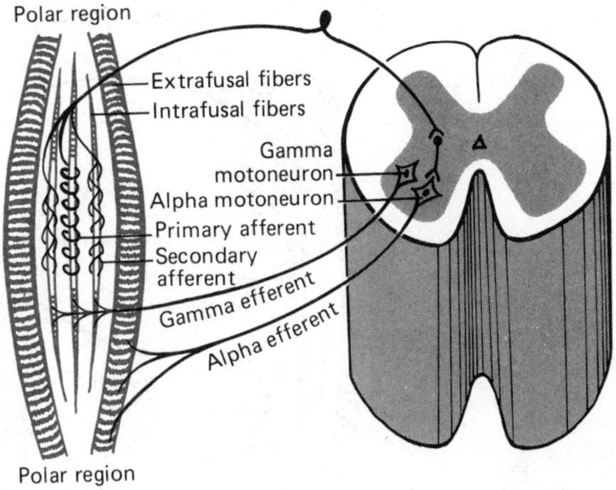

FIGURE 9.8 Schematic depiction of the pathways involved in the sensory control of muscle action. (See text and Figure 9.7 for further explanation.)

set of motoneurons (the gamma neurons) innervates only the sensory muscle fibers; the other motoneurons (the alpha neurons) innervate the muscle fibers that actually contract. Routinely, the feedback loops serve to maintain muscle tone and postural contractions.

Reflexes: Fundamental Building Blocks for Movement

The afferent-efferent loop described in the previous section involves what is called reflex action, a reflex being a preprogrammed motor response. That is, the afferent and efferent mechanisms are "wired" together such that excitation of the afferent mechanisms invariably influences the efferent mechanism. This concept will be elucidated by way of several examples.

The Stretch Reflex

When the afferent receptors in the muscle spindles are excited by the gamma fibers, the afferents in turn excite the alpha motoneurons, and this action causes muscle contraction by exciting extrafusal muscle fibers. This is called the stretch reflex because it is initiated by the stretching of the muscle spindle (see previous section). The knee jerk is an example of a stretch reflex. When a physician taps the knee tendon in order to test the patient's reflexes, the muscle fibers stretch slightly, and excite the muscle spindles, and the rest is now familiar to everyone.

The stretch reflex is an example of the simplest kind of reflex, called a *monosynaptic reflex*. This means that there is only one neural synapse involved from the beginning of the afferent to the end of the efferent

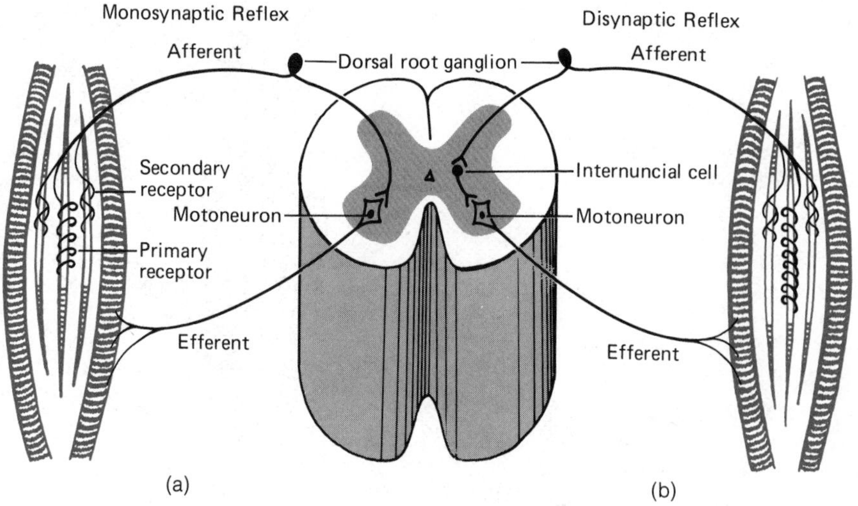

FIGURE 9.9 Monosynaptic and disynaptic reflexes. (See text for explanation.)

(see Figure 9.9(a)). Monosynaptic reflexes thus involve only two neurons—the sensory cell and the motor cell—and the one synapse between them. But the stretch reflex can also be two synapses (disynaptic), meaning that between the sensory and motor cell there is sometimes an interneuron. In the case of the stretch reflex, the interneuron is a spinal internuncial cell that is postsynaptic to the output of the dorsal root ganglia and presynaptic to the alpha motoneuron (see Figure 9.9(b)).

The Tendon Reflex

The tendon reflex is mediated by the Golgi tendon organ stretch receptors. It will be recalled that these receptors, unlike the muscle spindle receptors, are not in the muscles at all, but are in the tendons connected to the muscles. The tendon reflex is generally disynaptic. In this reflex, the Golgi tendon organ detects tension in the tendon caused by muscle contraction. The impulse of the sensory cell is in turn relayed to an inhibitory ternuncial cell, which synapses on the motoneuron. The net result of the tendon reflex is to inhibit the contracting muscle causing the tension in the tendon, so that the muscle will relax and the tension will be released. Thus, while the stretch reflex is excitatory, the tendon reflex is inhibitory.

Extreme tension elicits an extreme inhibitory reflex, which causes a sudden and complete relaxation of the entire muscle. For example, a person attempting to lift a weight that is too heavy may lose muscular control and drop the weight with a thud. The mechanism responsible for this embarrassing scene is the tendon reflex, which is believed to serve as a protective device to prevent damage to the muscle or tendon from straining too hard. When the tension reaches the danger level, the tendon reflex relieves the muscle through its inhibitory action.

Under normal conditions, the tendon reflex is important in controlling muscle tension. This automatic monitoring of muscle tension by the tendon reflex functions in a way similar to the gamma system, which automatically monitors muscle length.

The majority of neuromuscular reflexes, however, are not as simple as the stretch and tendon reflexes. The addition of many interneurons to the synaptic pathway of reflexes permits more complex influences on the reflex action, for the role of the interneuron system is to monitor afferent input and modulate efferent output. Through a process of algebraic summation, in which both excitatory and inhibitory inputs converge on the internuncial cells, modification of impulses from descending systems is effected. An excess of excitatory input will result in a reflex being activated, while an excess of inhibitory input will not trigger the reflex.

The internuncial system is also responsible for reciprocal innervation. That is, excitation of one muscle will automatically cause inhibition of the antagonist muscle. Reciprocal innervation through the internuncial cells also provides a means of communication in the spinal cord between one side of the body and the other. Activation of a reflex on one side of the body may call for a complementary reflex on the other side of the body. The flexor and crossed extensor reflexes, to be discussed next, illustrate how the efficiency of the reflexes is improved through the reciprocal innervation of the internuncial system.

The Flexor Reflex

A protective mechanism of the body is the flexor, or withdrawal, reflex. This reflex, generally elicited by a nociceptive stimulus, causes a body limb to pull back from the stimulus. It involves several internuncial cells as well as the sensory cell and motoneuron of the spinal cord. An important function of the internuncial cells in this reflex is to transmit the command for withdrawal to other muscles needed, for although the stimulus may affect only one finger, the muscles for the entire arm must be activated in order to withdraw the hand quickly.

The position the limb withdraws to depends on which nerve is stimulated. For example, stimulation of a nerve in the upper part of the arm will cause one final position, while stimulation of the wrist may cause the limb to be withdrawn to a totally different position. The limb will remain in this final position for several seconds after the flexor reflex is elicited. This persistence is another example of the body's protective mechanisms, for it automatically holds the limb away from the nociceptive stimulus, giving cortical control a chance to take over.

Crossed Extensor Reflex

Related to the flexor reflex is the crossed extensor reflex, which causes the extension of the limb contralateral to the limb withdrawn. For example, if the right arm is withdrawn in response to a painful stimulus, the left arm will extend (see Figure 9.10). The net effect of this reflex is to push the entire body further away from the stimulus. The reciprocal innervation system of the internuncial cells is responsible for activating

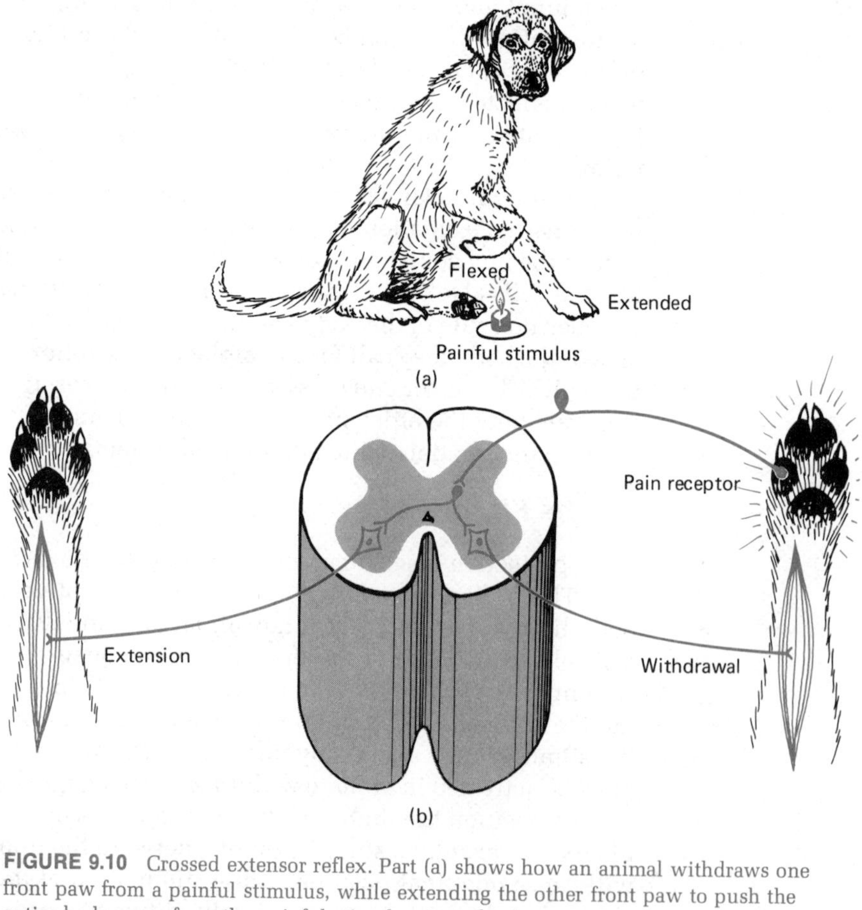

FIGURE 9.10 Crossed extensor reflex. Part (a) shows how an animal withdraws one front paw from a painful stimulus, while extending the other front paw to push the entire body away from the painful stimulus. Part (b) shows reciprocal innervation by spinal interneurons. (See text for explanation.)

the crossed extensor reflex. In other words, interneurons along the path of the flexor reflex send signals across the spinal cord to the other side and elicit the opposite reaction in the other limb.

Spinal Shock

Spinal cord reflexes, though seemingly simple, are nevertheless under the influence of higher cerebral centers. This is dramatically demonstrated in what is called a "spinal animal." The spinal animal has undergone surgical transection of the spinal cord. Immediately after the transection, all reflexive functions controlled by the spinal cord segments below the level of the transection are depressed. For example, skeletal reflexes, such as the stretch and tendon reflexes, are absent, as are a number of visceral reflexes mediated at the spinal level. But within a few weeks, the "shock" wanes and the spinal reflexes below the transection are maintained but without cerebral influence.

A person whose spinal cord has been severed is in grave danger, for the very basic functions served by the lower spinal cord are absolutely essential for life. Take the case of Greg, for instance. Greg was a talented but "flaky" architectural student. The appellation "flaky" came not only from friends but also from professors. The usual three years of course work had occupied Greg for five years, but not because of any failures; in fact, he graduated finally with honors. Many interests occupied his every waking moment, and he was always short of cash. Writing articles for architectural journals, finishing a book on Le Corbusier, and even moonlighting by designing a downtown disco never put a time squeeze on the betting at eight ball, or on the all-night bridge games.

His latest interest, though, was a beautiful and talented woman, and to see her he would often travel for hours at any time. The problem, inevitable as it may have seemed, was money. She had been recently discovered and now was being billed as the new opera diva of the decade. As the season opened in the fall, Greg concocted a painting firm, where he sold high-price designs for the outsides of town houses in the city's bohemian section. Fabulous success followed until one day he slipped on a third-story scaffold and fell to the ground. Fortunately, he was painting the rear face of the house, for if it had been the front facing, he would surely have been killed on the fancy iron grillwork fence. As luck would have it, he landed on the plush lawn—something of a cushion.

Lying flat on his back after the impact, he was in shock; in fact, he was in spinal shock. There was no loss of consciousness and the head trauma was minimal, for his complete thoracic and lumbar spine had absorbed the trauma of the fall. He suffered a flaccid and complete paralysis from his chest to his toes. Of course, he was rushed to the hospi-

tal. Complete examination revealed he had not ruptured any internal organs but his vertebral column was fractured at the eleventh thoracic vertebra. His neurologic exam revealed a flaccid paraplegia with decreased reflexes initially. The condition of decreased reflexes, or hyporeflexia, was due to spinal shock, a result of the abrupt dysfunction of spinal reflex arcs.

The gravity of Greg's situation was indicated by the exhibition of an upgoing Babinski response (recall Chapter 1). Normally, stimulation of the sole of the foot results in flexion of the toes toward the sole of the foot, called a plantar flexion. Greg was paralyzed, with spinal cord shock, so strong stimulation led to the development of what is called the full Babinski response—upward extension of the great toe with fanning and plantar flexion of the other toes. This response suggested corticospinal tract damage, or the possibility that cord transection had occurred.

Because Greg displayed no feeling for any sensory modalities below the eleventh thoracic level, immediate x-ray studies of his spine were done. They revealed a subdural collection of blood around the fracture. He was taken within one hour for a neurosurgical decompression, to remove the blood and relieve the pressure on the spinal cord.

If this neurology service had not been so efficient, Greg would have been paralyzed forever. In this state of cord transection there would have been many effects. There would have been retention of urine with painless distension of his bladder until overflow pressure overcame the reflex closing of the bladder sphincters. As time progressed in this paraplegic state, the threshold for eliciting the Babinski reflex would have decreased. Only moderate stimulation would have provoked withdrawal of the entire limb. Thresholds for reflexes would have fallen until the state of hyperreflexia typical of an upper motor lesion would have appeared. Hyperreflexia is a condition in which reflexes are hyperactive and spastic; that is, the deep tendon reflexes are exaggerated. The lower motor neuron, now without time inhibitory influence, would have set the reflex arc to a hypertonic or overly tense posture, and the overall reflex orientation would be typified by the mass flexion reflex. Mild plantar stimulation would have induced strong involuntary withdrawal of both limbs accompanied by a variety of autonomic reactions—piloerection (commonly known as "goose pimples"), sweating and involuntary evacuation of bowel and bladder. Over months of paraplegia Greg would have evolved to a state of tonic flexion with markedly intensified stretch reflexes so that clonus, a series of spasmodic reflex contractions following sudden stretch of a hyperreflexic muscle, would have appeared. Clonus is largely due to increased sensitivity of the muscle spindle. In the spastic state that might have evolved, fusimotor tone would have been heightened with subsequent increase in spindle sensitivity. Sudden stretch of the spastic muscle would have caused a huge spindle afferent barrage, which would have given rise to a powerful reflex contraction and shortening of the extrafusal muscle mass. This sudden shortening would release the pressure on the spindle, and silence the afferent discharge. This powerful contraction, and sudden release is called clonus, and it would have begun again setting up a repetitive series of discharges that might last for some time.

But none of this did develop; the operation saved Greg's spinal cord and over a three-week convalescence he regained full motor power of his legs, full control over bladder, bowel, and sexual function. He did lose the girl—she married her agent—but the depression made him focus on his degree and he finally graduated.

Autonomic Reflexes

Greg's fall could easily have damaged his autonomic reflexes. The autonomic nervous system, it will be recalled (see Chapter 2), is the visceral efferent system. This system, in response to excitation from visceral afferents, mediates a variety of life-sustaining reflexes. For example, as the bladder fills with urine, it begins to stretch. Afferent impulses are sent to the spinal cord and the visceral efferent fibers of the parasympathetic nervous system then cause the bladder muscles (smooth muscles) to contract, thus expelling the fluid. Obviously, however, the organism can learn to inhibit this reflex, and generally does learn during early childhood. Cerebral pathology that blocks the inhibitory messages from the higher brain centers results in incontinence (loss of bladder control). Other parasympathetic reflexes include the peristaltic reflex (which controls bowel movements), digestive reflexes initiated by appetizing odors, sexual reflexes (which result in penile erection and swelling of the clitoris), cardiovascular reflexes, and a variety of other wired responses required to maintain routine visceral function. In contrast, when the organism is in a nonroutine situation, the sympathetic reflexes take over until normality is again reached (Table 9.1).

TABLE 9.1

Organ	Sympathetic Effect	Parasympathetic Effect
Eye (pupil)	Dilation	Constriction
Sweat glands	Sweating	None
Heart (cardiac muscles)	Increase in rate and force of beat	Slowing of rate and force of beat
Gut	Decreased peristalsis	Increased peristalsis
Gall bladder	Inhibition	Excitation
Penis	Ejaculation	Erection

(Adapted from Guyton, 1976.)

Brain Stem Reflexes

Some of the autonomic reflexes are multisynaptic, suprasegmental reflexes. That is, nuclei in the brain stem are involved in the closed circuit. Certain cardiovascular and respiratory reflexes fall into this category. For example, heart rate is controlled by a feedback system involving afferents from the heart that ascend in the spinal cord to the "solitary nucleus" of the medulla. This nucleus, in turn, is connected to the vagal nucleus, also in the medulla. The vagal nucleus gives rise to the vagus nerve (cranial nerve X), which is a visceral efferent that descends to the cardiac muscles of the heart.

In many ways, the functions of the brain stem are similar to those of the spinal cord, at least with regard to reflexes. The head and neck regions, it will be recalled, are supplied by the cranial nerves rather than the spinal nerves, and the brain stem serves as the integrating center for the reflexes involving these nerves. For example, pupillary constriction occurs when a light is flashed to the eye. The visual receptors (rods and cones) detect the change, and afferent fibers that make up part of the tectal projection (see Chapter 7) terminate in the pretectal region of the brain, which is just anterior to the superior colliculus. Internuncial cells in the pretectal region are excited, and they in turn excite the accessory oculomotor nucleus, the efferent fibers of which complete the circuit of pupillary constriction in response to the flash of light. Similar reflex circuits are involved when the head and neck reflexively turn to a sudden noise or a visual stimulus. Later, we shall examine the complex reflex activities involved in coordinating eye and head movements in such turning responses. In addition, we shall look at the reflexive function of the vestibular system, through which our sense of balance is maintained.

Cerebral Motor Mechanisms

Now that we have seen how reflexes are handled by the spinal cord and brain stem, we shall consider how more complicated actions are initiated and controlled by the higher brain centers. As is clear by now, motor control cannot be considered independent of sensory input, for movements are not purely "motor." Sensory feedback is an integral part of the process of coordinating movement, and each of the major cerebral motor regions receives sensory input as part of the feedback loop for initiating and controlling actions.

The three cerebral areas generally thought to be most involved with motor activities are the cerebellum, the basal ganglia, and the cerebral cortex (see Figure 9.11). Traditionally, the cerebral cortex has been

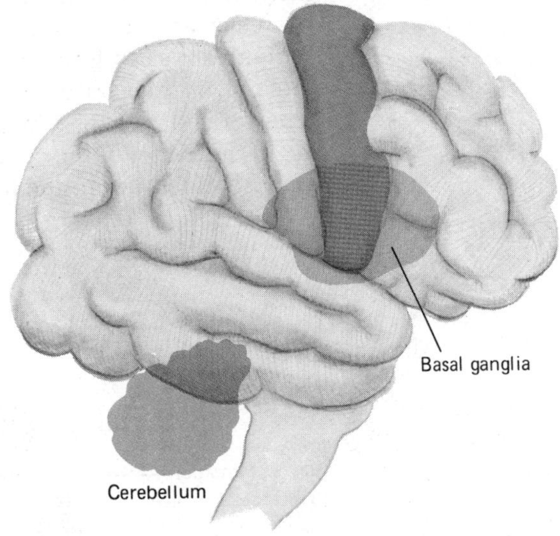

FIGURE 9.11 Cerebral motor mechanisms. The main brain areas that control motor output are the cerebellum, the basal ganglia, and the cortical motor areas.

considered to be the locus of the highest motor function, that is, the place initiating voluntary movements. However, recent findings indicate that the cerebellum and the basal ganglia also play important roles in initiating nonreflexive motor activity. Electrical recording has failed to isolate the exact place in the brain where volitional motor commands first arise, but it seems that the cerebellum and basal ganglia are involved in specifying the gross pattern of movement needed. The motor cortex, on the other hand, seems to be more involved with perfecting movements, refining the execution of the gross pattern sent up by the lower brain structures. Furthermore, the cortex is responsible for sending the bulk of the efferent command down to the spinal cord, having more direct spinal connections than either the cerebellum or basal ganglia. The particular functions of each of the three cerebral motor mechanisms will be discussed below.

The Cerebellum: Coordinating the Command

Movement without a functioning cerebellum is uncoordinated and awkward, for the cerebellum serves as one of the control centers of the motor system, coordinating sensory input and motor output. The cerebellum operates at a subconscious level to regulate the motor system. It performs a number of complicated tasks, ranging from inhibiting an overzealous motor cortex to "preprogramming" routine movements.

As noted in Chapter 3, the cerebellum has a cortical layer that covers its underlying white matter (fiber tracts) and deep nuclei. The three lobes of the cerebellum make up the cerebellar cortex, which is not to be confused with the cerebral cortex. The cerebellar cortex is shaped in such a way as to form convoluted folds called folia. The folia contain three cortical layers, and within these layers, as many as seven different types of cells can be identified (see Figure 9.12). Deep below the cortex in the center of the cerebellum are the cerebellar nuclei: the dentate, globose, emboliform, and fastigial nuclei.

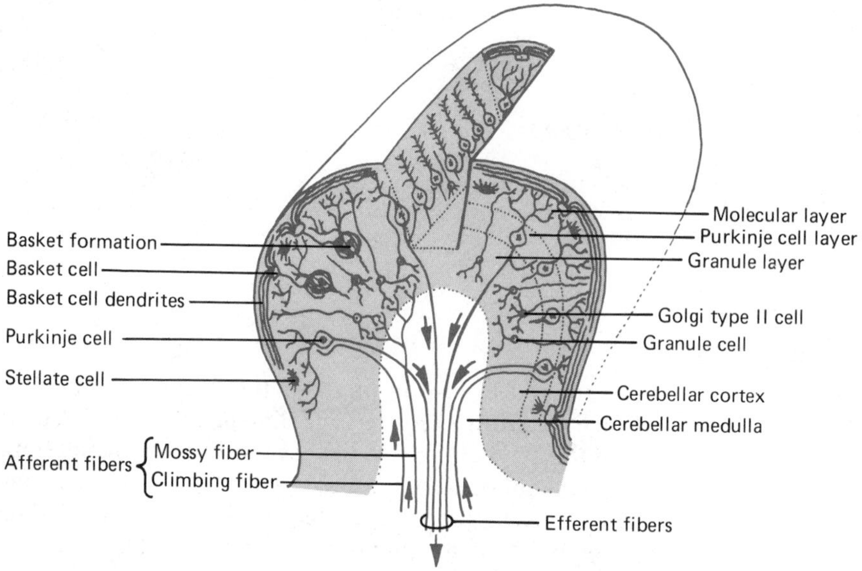

FIGURE 9.12 The cerebellar cortex is convoluted. One folium is shown in the figure. The three lamina of the cerebellar cortex are identifiable, as are numerous cell types, some peculiar to the individual layers. (Adapted from Rubinstein, 1953.)

There are at least a dozen afferent pathways to the cerebellum, bringing input from all parts of the central nervous system (see Figure 9.13). Afferent input from the sensory areas of the cerebral cortex goes directly to the cerebellar cortex by way of descending fibers to the pons and then to the pontocerebellar tract. The cerebellar cortex receives afferent input from the reticular formation and the spinal cord via the reticulo-cerebellar tract. The vestibulo-cerebellar tract carries vestibular information and accounts for the cerebellum playing a major role in the maintenance of equilibrium.

Sensory information from muscle spindles and Golgi tendon organs, as well as from cutaneous receptors, ascends to the cerebellum through the spinocerebellar tracts. The speed of conduction in these tracts is quite fast—100 meters per second—thus facilitating rapid integration of

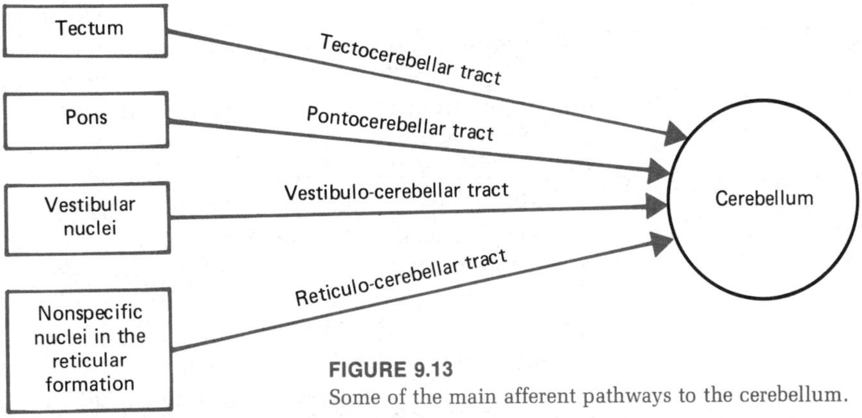

FIGURE 9.13
Some of the main afferent pathways to the cerebellum.

sensory and motor information by the cerebellum. Auditory and visual information is transmitted from the inferior and superior colliculi of the tectum by the tectocerebellar tract, and fibers from the motor cortex traveling to the spinal cord project collaterals directly to the cerebellum so that signals on their way to the muscles can be monitored by the cerebellum.

Of course, the efferent pathways from the cerebellum are an integral part of the feedback role it performs (see Figure 9.14). The efferent fi-

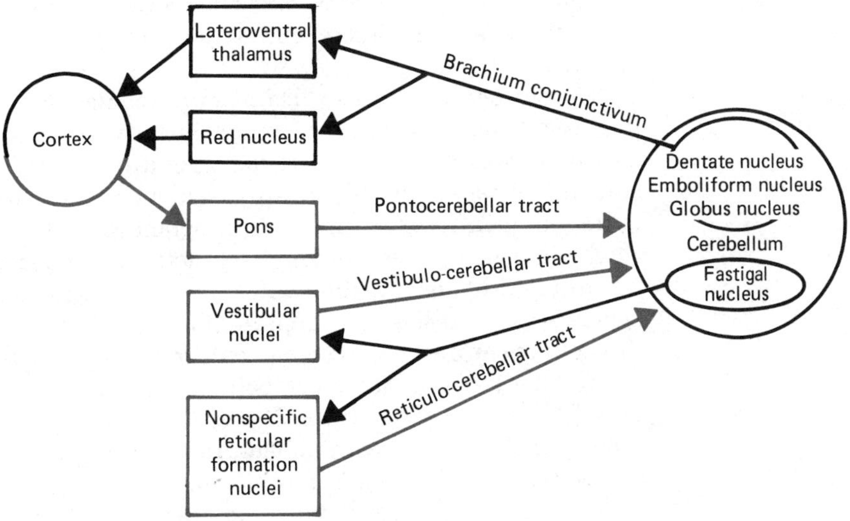

FIGURE 9.14 Afferent-efferent loops of the cerebellum and related structures. Output of the cerebellum mainly goes to cerebral areas reciprocally connected with the cerebellum. Some of the loops, such as those involving the cerebral cortex, are multisynaptic. Others, such as those involving the vestibular nuclei, are monosynaptic.

bers all originate in cerebellar nuclei. The dentate, globose, and emboliform nuclei project their efferent fibers by way of a tract called the brachium conjunctivum to the red nucleus and the lateroventral thalamus. These areas in turn project to the motor cortex, and then by way of the cortico-pontocerebellar tract, the loop is completed. These pathways between the cerebellar and the motor cortex provide many opportunities for modification of signals along the way. The output of the fastigial nucleus goes to the vestibular nucleus of the brain stem, as well as to a variety of nuclei in the reticular formation. By way of afferent pathways described earlier (vestibulo-cerebellar and reticulo-cerebellar tracts), these feedback circuits are maintained.

As noted, in addition to receiving a multitude of sensory signals, the cerebellum also receives collaterals from cortical motor fibers headed for the spinal cord. Then, once movement is initiated at the muscular level, signals are instantly transmitted from the muscle spindle and tendon organs (by way of the spinocerebellar tracts) to the cerebellum, so the cerebellum is well suited for performing its important function of monitoring movement and integrating sensory feedback.

One aspect of the cerebellum's integrating function is "error control." For example, the motor cortex overstimulates the muscles, sending more impulses to the spinal cord than necessary as a safety factor for insuring that the movement gets executed. The cerebellum must monitor the movement and inhibit the muscles when they have moved far enough. All output from the cerebellar cortex is inhibitory, whereas output from the rest of the cerebellum (the nuclei) is excitatory (Henneman, 1974a).

The cerebellum can also "learn" movements. For instance, if the door to a particular classroom is extremely heavy, a student going to that classroom will soon anticipate the weight of the door. As a result, the student's cerebellum will "learn" that more force than normal is required to open the door, and will program the action accordingly. The cerebellum also serves a predictive function, subconsciously computing where a rapidly moving limb will stop, and exciting the antagonist muscles as the limb reaches the appropriate spot. Using vestibular input, the cerebellum can also predict what to do to maintain equilibrium.

Another function of the cerebellum is to stop movement. Antagonist muscles are automatically excited by the cerebellum, while at the same time agonist muscles are inhibited. Along the same lines, the cerebellum serves to "damp" muscular movements. That is, not only does the cerebellum cause the movement of a limb to stop at the appropriate point; it also prevents the tendency of the limb to oscillate back and forth as it would if cortical impulses were not inhibited and the momentum of the limb allowed to take its natural course.

Lesions of the cerebellum produce errors in movement. Although a number of terms exist for particular syndromes, all impairments may be categorized as "ataxia," which means simply uncoordinated movement. A patient with cerebellar dysfunction does not lose the capacity for movement, but loses much of the ability to control movement, even at a rather gross level (see Smithie in Chapter 12). The patient experiences no loss of sensation, for cerebellar activities are normally carried out subconsciously. Fortunately, recovery from small cerebellar lesions is fairly complete. Patients with injury to the cerebellar nuclei, however, demonstrate a lesser degree of recovery. Finally, it should be noted that cerebellar lesions result in an intention tremor, that is, a person shakes when trying to perform a voluntary act, as opposed to basal ganglia lesions, which cause a person to tremble when resting.

Basal Ganglia: Refining Efferent Programs Further

The cerebellum coordinates movements in a refined and important manner. But all movement proceeds upon a specific background of muscle posture and tone. The basal ganglia establishes these set points. This stability at rest with easy progression to the initiation of movement is one of the functions of the basal ganglia. Van's story illustrates the importance of the basal ganglia:

Van had been an outstanding polo player in his day. In fact, there had been a time in his life during which he had done little except play polo. Running the business started by his great-grandfather had amounted to money managing, and Van was good at picking profitable investments. Now, in his early sixties, his appetite for riding horses was undaunted, although competitive polo, even frequent riding for pleasure, was out of the question. Those occasional horseback riding jaunts and making money provided him with a full existence.

Recently, though, he was spending more time in pensive solitude. Advancing years seemed to render his spine and limbs less pliable. These episodes of stiffness and soreness, especially in shoulders, back, and hips, now occurring whether or not he had ridden, were attributed to his age and degenerative arthritis. But age alone could not explain the new resting tremor in his hands. This was a 4-cycle-per-second tremor of the thumb and fingers that was present when the hand was not used in voluntary movement; hence the term resting tremor. In association with this tremor was a curious decrease in blinking, now less than 10 times per minute, and a general paucity of facial expression as well as movement in general. Sadly, these early and subtle changes in Van's manner could only represent the beginning of a condition named by James Parkinson in 1817—paralysis agitans.

Van will find that as the movement disorder worsens, all accustomed activities will show the effect. First, he will be afflicted with a general poverty of movement, then a progressive loss of facial expression. But perhaps the inevitable changes in gait will represent the greatest debility. Stiffness will cause forward bending of the trunk. The stance will have a narrow base. The arms will be carried ahead of the body and will not swing. The steps will be short, the feet will barely clear the ground; truly, a shuffling gait. Bradykinesia, defined as difficulty initiating or altering movement, will complicate his locomotion. That is, once directional movement begins and the upper part of his bent body advances ahead of the lower part, it will seem as though he is chasing his center of gravity. His steps may become more and more rapid so that he might fall if not assisted. This really describes the involuntary hastening of gait that occurs commonly in patients with Parkinson's disease.

Other aspects of his motor activities that may become more difficult to control include his handwriting, which may become small and cramped (micrographia). His voice will soften to a whisper, and he will drool because of swallowing inability. All these dreadful possibilities are in the future for Van. But hope exists in the form of a medicine called L-dopa. Now there are many forms of this drug, each one slightly more effective in relieving the cardinal symptoms of Parkinson's disease. Rigidity and bradykinesia can often be controlled; tremor is much more difficult to control. Excessive salivation and sweating are often controlled too. And even newer drugs are appearing on the market, so in spite of the inability to halt or reverse the neuronal degeneration that underlies this condition, available methods offer considerable relief.

The basal ganglia constitute a major portion of the descending motor systems, functioning both as part of a maintenance loop that begins and ends at the motor cortex, and as the source of a motor pathway that ultimately leads to the motoneurons in the spinal cord.

The basal ganglia are intimately connected with the cortex. The motor cortex sends information to the caudate and putamen of the basal ganglia (see Figure 9.15). This information is then relayed by the globus pallidus to the ventrolateral nucleus of the thalamus. The thalamus forwards the information, which by now has probably been transformed in some way, back to the cortex, where presumably the same process could again be initiated. Cortical sensory input to the basal ganglia is from the visual, auditory, and somatosensory cortices, and while the functional significance of the basal ganglia as a pivot point for such information is not fully known, undoubtedly the basal ganglia are an important stop in the sensory-motor loop. Subcortical input comes to the basal ganglia from the thalamus and substantia nigra via the thalamostriatal and nigro-striatal pathways.

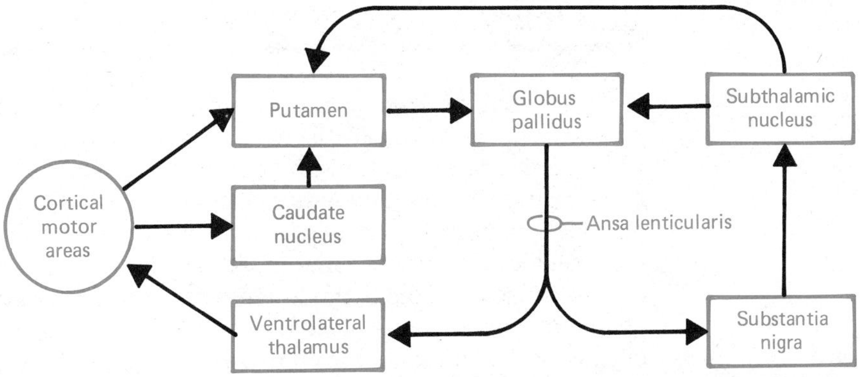

FIGURE 9.15 Feedback loops of the basal ganglia. The precise nature of these loops, that is, whether there is facilitatory or inhibitory activity, is an active area of present investigation.

Most of the efferent connections leaving the basal ganglia pass through the fiber tract called the ansa lenticularis, which is the output of the globus pallidus. These efferent fibers then make connections with the substantia nigra, red nucleus, subthalamus, hypothalamus, thalamus, and reticular formation, which, in turn, contribute fibers to the various subcorticospinal tracts.

Because lesions of the basal ganglia tend to produce varied results, their exact functions are not known. Chorea, an inherited disease with lesions in basal ganglia, is marked by random movements occurring spontaneously and continuously (one form of this disease, Huntington's chorea, affected Allen in Chapter 4). However, victims of Parkinson's disease, which is also characterized by basal ganglia lesions, show a tremor when resting and find it difficult to initiate slow movements. From such evidence, we can deduce that the basal ganglia are involved in the control of posture and tone. Recording from cells in the basal ganglia gives further evidence that these nuclei are involved in the initiation of movements, for these cells show activity before a muscle is actually contracted.

A recent discovery that has both helped Parkinson's disease patients and revealed something about how the basal ganglia operate is that many patients with Parkinson's disease have been successfully treated with L-dopa, a chemical compound that is very similar to dopamine (see Chapter 5), one of the neural transmitters of the brain. It is believed that cells ending in the basal ganglia secrete dopamine, and thus administration of L-dopa compensates for the missing transmitter normally utilized by the basal ganglia nuclei.

Summary

The elaborate sensory physiology studied so far informs the human organism of its physical disposition in the surrounding environment. This chapter details the culmination of this sensory system, for response systems allow interaction with that environment. Humans can alter their physical place, and so not only perceive the world about them but also effect change through action upon it.

The muscles of the body do the work and are organized according to anatomic types responsible for visceral organs as well as peripheral muscles: smooth and striated. And this striated group is organized according to fiber groups—type A, type B, type C; and into intrafusal groups and extrafusal groups. The type A, B, and C fibers vary according to concentration of mitochrondria and metabolic function. The extrafusal fibers do the main work of contraction, and thus are the efferent system, while the intrafusal group contain the muscle sensory receptors, and thus are the afferent system.

Active muscles exert force only by contracting and therefore pulling. To effect a complex movement then, such as playing polo, muscles are organized into functional groups around limbs and joints. Synergistic muscles work together to pull the limb in one direction, while antagonistic muscles able to pull in the opposite direction are relaxed.

To ensure precision in this action each skeletal muscle is controlled by a group of efferent neurons transmitting command signals only to that muscle. Each muscle may contain thousands of muscle fibers, and a single skeletomotoneuron, the alpha motoneuron, controls only a fraction of the total number of muscle fibers. The basic element of the response system then is the motor unit, consisting of a skeletomotoneuron and the group of muscle fibers it innervates. This motor unit is the final common path for CNS command signals to muscles.

Commands from neuron to muscle fibers are relatively simple; the fibers can be directed to contract or not to contract. After the sensory impulses have been analyzed and integrated at various levels of the neuraxis the response system must translate this complex information into on or off commands to individual motor units. Humans perform harmoniously and with organized movements by changing the rate of these commands to the motor units of different muscles, and this rate of temporally and spatially summated "on" signals determines the tension produced by the muscle fiber. Tension and length of a muscle are intimately linked.

The first integration of the sensory information occurs at the spinal cord. Isolating the actions and integrating ability of the spinal cord has evolved from experiments in which the sensory information to, and response command from, the brain are interrupted. Sensory impulses then initiate a series of somatic spinal responses which may be divided into a number of individual reflexes. The stretch tendon, flexor, and crossed extensor reflexes may each be considered a functional entity. However, the cardinal rule in spinal reflex organization is to understand the integration of the several reflexes. The normal response system of humans does not use any one of these reflexes to the exclusion of all the others. Greg's saga of spinal shock after trauma to his spinal cord serves to illustrate the interdependence of spinal reflexes and emphasizes two anatomic and physiologic points. First, in the periphery, two reflexes may share the same afferent receptor population, and in the spinal cord the same motor neuron (efferent) may serve more than one reflex. Second, muscle contraction, which is the end product of any single spinal reflex, may initiate other reflexes by virtue of subsequent muscle and joint stimulation.

In Greg's case spinal shock resulted from a fall and led functionally to a loss of descending input from higher centers. Certain brain stem centers exert a tonic, low-level facilitatory influence on spinal cord extensor alpha motoneurons. Descending extensor-bias exists to maintain posture against gravity. The normal upright posture of standing, or the maintenance of posture when walking or running, are both predominantly extensor functions. It came as no surprise for Greg that interruption of all descending impulses from higher centers left the extensor reflexes most markedly depressed, and that flexor reflexes emerged as the first signs of recovery.

The aberrant plantar reflex, demonstrated by fanning of the little toes and upward movement of the big toe, and the normal plantar reflex share the same afferent path. The end product of this reflex—muscle contraction—initiated action at several parts of Greg's limb, which were imperfectly coordinated into primitive flexor withdrawal response.

Integration proceeds at brain stem, cerebellar, and cortical levels as well. And just as the multiple sensory messages to the spinal cord are integrated before activating the response system, each sensory impulse also travels to higher centers and influences other impulses, and the resultant command signal is translated into movement by the motor systems. The next chapter focuses on this integration of sensory and response systems.

References

Altman, J. 1967. *Organic Foundations of Animal Behavior.* New York: Holt, Rhinehart and Winston.

Barker, D. 1948. The innervation of the muscle spindles. *Quart. J. Micr. Sci.* 89:143–186.

Brinkman, J., and H. G. J. M. Kuypers. 1972. Splitbrain monkeys: Cerebral control of ipsilateral and contralateral arm, hand, and finger movements. *Science 176*:536–539.

Curtis, B. A., S. Jacobson, and E. M. Marcus. 1972. *An Introduction to the Neurosciences.* Philadelphia: Saunders.

Evarts, E. V., Chairman. 1971. Central control of movement: A report based on an NRP work session. *Neuroscience Research Program Bulletin.* Vol. 9, No. 1, Jan. 1971.

Evarts, E. V. 1976. Brain mechanisms in movement. In: *Progress in Psychobiology.* San Francisco: Freeman.

Griffin, D. W. 1962. *Animal Structure and Function.* New York: Holt, Rinehart and Winston.

Guyton, A. 1976. *Textbook of Medical Physiology.* Philadelphia: Saunders.

Henneman, E. 1974a. Motor functions of brainstem and basal ganglia. In: V. B. Mountcastle, ed. *Medical Physiology.* St. Louis: Mosby, pp. 678–703.

Henneman, E. 1974a. Motor functions of brainstem and basal ganglia. In: V. B. Mountcastle, ed. *Medical Physiology.* Vol. I. St. Louis: Mosby, pp. 678–703.

Mountcastle, V. B. 1957. Modality and topographic properties of single neurons of cat's somatic sensory cortex. *J. Neurophysiol. 20*: 408.

Myers, R. E. 1961. Corpus callosum and visual gnosis. In: J. F. Delafresnaye, A. Fessard, R. W. Gerard, and J. Konorski, eds. *Brain Mechanisms and Learning.* Oxford: Blackwell Scientific.

Paillard, J. 1960. The patterning of skilled movements. In: J. Field, H. W. Magoun, and V. E. Hall, eds. *Handbook of Physiology.* Vol. III. Baltimore: Williams & Wilkins, pp. 1679–1708.

Rubinstein, H. S. 1953. *The Study of the Brain.* New York: Grune and Stratton.

Von Economo, C. 1929. *The Cytoarchitectonics of the Human Cerebral Cortex.* New York: Oxford University Press, p. 16.

CHAPTER

10 Sensory-Motor Integration

Traditional thinking had always held that the highly developed cerebral cortex initiated movement, and that subcortical structures such as the cerebellum and basal ganglia served only a regulatory function for movement. Electrophysiological recordings, however, have shown that cells in all three motor areas fire *prior* to movement. The locus of initiation of movement is still not known, but we do know that interaction among these areas is essential for well-coordinated movement. This is what sensory-motor integration is all about. Anatomically, there are vast interconnections between the cortex and the cerebellum and basal ganglia.

The Motor Cortex

The three cortical areas that are concerned mainly with motor functions are the primary motor cortex (area MI), which is the precentral gyrus, the supplementary motor cortex (MII), and the premotor region, all of the areas being in the frontal lobe (Woolsey et al., 1950). Like the somatosensory cortex, the motor cortex may be mapped according to the area of the body it innervates. Each of the three cortical areas has a distinct topographical representation of the body. Much of the essential integration of sensory and motor information takes place in the cortex, since studies have shown that the somatosensory and motor representations in MI and SI are virtually mirror images of each other (see Figure 10.1). In both, the representation of different parts of the body varies according to the density of innervation. For example, the cortical area corresponding to the thumb is much larger than the area devoted to a region of the arm that is actually larger in skin surface than the thumb.

As in some other cortical areas (such as the visual cortex and the somatosensory cortex), the cells of the motor cortex are arranged in columns, each of which may contain thousands of cells (Henneman, 1974).

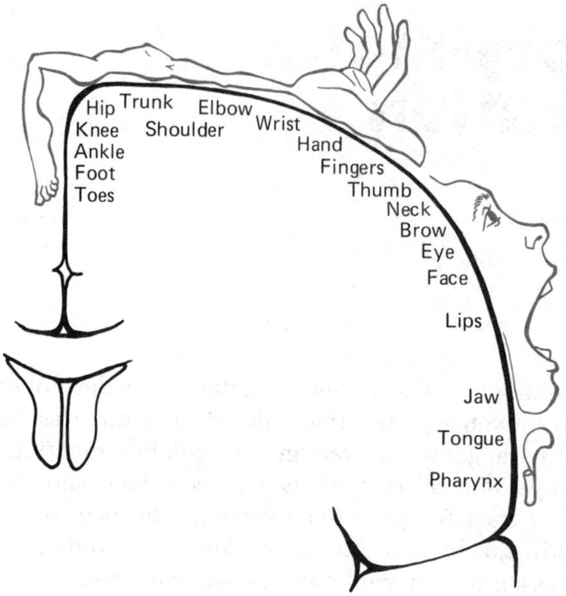

FIGURE 10.1 Density of innervation and topographic representation of the body in the primary motor cortex.

There are six layers of cells (as in all cortical regions), and the input each layer receives is neatly organized. Each cell in a particular column receives somatosensory input from the same area of the body, but in contrast to the somatosensory areas, a single motor column may receive more than one modality of somatosensory input.

The afferent impulses to the primary motor and secondary motor areas come from other regions of the cortex, particularly the zone called the premotor cortex, which is believed to serve as a motor association area (Geschwind, 1965). Admittedly, "association area" is a somewhat vague term, but it is used because no specific function of this area has yet been specified. The area is known to receive indirect projections from the visual, somatosensory, and auditory systems by way of the prefrontal connections, and it projects to MI and MII. Thus MI and MII are influenced by cortical sensory information via a premotor relay.

Lesions of the motor cortex are generally characterized by muscular paralysis, or in some cases, spasticity. When the subcortical structures, particularly the caudate nucleus, are not affected by the lesion, the patient is capable of gross bodily movements but loses the fine control of movement. This suggests that subcortical structures such as the cerebellum and basal ganglia are able to coordinate gross motor activity, but it is the role of the cortex to impose the final ordering scheme. An anatomical indication that the cortex is responsible for the final integration of sensory-motor impulses is the fact that the cortex has more direct access to the motoneurons of the spinal cord than either of the subcortical motor mechanisms. One event that often results in lesions of the cortex is a stroke, or a sudden rupture or obstruction of the blood supply to the brain. In the following example, we shall see some effects of a stroke focused in the motor area of the cortex.

Frank bought and sold major shipments of domestic grapes for a large West Coast firm. This man grew up in the fine wine-making regions of France and some said it was in his blood. He was one of the world's experts on the wines of many areas, but became tired of writing books and sought the more glamorous West Coast manner. He worked very hard at his business but not without paying a price. Heart disease and hypertension were major risk factors for stroke. Frank didn't help matters by continuing to smoke a pack of cigarettes a day.

His first heart attack struck when he was only 52; afterwards he was placed on medicine to control his blood pressure. His compliance to medical schemes was reluctant. Even a year later when he began experiencing transient ischemic attacks, denial and reluctance continued. A transient ischemic attack (called a TIA) is an episode of focal neurologic deficit lasting less than a day and sometimes only a few minutes. Frank's attacks suggested compromised blood supply from the right middle cerebral artery to the cortex. He suffered a transient left hemiparesis more dense in hand and face than leg. He had no speech difficulties during the attack, and no visual symptoms, and neither blurred vision nor blindness complicated this picture. The attacks lasted 10 minutes and were occurring every other day.

When the attacks increased in frequency to two or three per day, he sought medical attention. During his appointment the exam was completely normal, but he left scheduled for hospital admission later that afternoon. In the cab home he had another attack, this one dramatized by headache and dense paralysis of the entire right side of his body. The cabbie took him to the hospital, where on arrival he appeared to have suffered a stroke, an acute loss of the blood supply to a large area of cortex and subcortex. As is common in paralyzed patients, his reflexes on the right side were hyperactive, and his plantar reflex on the right was extensor (a positive Babinski response). For some reason, muscle tone was increased on this weakened side. There was no motor activity in the distal parts of the right-sided extremities although some slight shoulder movement remained. The right lower half of his face was paralyzed but the upper half around the eyes and the forehead was intact. This was certainly due to the bilateral hemisphere innervation of the upper half of the face, as opposed to the single contralateral cortical innervation of the lower half of the face.

Thus, the percentages had finally caught up with Frank. His style of life had perhaps predisposed him to vascular disorders, and now the odds were greater than 20% that he would suffer a stroke in the same distribution within two years. This stroke, affecting one of the main arteries supplying the brain, had, because of the proximity of the artery to the motor areas, damaged Frank's motor functions.

Damage to motor functions is commonly an effect of strokes, since there are many cerebral areas involved with motor functions. Additionally, motor deficits are one of the most obvious effects. More subtle effects, such as memory or language, are harder to assess.

In the following section, we shall investigate further the cortical influences on the sensory-motor system.

The Descending Pathways

Up to now, we have dealt with the cerebral motor mechanisms in terms of afferent-efferent loops that interconnect the cerebellum, basal ganglia, and motor cortex. These loops make up the complex circuitry of motor control in the brain. However, the actual realization of motor control through muscle contraction has only been implied. This last step in sensory-motor integration is mediated by the descending efferent pathways from cortical and subcortical cell groups.

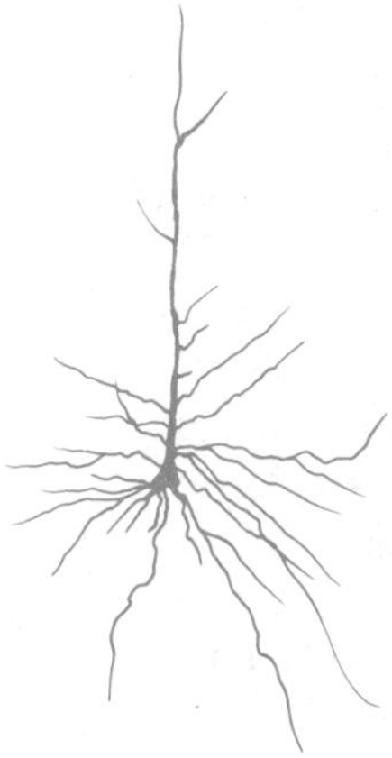

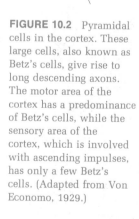

FIGURE 10.2 Pyramidal cells in the cortex. These large cells, also known as Betz's cells, give rise to long descending axons. The motor area of the cortex has a predominance of Betz's cells, while the sensory area of the cortex, which is involved with ascending impulses, has only a few Betz's cells. (Adapted from Von Economo, 1929.)

Layer V of MI contains pyramidal (or Betz's) cells, which are large neurons that give rise to a small number of long, fast-conducting axons that descend without synapse to the spinal cord (Figure 10.2). These fibers are in some cases greater than 3 feet in length. It has been estimated that 80 percent of these long descending axons cross the midline in the pyramid of the medulla and descend to motor neurons and interneuronal cell groups in the contralateral ventral horn of the spinal cord, while the remaining 20 percent descend ipsilaterally (Kuypers, 1960).

The majority of cells in MI, as well as in MII and the premotor region, give rise to short axons that descend to various subcortical nuclei. These nuclei, in turn, give rise to axons that either synapse on other subcortical cell populations or descend bilaterally to the interneurons of the spinal cord.

This anatomical arrangement led to the classical notion that the motor system is composed of two components—a pyramidal and an extrapyramidal division. In this scheme, the pyramidal division included the direct projections from the pyramidal cells in MI to the contralateral spinal cord, as well as multisynaptic projections originating in MI, but synapsing in one or more subcortical nuclei prior to decussating in the medullary pyramids. This system was believed to control discrete movements of the contralateral body. In contrast, gross bilateral movements were believed to be carried out by the extrapyramidal division, which was described as being under the cortical control of MII, the premotor region, and other cortical areas. The extrapyramidal cortical cells were known to project short axons to subcortical neuronal populations (such as the basal ganglia, the vestibular nuclei, the red nucleus, and various reticular formation nuclei), which, on the basis of clinical observations, were attributed a critical role in motor function. These cortical and subcortical nuclei composed multisynaptic extrapyramidal pathways that were believed to project bilaterally to the spinal cord.

The pyramidal-extrapyramidal terminology proved to be troublesome. In the first place, it was never clear whether "pyramidal" referred to fibers arising from pyramidal cells in MI, or to fibers crossing the midline in the medullary pyramids, or to both. In addition, the subcortical components of the two systems were not mutually exclusive.

Lawrence and Kuypers (1968) redefined the motor system in terms of the origin of the final axon, rather than in terms of the origin or course of sequential fibers. Using the monkey, they made discrete lesions at various levels of the central motor system and examined degeneration products in the spinal cord. They found that lesions of MI produced fairly dense degeneration in the contralateral anterior motoneuronal cell groups and sparse degeneration in the ipsilateral interneuronal area. They referred to these projections as the corticospinal motor system (see Figure 10.3). Using a similar approach, Lawrence and Kuypers

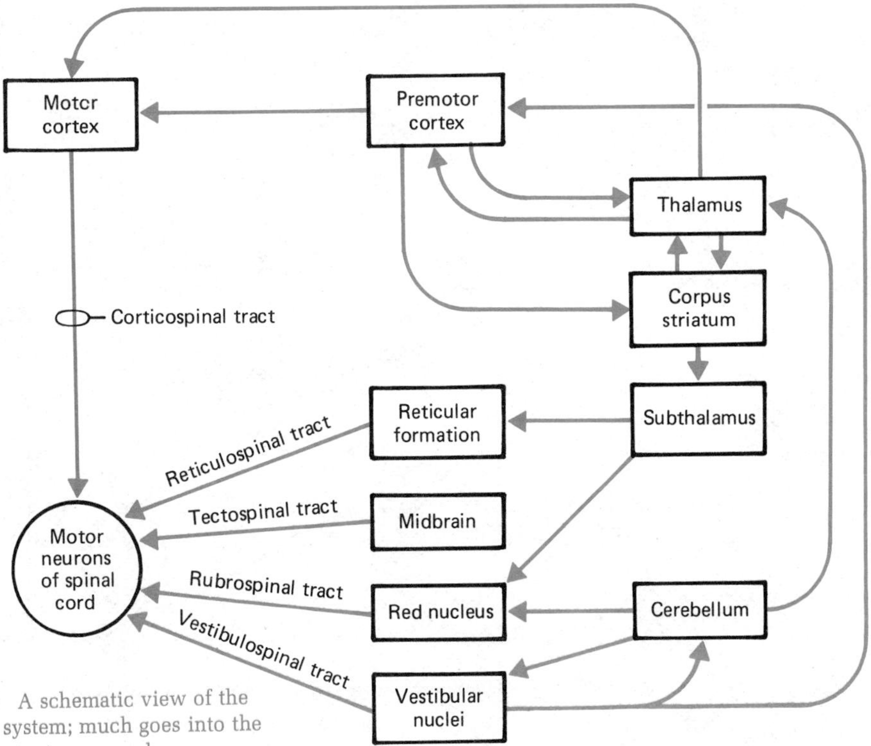

FIGURE 10.3 A schematic view of the corticospinal system; much goes into the basic motor output command.

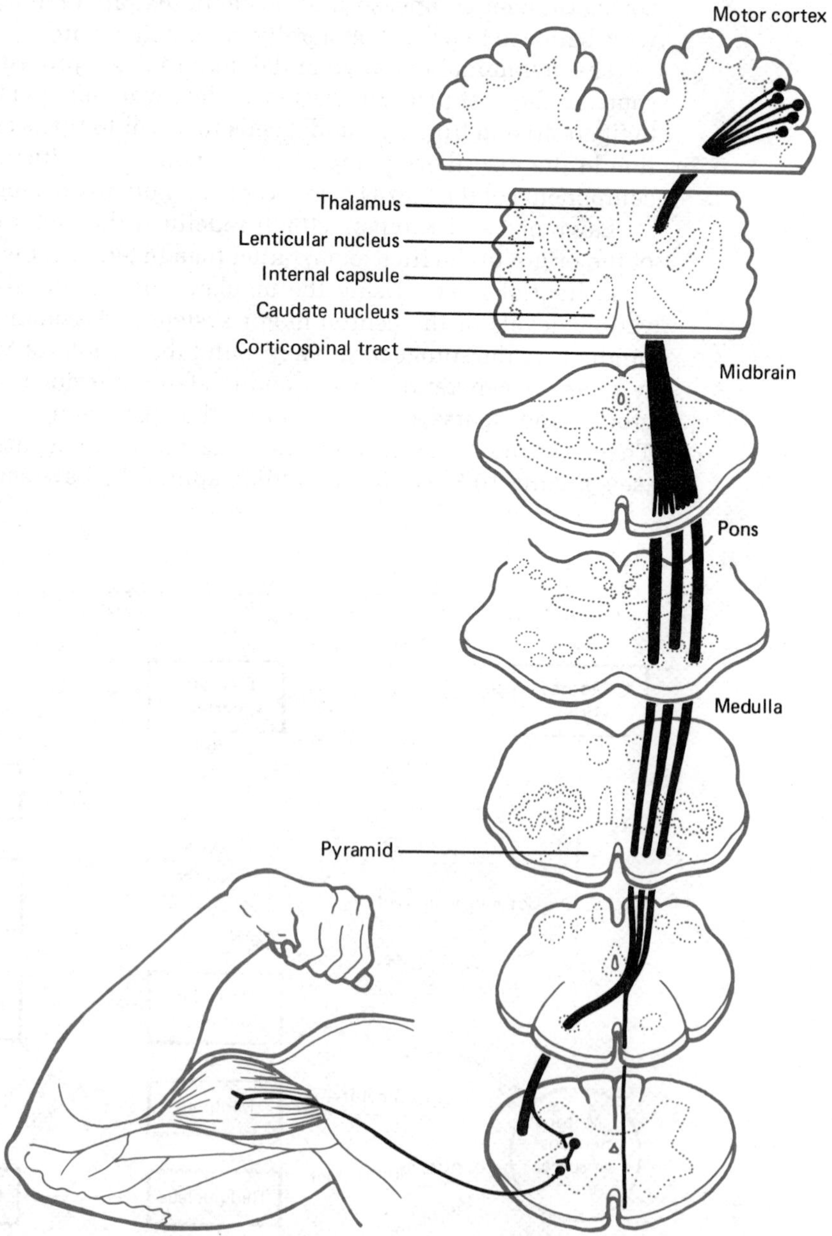

FIGURE 10.4 The neuroanatomy of the cerebral motor mechanisms in summary.

went on to identify two subcorticospinal motor systems. The medial system terminates in the medial internuncial zone and is composed of several tracts. One originates in the tectum (tectospinal tract), one in the brain stem vestibular nuclei (vestibulospinal tract), and a third in the reticular formation (reticulospinal tract). The lateral system, which terminates in the lateral internuncial zone, arises in the red nucleus and is called the rubrospinal tract.

On the basis of behavioral observation of monkeys with damage to different descending pathways, Lawrence and Kuypers inferred the function of the various systems. They concluded that the medial system (tectospinal, vestibulospinal, and reticulospinal tracts) is the basic system by which the brain controls movement, and that this system controls posture and bilaterally integrates trunk and limb movements with the course of progression. The lateral system (rubrospinal tract) superimposes upon these basic movements the capacity for independent use of the extremities, especially the contralateral hands. Finally, the corticospinal system provides for speed and a high degree of discrete contralateral finger movements by its direct connections to the spinal motor neurons. The corticospinal system also influences brain stem control by its collateral connections with the cell bodies of origin of the medial and lateral systems.

The "final axon model" of the descending motor pathways, when combined with the cerebral sensory-motor loop model involving the cerebellum, motor cortex, basal ganglia, and their afferent and efferent connections, provides a useful way of understanding the complexity of motor organization in the central nervous system. These relations are summarized in Figure 10.4. Given the overview, we shall now turn to a consideration of several real-life examples of sensory-motor integration.

Sensory-Motor Integration in Action

Whack! In a major league baseball game, a fastball is thrown, and the batter strikes the ball solidly, sending it well over the right field fence for a home run. Such a feat is an amazing example of sensory-motor integration. That a baseball player can coordinate the timing of his swing with the arrival of the baseball, which is sometimes hurled at speeds as fast as 90 miles an hour, is nothing short of remarkable. To accomplish this act, the batter must use his visual sense to watch the ball and his proprioceptive sense to tell him how to move his body and limbs, and then the sensory feedback mechanisms of the muscles must interact to insure that the bat will indeed collide with the leather sphere. Similar sensory-motor integration is required in fielding a ball (Figure 10.5).

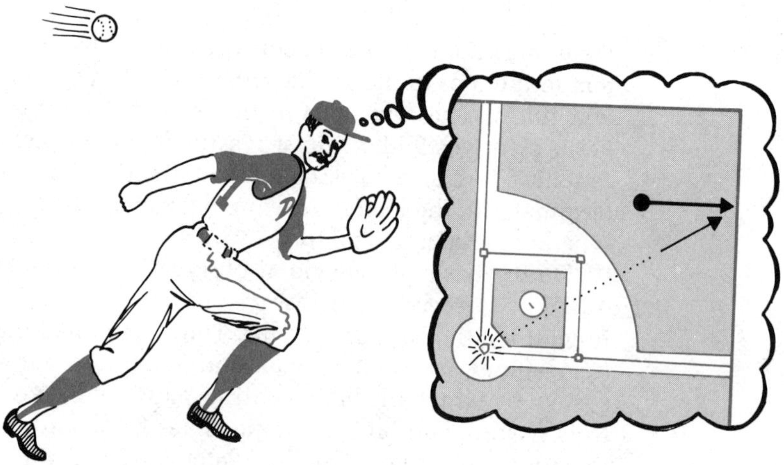

FIGURE 10.5 Catching a fly ball hit hard and traveling at a high rate of speed requires tremendous sensory-motor coordination.

Not everyone is able to hit a baseball, but even the basic process of reaching forward with your hand to grasp an object involves many computations. A complex motor response must be organized to exclude the multitude of other possible arrangements of muscular contraction. Such organization is supplied by information from sensory receptors that guides motor movements to the correct place.

The interdependence of sensory and motor mechanisms has been apparent throughout this chapter. The feedback loops involving the sensory receptors of the muscles, as well as other reflex actions, are prime examples, as are the central feedback circuits involving the cerebellum, basal ganglia, and motor cortex. In this section we shall examine how studies of sensory-motor integration are beginning to identify the brain mechanisms of certain behaviors, such as eye-hand coordination, prism adaptation, posture, and eye-head coordination.

Eye-Hand Coordination

One of the biggest myths concerning brain organization is that each hemisphere has exclusive sensory-motor control over the contralateral side of the body. As we noted in our discussion of the somatosensory pathways, only some modalities within somatosensation are crisply lateralized, and it is mainly the representation of the distal extremities that is lateralized in any modality. The same is suggested by the anatomical organization of the descending motor pathways. Each hemisphere has the connections that would allow for exclusive control over the contralateral fingers (corticospinal tract) and hand (rubrospinal tract). However, the various tracts of the medial subcorticospinal system give each hemisphere the ability to control arm and trunk movements, regardless of the body side in question. Thus, the exclusive control exercised by a hemisphere is limited to the hand and fingers only. This is clearly demonstrated in studies of split-brain subjects.

In split-brain monkeys, visual input can be restricted to one hemisphere by surgically sectioning the optic chiasm and covering one eye. When this is done, the input from the exposed eye goes entirely to the ipsilateral hemisphere (see Figure 10.6). With visual input restricted to one hemisphere, split-brain monkeys are able to carry out normal body movements in response to visual stimuli. They are not limited to using only the opposite body side, when, for example, walking over to pick up a piece of banana. Moreover, with visual input restricted to one hemisphere, a split-brain monkey can reach with either arm to grab a piece of food held out on a stick (Gazzaniga, 1970). However, if the animal is required to remove a piece of food from a small groove using its thumb and forefinger, the monkey will perform with the hand contralateral to the visually exposed hemisphere, but will be extremely inept

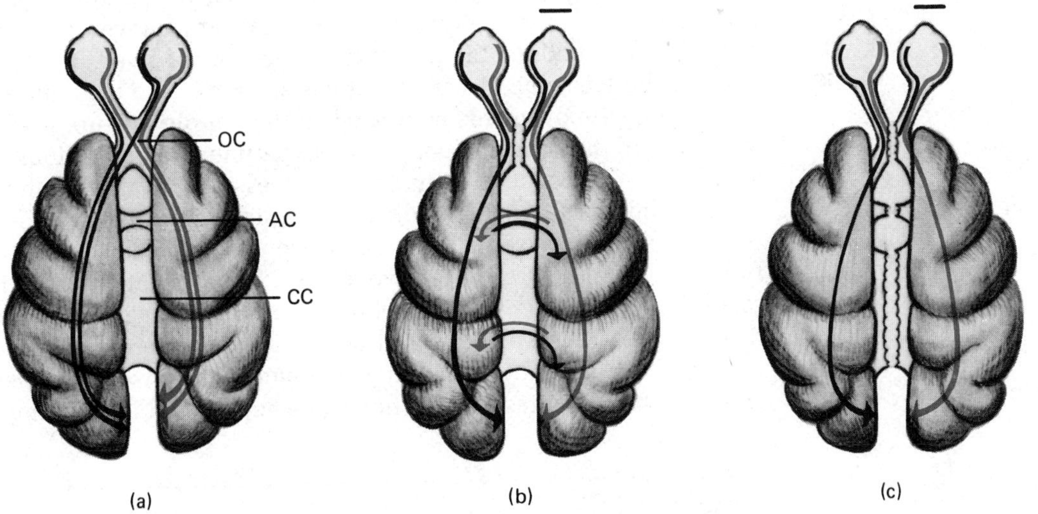

FIGURE 10.6 The split-brain animal. The normal visual projection system is depicted in part (a). The key features in this part are the optic chiasm (OC), the corpus callosum (CC), and the anterior commissure (AC). After the crossed optic projectors are severed, only the uncrossed projections remain (b). Each eye then projects to the ipsilateral hemisphere, so covering of one eye leads to monocular exposure of the hemisphere ipsilateral to the open eye. When the interhemispheric pathways (corpus callosum and anterior commissure) are subsequently sectioned (c), the hemisphere undergoing monocular exposure has exclusive access to the visual inputs.

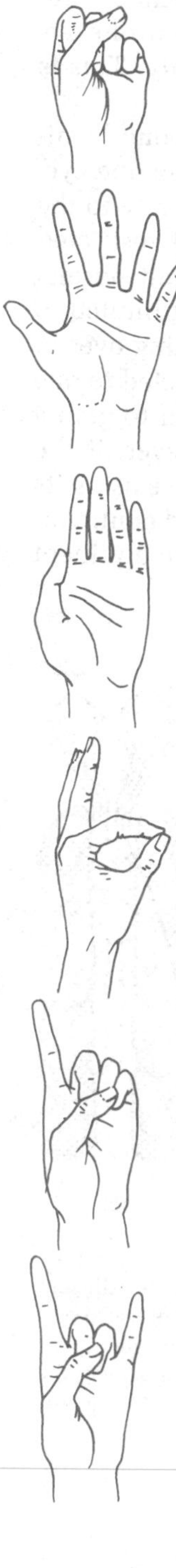

with the ipsilateral hand and fingers (Haaxma and Kuypers, 1975). Similiarly, if finger postures are exposed to one hemisphere of a split-brain human, the patient will be able to mimic the postures with the contralateral but not the ipsilateral hand (Gazzaniga, 1970) (see Figure 10.7). Thus, the behavioral data support the anatomical circuitry that suggests that each hemisphere is wired to control body and arm movements on either side, but controls only contralateral hand and finger movements.

Prism Adaptation

An interesting case of sensory-motor integration occurred in an early series of experiments involving prism adaptation. Adaptation to the visual distortion was complete and rapid: After some practice, a subject looking through a glass prism that displaced images to his right was able to reach correctly for an object with his eyes closed. Upon removal of the prism, the subject invariably missed the object when he reached for it with his eyes closed, because he retained the corrective reaching to the left that was necessary when looking through the prism (Helmholtz, 1867). Further experiments showed that the subject must move his arm voluntarily when practicing with the prism if a strong aftereffect is to be produced (Held, 1965). Simply seeing one's arm moved by somebody else does not produce the perceptual learning involved in this experiment. Although some disagreement has emerged as to the importance of self-produced movements compared to the simple pickup of visual information in the course of adaptation experiments, it is obvious that the subject must associate what he actually does with what he intends to do. That is, one must get some feedback if adaptation is to occur.

One question raised in these experiments was whether the adaptation is a visual or proprioceptive change. Experiments with split-brain monkeys (Hamilton, 1964) suggested that the change was proprioceptive. Visual input was restricted to one hemisphere (as described earlier), and the monkeys used only one hand while wearing prism goggles. In subsequent tests, they showed an adjustment in reaching for tar-

FIGURE 10.7 Finger postures used to test visual-motor coordination in split-brain humans. Because the optic chiasm is not included in the human surgery (there is no medical justification for chiasm sectioning), visual exposure of a single hemisphere is accomplished by taking advantage of the visual field effects described in Chapter 7. If a stimulus, such as one of the finger postures, is briefly presented in the left visual field, then the right hemisphere selectively receives that information (remember right visual field exposure lateralizes input to the left hemisphere). In general, the split-brain patients are able to mimic the finger postures only with the hand contralateral to the exposed hemisphere, thus demonstrating the crossed nature of the motor control over the distal extremities. (Adapted from Gazzaniga, 1970.)

gets seen with either eye, but only when they used the practiced hand. In other words, adapting to prisms was nothing like learning a new visual discrimination. In fact, there was no change in the monkeys' visual perception at all, because if there had been the monkeys would have reached the same way with either hand when the practiced eye was tested. Thus, proprioceptive, not visual, feedback seems to be involved in prism adaptation. (It should be noted that unlike motor control, proprioceptive feedback from the arm is crisply lateralized to the contralateral hemisphere).

Similar results were obtained in experiments on normal humans. When the subjects used only one hand while wearing prisms, only that hand manifested any adjustment to the prisms. Rather than any change in vision, there was a change in the position sense of one arm.

It is clear, then, that changes occur more readily in the proprioceptive sense than in vision. The position sense is "learned" only if motor movements are actually executed, when the feedback from the sensory-motor loop can be taken into account and used in programming further movement.

Vestibular Control of Balance

The vestibular system is a fine example of sensory-motor integration, for it is the vestibular system that gives us our sense of balance, and coordinates sensory input and muscular contraction to maintain the correct posture. Because the vestibular system has direct contact with the motoneurons of the spinal cord, it is able to coordinate muscular activity that requires fast integration of movement, such as gymnastics and acrobatics.

The anatomy of the vestibular receptor apparatus is somewhat similar to that of the auditory system. Located adjacent to the auditory receptor system, the vestibular system consists of five fluid-filled cavities. These cavities are connected to the ear through a tiny opening at the basal end of the auditory canal. Two of the cavities, called *otoliths*, are the *utriculus* and *sacculus;* they are oval-shaped. The other three are *semicircular canals.* As in the auditory system, the receptors are hair cells, which are bent by the motion of the fluid whenever the head is turned or the body moves and experiences a change in gravity. Although the canals and otoliths both contain hair cells, their structures are slightly different, and thus they are somewhat differentially sensitive to movement.

The structure of the canals is quite similar to the structure of the inner ear. Each of the fluid-filled semicircular canals curves up from the cochlea and then terminates on the utriculus. The termination point of each canal is a somewhat enlarged bulb-shaped area, the *ampulla.* Inside the ampulla are the receptor cells, which are hair cells embedded in the *cupula*, a mass of gelatinous substance. This gelatinous substance is of approximately the same density as the endolymph and thus absorbs and transmits the force passed on by the fluid of the canals.

The utriculus and sacculus have a similar structure for hair cells, but their gelatinous substance includes a thin layer of calcium salts known as otoconia. Because the mass with the otoconia is much denser than the surrounding fluid and tissues, it is displaced by gravity or linear acceleration and thus stimulates the underlying hair cells.

The canals and otoliths are differentially sensitive to aspects of balance, the canals being more sensitive to angular motion, and the otoliths more sensitive to linear motion. In either case, the transduction mechanism is the hair cell, which synapses with second-order axons from the vestibular ganglion just outside the medulla. The ganglion sends its fibers into the medulla, where they branch into four different pathways and form the four *vestibular nuclei:* the superior, medial, lateral, and spinal nuclei. The superior nucleus has only ascending projections, which go to the ipsilateral oculomotor and trochlear nuclei of the cerebrum. The medial nucleus bifurcates and sends ascending fibers to the contralateral oculomotor and trochlear nuclei of the cerebrum. The medial, lateral, and spinal nuclei have descending fibers to the spinal cord. The ascending pathways of the vestibular nuclei largely control eye movements, while the descending pathways have direct contact with the motoneurons. The medial vestibular nucleus and the spinal nucleus send fibers through both the ipsilateral and contralateral medial longitudinal fasciculi to synapse with the motoneurons of the ventral roots, thus controlling the skeletal muscles. The lateral nucleus projects ipsilaterally through the lateral vestibulospinal tract, and thus also has influence on motoneuron activity.

The vestibular system detects changes in orientation and movements of the head only. On the basis of the sensory information from the head, the vestibular system can "register" either a normal state or an abnormal state: that is, disequilibrium for the body. Information from neck proprioceptors is of fundamental importance to the vestibular system's maintenance of equilibrium. For instance, if the head is tilted to one side, the vestibular apparatus notes a change in equilibrium, but input from the neck receptors corrects the notion that the body is off balance.

Neurons of the vestibular system are quick to adapt, and they are likely to retain the adaptation for a time through a process called habituation. Spending considerable time aboard a boat, for example, generally results in habituation to the rolling motion of the deck of the boat, and the sensation of being on the water may persist for a few days afterward (Young, 1974).

Similarly, through repeated exposure, the vestibular system is capable of *learning* to adapt quickly to movements that normally would upset one's sense of balance. A person who regularly does gymnastics, whirls and turns as a ballet dancer, flies a stunt plane, or participates in any such unsettling activity, does not feel dizzy even after many dives and flips. The ability of persons to control the responses of the vestibular system suggests that habituation may be under central control.

Eye-Head Coordination

Another function of the vestibular system is to help coordinate eye and head movements, for whenever the head is turned, eye movements must adjust accordingly. Eye-head movements range from a gradual shift of the head while looking at an object straight ahead to turning the head quickly to catch sight of a sudden stimulus, triggered perhaps by an unexpected noise.

These "triggered" eye-head movements usually elicit a series of three steps: first, there is a quick saccadic or high-velocity eye movement to focus the fovea on the image. Next, the head turns toward the object. Finally, there is a compensatory eye movement to bring the eyes back to the target after the head moves.

Such movements require sensory-motor integration through both central programming and peripheral feedback. Recordings made from animals trained to respond to a target light were used to investigate this integration. These studies revealed that central control of movement is effected through several programs (Bizzi, 1975). First, agonist neck muscles fire, and all activity in antagonist neck muscles is suppressed (agonist muscles are the ones that will contract to move the head in the proper direction, and antagonist muscles are those in opposition to them). The second electrical activity noted is in the eye muscles, about 20 milliseconds after the initial burst of activity in the neck muscles. However, the eye muscles are able to move faster than the neck muscles, so the eyes move before the head. Peripheral input from the receptors of the neck and the vestibular system exert an influence on the programmed movements, through a sort of reflex action. For example, the eyes reach the target before the head because they move faster, but even while the head is turning, the eyes remain fixed on the target through compensatory eye movements, which are mediated by visual, vestibular, and proprioceptive reflexes rather than central programming. The saccadic movements of the eye, on the other hand, are centrally programmed, but are modified by the vestibular reflexes.

Summary

Sensory-motor integration, then, is a complicated, well-ordered process. Motor function depends first on the sensory innervation of muscle fibers, and subsequently on the processing ability of the spinal cord and brain. Thousands of neurons must work together to achieve an act so simple as reaching out to pick up a pencil. Even a minor muscular movement requires that the entire well-ordered sequence of steps be executed.

Information from touch and proprioceptive afferents in the skin and joints and from sensory afferents in muscle spindles is conveyed to the spinal cord. From there the information is transmitted through the lemniscal pathways to the thalamus and finally relayed to the cortex. Integration of all afferent systems also includes visual and auditory information, for they are just as important in motor programming as touch information. Much evidence supports the importance of integrated sensory information and further sensory feedback in eliciting, maintaining, and refining the motor output.

The subsequent neural activity consists of organizing a motor response. Some researchers hold that the central nervous system contains all the information necessary for spatially and temporally organized motor response patterns. Although there are numerous instances of centrally patterned motor outputs not dependent on sensory input, much experimental evidence suggests an interaction between central activity and peripheral sensory afferent information (Bizzi, 1971).

The neural command issues from the brain, influenced by the multiple other areas of central nervous system. The basal ganglia, the cerebellum, and the vestibular system provide the major coordinating activity for the efferent command. In this manner, the voluntary act, as in the case of the conscious decision to scratch your leg, is executed smoothly, efficiently, and without loss of balance in your bending and stretching.

Involuntary activity is represented by a reflex action, as in blinking the eyes, or recoil from pain. Reflex movements are slightly different in that cerebral intervention is not absolutely essential for movement, although it is needed to refine the movements and certainly receives sensory information and modifies motor programming subsequent to the reflex. Reflex activity often begins with stimulation of the gamma motoneurons. The gamma fibers then send impulses to the muscle spindles, the sensory endings in the muscle fiber. As the muscle spindles shorten, they send a message back to the spinal cord, stimulating the alpha motoneurons. The alpha neurons then cause the larger fibers to contract, and muscular movement takes place, for example, a finger is quickly pulled away from a hot iron. Reflex activities also occur when the visual system afferent information is perceived in such a manner as to initiate muscular action to turn the head. Here subsequent information from the vestibular system plays an important role. All of these complex neural actions, whether voluntary or involuntary, take place instantaneously.

References

Bizzi, E. 1971. Eye-hand coordination in monkeys. *Science 173*:A52.

Bizzi, E. 1975. Motor coordination central and peripheral control during eye-head movement. In: M. S. Gazzaniga, ed. *Handbook of Psychobiology*. New York: Academic Press, pp. 427–440.

Gazzaniga, M. S. 1970. *The Bisected Brain*. Englewood Cliffs, N.J.: Prentice-Hall.

Geschwind, W. 1965. Disconnexion syndrome in animals and man. I. *Brain 88*:237. II. *Brain 88*:585.

Haaxma, R. and H. G. J. M. Kuypers. 1975. Intrahemispheric cortical connexions and visual guidance of hand and finger movements in the Rhesus monkey. *Brain 98*:239–260.

Hamilton, C. R. 1964. Intermanual transfer of adaptation to prisms. *Amer. J. Psychol. 77*: 457–462.

Held, R. 1965. Plasticity in sensory-motor systems. *Sci. Amer. 213*(5):84–94.

Helmholtz, H. von. 1867. *Handbuch der Physiologischen Optix*. Leipzig: Voss.

Henneman, E. 1974. Motor functions of the cerebral cortex. In: V. B. Mountcastle, ed. *Medical Physiology*. Vol. 1. St. Louis: Mosby, pp. 747–779.

Kuypers, H. G. J. M. 1960. Central cortical projections to motor and somatosensory cell groups. *Brain 83*:161.

Lawrence, D. B., and H. G. J. M. Kuypers. 1968. The functional organization of the motor system in the monkey. II. The effects of lesions of the descending brainstem pathway. *Brain 91*:15–36.

Von Economo, C. 1929. *The Cytoarchitectonics of the Human Cerebral Cortex*. New York: Oxford University Press, p. 16.

Woolsey, C. N., H. Paul, R. M. Settlage, W. Sencer, T. P. Hanery, and A. M. Travis. 1950. Patterns of localization in precentral and "supplementary" motor areas and their relation to the concept of a premotor area. Vol. XXX. Patterns of Organization in the Central Nervous System. *Proceedings of the Association for Research in Nervous and Mental Diseases*. December 15, 16. New York.

Young, 1974. Role of the vestibular system in posture and movement. In: V. B. Mountcastle, ed. *Medical Physiology*. Vol. 1. St. Louis: Mosby, pp. 704–721.

CHAPTER 11

Motivation and Emotion

Why do we do what we do? Scientific accounts of behavior assume that behavior has identifiable causes, and the study of motivation is the study of the factors that determine or motivate behavior. *Motivation*, then, refers to an organism's tendency to behave. When an organism is highly motivated, we say it has a high likelihood or probability of responding. If a motivated animal is said to have a high tendency to perform a behavior, then the ultimate task of any proposed explanation of motivation is to allow predictions to be made about the occurrence of the behavior. Whatever one's idea of motivation is, it is not scientifically useful unless it can forecast or predict such things as (1) when a behavior will occur, (2) how long it will last, or (3) how vigorously it will be performed. The task of the theorist-researcher in motivation is to discover how to make meaningful predictions about the occurrence of behavior. It is no longer adequate to state that a person does something because he or she *wants* to. We must be able to say that, given the proper conditions, the person will or will not engage in a particular behavior—or at least will or will not do so with a given probability. Motivation then, is the tendency to behave, and the study of motivation is the study of ways in which that tendency can be reliably and predictably changed.

Motivation and Homeostatic Mechanisms

Regulation of the Internal Environment

Behavior is often motivated by regulatory mechanisms. Dehydration of bodily tissues will cause an organism to seek out water. Many of the body's basic organic functions seem to be controlled in such a way. An optimal physicochemical balance is needed for the body to function, and when that balance is upset, steps must be taken to restore the balance. The general term for this equilibrium-preserving tendency is homeostasis (Cannon, 1927).

Homeostatic mechanisms depend on the presence of a means of detecting disturbed equilibrium through a sensory mechanism, a means of restoring equilibrium by an effector, and a control center for integrating sensor and effector processes. These are feedback mechanisms that maintain critical balance in a manner not unlike that of the thermostat of an air conditioning unit. If a thermostat is set at a fixed temperature, the "set point", significant changes in either direction are detected by the sensor. The control unit then turns on the effector mechanism until the sensor indicates that the "set point" has been restored.

When the dysequilibrium detectors of the body sense that some critical balance has been upset, one or both of two possible homeostatic mechanisms can be employed by the organism to restore the equilibrium state. The first solution is a physiological one. The body, having detected a system out of balance, can make use of hormones and other built-in metabolic mechanisms to release stored substances or institute conservational measures. Alternatively, behavioral solutions can be used. Both types of solutions are well illustrated by the example of thermal regulation.

Thermal Regulation

One of the basic physiological requirements of warm-blooded animals is to maintain a body temperature of 98.6° F (37° C). Different species have their own specialized strategies for coping with the onset of temperature changes. Some species migrate, others shed their fur. But of more interest to us than these seasonal control mechanisms are the mechanisms involved in controlling temperature from moment to moment.

The law of thermodynamics states that given two objects of different temperatures, heat will be transferred from the warmer to the cooler object. This means that as external temperature drops, the tendency of the body of a warm-blooded animal is to lose heat to the environment. As this occurs, sensory receptors in the skin detect the change and send messages to the brain.

The control center for that regulation is in the hypothalamus. Somehow, the ideal temperature is set in the hypothalamus, and when the peripheral input suggests that body temperature is deviating from this "set point," measures to restore equilibrium are instituted. In response to heat loss, the hypothalamus turns on "effector" mechanisms, initiating metabolic changes to restore the balance. By increasing the basal metabolism rate, the body produces more heat. In addition, conservation measures are used. Blood flow through the peripheral vessels slows down through vasoconstriction, thus reducing the rate at which internal heat from the blood reaches the periphery where it dissipates. On the behavioral level, the organism seeks a warmer set of circumstances. A ground squirrel may snuggle in its nest. A human adds another layer of clothes. Once the hypothalamus determines that the heat balance has been restored, it "turns off" the effector mechanisms. The importance of the hypothalamus in thermal regulation is suggested by the observation that, following damage to the hypothalamus, both physiological and behavioral temperature regulation are largely absent (Keller, 1950; Murgatroyd, 1958).

Thermal regulation is thus an instructive example of how critical balances are maintained. Obviously, however, only the behavioral restoration of homeostasis is representative of motivated behavior. In the following, we shall examine one class of homeostatic mechanisms that are almost exclusively maintained through behavior.

Regulation of Feeding

The body continually requires energy (calories) in order to renew itself. Calories are usually obtained by carbohydrate (glucose) metabolism, but lipid (fat) metabolism also plays a role. When more calories are needed, what sort of cues signal the organism to look for food? As with thermal regulation, the detector mechanism of caloric regulation is not well understood. Some evidence suggests that there are receptors that fire when the level and utilization rate of glucose in the blood fall too low. This monitoring system thus operates as a "glucostat." Other evidence suggests that there are receptors that fire when fat deposits and lipid levels in the blood diminish too greatly. This monitoring system could be termed a "lipostat." Other systems may operate upon the basis of the amount of heat the body has the energy to generate, a thermostat, or upon whether, in the time since the last meal, the stomach has emptied itself enough to terminate the activation of stretch receptors that are inhibitory to hunger.

In addition to caloric regulation, feeding behavior can be initiated by a host of psychological factors, especially in humans. In the absence of caloric needs, people eat because food is available, because it is "time" to eat, because ice cream tastes good, and on and on. Little is known about the detector mechanisms involved in the psychological initiation of feeding behavior.

In contrast to thermal regulation, homeostatic regulation of hunger is almost entirely through behavior. The motivated (hungry) organism engages in the search for food. Feeding, then, is a prime example of motivated behavior. In the following section, we shall examine the studies that have implicated the hypothalamus as the central control unit of feeding.

Hypothalamus and Feeding

In the effort to understand how the needs for food are apprehended and translated into appropriate action, the behavioral effects of experimentally manipulating the nervous system in various ways have been studied. Although the emphasis has been on the hypothalamus, caution must be exercised in concluding that the hypothalamus is the center for total regulation of feeding. One example of the many effects of hypothalamic damage or pressure can be seen in the following case history of Pat.

Pat had finally completed the large government bond issue that would give his shipping firm money for major expansion. It culminated five days and nights of difficult legal argument, each point of which Pat needed to prove over and over again. Government lawyers are very careful people. The final night of negotiating ended at 2 a.m., and each point of the contract was agreed upon. The papers were to be signed by 11 a.m. so that Pat could signal his men at the exchange to start selling the issue. So many millions of dollars were involved that even a single day lost represented a major loss of interest revenue. Thus if the bond were not completely signed at 11 a.m. it would have to be held until the following day. The government agent knew this, and Pat was prepared for his stalling techniques.

Pat was not prepared for the recurrence of a headache and vision problem that had plagued him for months. The contract signing marked the third episode of headache and visual loss. The morning was more aggravating than usual, so Pat attributed the headache to tension. The signing was done by 11 a.m. and all retired to celebrate the triumph. Pat's headache raged unabated, and soon was accompanied by frightening visual loss in the outer (temporal) aspect of each visual field. He was rushed to the hospital where certain diagnostic maneuvers revealed an obstruction of the visual pathway. Pat had a tumor that deformed the optic chiasm, and he was rushed to surgery, where the tumor was removed, and his vision was saved.

His postoperative course was most remarkable. Visual fields returned almost to normal and the headaches ceased. The surgeons were most pleased with how quickly Pat assumed normal activities after the operation. They further beamed at the so-called excellent surgical cure when it seemed Pat would eat anything and everything on the tray. One week later, when he had gained 30 pounds—mostly due to the extra food Pat had coerced his friends to bring—the physicians realized that Pat was suffering with bulimia, a symptom that entails insatiable hunger and the ingestion of food far in excess of metabolic needs. A diet was worthless, for in the wee hours of the morning he was discovered, quite like a rotund bear now, drinking a jar of honey taken from the hospital commissary.

The seriousness of this symptom was difficult to face, for Pat really had no sense of limit to his appetite and no insight into his bulimia. The origin of this symptom was speculative but dealt with the sudden re-

lease of pressure from the hypothalamus. Pat's visual problems and the appetite problem that plagued him after surgery were not unrelated. In Pat's case, it was likely that during removal of the tumor on the optic chiasm, the hypothalamus had been nudged, since there was no evidence for regrowth of the tumor. Fortunately, and for completely unknown reasons, after three months and 80 pounds, the bulimia ceased. Four years passed and he continued to do well, and even lost some of the weight. The cause for his transient bulimia was never fully explained.

Clinical data during the 1930s and 1940s repeatedly showed the occurrence of two syndromes in hypothalamic patients. Some patients with hypothalamic damage would grossly overeat; others would literally starve to death if allowed to regulate their own caloric intake. When experimental psychologists later began their lesion work with animals, they were able to explain both syndromes. There were in fact two areas in the hypothalamus that were involved with feeding: the medial and the lateral hypothalamus.

The Medial Hypothalamus and Hyperphagia By electrically lesioning the medial core of the mammalian hypothalamus, researchers discovered that the mammals would overeat until they became quite fat (Hetherington and Ranson, 1940), a phenomenon labeled hyperphagia (see Figure 11.1). Since it was discovered that an increase in meal size rather than in number of meals per day accounted for this hyperphagia, it was concluded that there was no ability to judge from stomach stretch-receptor signals when an appropriate amount of food had been eaten. In other words, a satiety metering mechanism had been impaired, so the body's conception of its appropriate size was adjusted to some more sluggish and higher homeostatic set point (Teitelbaum, 1955, 1961) (see Figure 11.2).

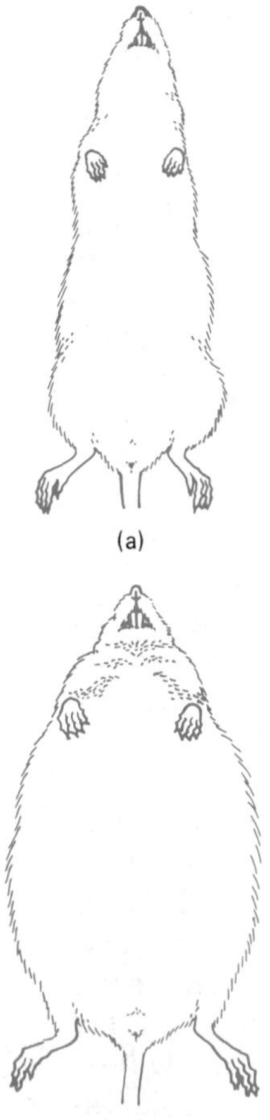

(a)

(b)

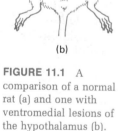

FIGURE 11.1 A comparison of a normal rat (a) and one with ventromedial lesions of the hypothalamus (b).

Other effects, however, complicate the simplicity of this interpretation. Rats made obese by this technique of destroying the medial hypothalamus, in particular the ventromedial nucleus, became much more finicky about what constituted palatable food (Teitelbaum, 1961). As compared to normal rats, they would overeat when presented with delectable foods but undereat when given substandard fare. It was as if they had been left much more to the hedonistic mercies of their external sensory receptors in judging what they should eat and much less to the pragmatic mercies of internal need state receptors in making these decisions. In other words, without their medial nuclei, animals eat mainly what tastes good rather than what is good for them. It is interesting to note that Schachter and his colleagues have shown that normally obese human subjects behave in much the same way (Schachter, 1971b).

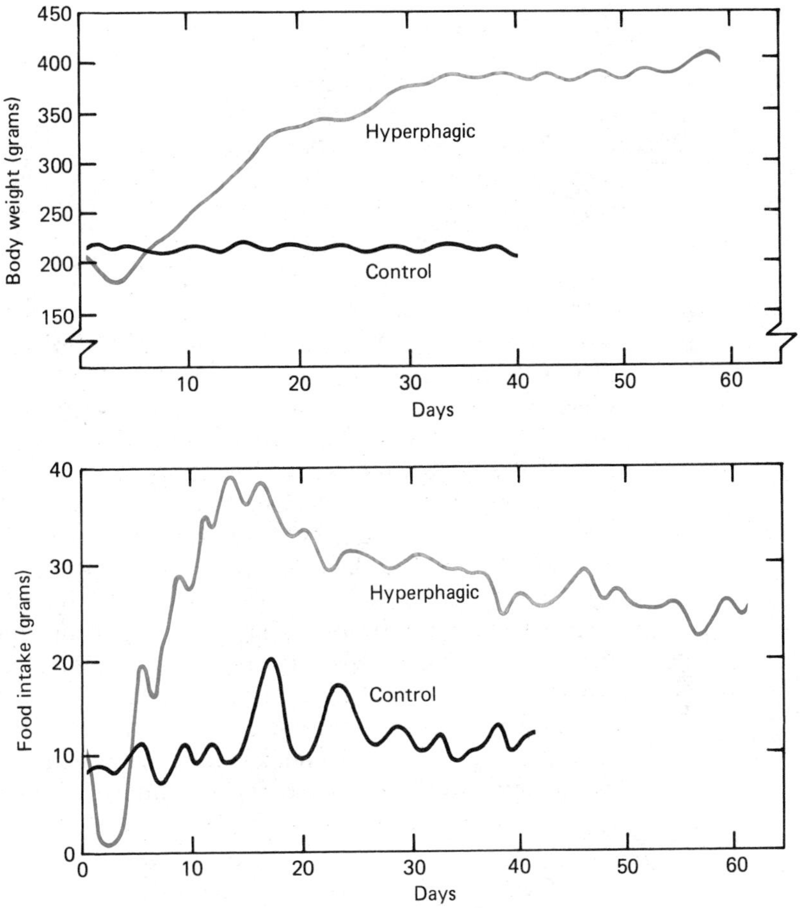

FIGURE 11.2 The amount of real weight put on by a hyperphagic animal is dramatic. Within a month, the rat doubles in size.

Brain lesion and brain stimulation approaches usually have opposite effects of behavior. If destruction of the medial hypothalamus causes overeating, then stimulation of the same region is expected to cause a hungry animal that is eating to stop eating, presumably by eliciting a state of satiation. This is exactly what happens (Wrywicka and Dobrzecka, 1960), although one might quibble with the interpretation as to why, since the stimulation may be merely detraction in some way. However, the fact that ventromedial stimulation in normally satiated rats is followed by a brief "rebound" eating effect upon termination strengthens this argument.

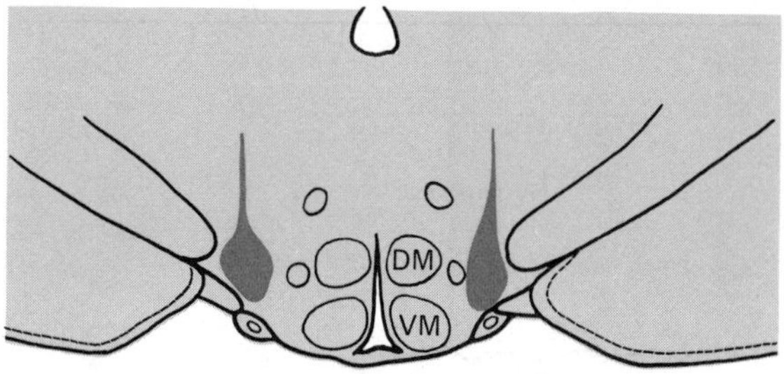

FIGURE 11.3 A schematic cross section of a rat's hypothalamus. The heavily shaded regions represent lesions in the lateral hypothalamic area that produce aphagia and adipsia. DM, dorsomedial nucleus; VM, ventromedial mucleus.

Aphagia and Adipsia: The Lateral Hypothalamus Destruction of the lateral hypothalamus on either side of the medial nucleus produces animals that temporarily are aphagic (Anand and Brobeck, 1951); they no longer initiate feeding behavior and will actually starve to death (see Figure 11.3). Much more drastically, however, the animals are adipsic, that is, they will not drink water. Since an animal long without water will not eat, the effect is to produce an extended aphagia. That is, the aphagia seems to be only secondary if the animal is kept artificially hydrated by water injection (Teitelbaum and Epstein, 1962).

Recovery from primary aphagia usually occurs within a few days, but the recovery from adipsia is much more prolonged and may never be complete if the area of destruction is too large. Even after apparent recovery, however, the animal may regulate its water intake in an abnormal way (see Figure 11.4). A rat's drinking response to a sudden overload of salt or depletion of its body of fluid volume may not be normal. It may be

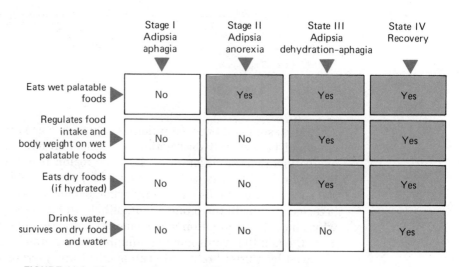

	Stage I Adipsia aphagia	Stage II Adipsia anorexia	State III Adipsia dehydration-aphagia	State IV Recovery
Eats wet palatable foods	No	Yes	Yes	Yes
Regulates food intake and body weight on wet palatable foods	No	No	Yes	Yes
Eats dry foods (if hydrated)	No	No	Yes	Yes
Drinks water, survives on dry food and water	No	No	No	Yes

FIGURE 11.4 The stages of recovery following lesions in the lateral hypothalamus. It is still not known where compensation occurs in the brain.

successfully regulated by the rat's taking water with meals; if food is removed, the rat may fail to drink. It is as if the rat had learned to rely on dry-mouth cues associated with food intake as the only way to successfully steer an approach to water. Evidently, some but not all of the receptors for thirst or the pathways leading from these receptors to the regulatory response mechanism have been destroyed by the lateral hypothalamic damage.

Coons et al. (1965) observed that rats that were electrically stimulated in their lateral hypothalamus often would immediately start engaging in food seeking and eating behavior, even though entirely satiated beforehand. This behavior was stimulus bound in that it generally would terminate immediately with the offset of electrical current. The eating behavior elicited had most or all of the characteristics associated with normal hunger according to a battery of tests. For example, while being stimulated, an otherwise satiated animal would press a bar in order to receive food, thus suggesting that the stimulation elicited the psychological consequences of hunger.

The Trigeminus and Feeding

The trigeminal nerve continues a system of orosensory (mouth sensory) input that has been overlooked by researchers of hunger mechanisms. What is of interest is that the trigeminal nerve, on its way to the thalamus (from the mouth and face), passes in the vicinity of the lateral hypothalamus. The fibers of this nerve, it turns out, are generally severed when the lateral hypothalamus is lesioned. When lesions are carefully placed so as to damage only the trigeminal system but not the lateral hypothalamus, two points become apparent. The lateral hypothalamus is not as potent a feeding "center" as had been assumed and the trigeminal system is part of a neural circuit that plays an important role in controlling feeding behavior (Zeigler and Karten, 1974). Thus the classic lateral hypothalamic syndrome described earlier is partly attributable to disruption of these circuits and not wholly to hypothalamic damage per se.

Nonhomeostatic Motivation: Sexual Behavior

The fact that animals work to reduce their physiological needs (hunger, thirst, thermal regulation, etc.) led many to suppose that need satisfaction formed the basis for motivations; those behaviors that reduced a need were assumed to be motivated. However, not all types of motivated behaviors satisfy physiological needs in apparent ways. Indeed, not all needs will eventually cause harm to the organism if unattended.

Sexual behavior, for example, clearly is motivated, but no harm is done when sexual desires remain ungratified. At least no harm is done to the *individual*; nongratification of sexual needs could eventually be deleterious to the species, but has no obvious harmful effect on an individual organism.

Further evidence that sexual behavior is clearly motivated but not in any homeostatic sense is provided by Sheffield's study (Sheffield et al., 1951). He trained male rats to negotiate a maze in order to gain access to female rats, even though they were prevented from copulating. If sexual motivation was homeostatic, it would presumably be reduced by copulation. Being prevented from copulation after contact would, if anything, *increase* the motivation, not reduce it. Yet such abbreviated contact was an effective reward, with the rats vigorously maintaining the behavior over a long period of time.

Much of what is known today about the biological basis of sexual behavior concerns the role of hormones. In the following, we shall examine these hormonal influences on sexual motivation.

Hormonal Influences on Sexual Behavior

An interrelated system of ductless glands known as the endocrine system is directly or indirectly involved in a great number of vertebrate behaviors. Glands in the endocrine system secrete hormones directly into the bloodstream, which transports the chemicals throughout the body to work their influence on various neural, muscular, or glandular tissues. In particular, hormones released primarily from gonadal glands influence sexual arousal and sexual behavior. The gonads in the male are called *testes* and in the female are called *ovaries*. These glands remain inactive before puberty, but at the onset of puberty, hormones released from the *pituitary* gland (a tiny endocrine gland located deep in the brain slightly below the hypothalamus) stimulate cells in the gonads to produce their own hormones. Ovaries produce two main classes of sex hormones, *estrogen* and *progesterone*, and the testes manufacture and secrete *testosterone*. In turn, the sex hormones induce the formation of such secondary sex characteristics as the growth of body hair and lowering of the male's voice. As a result of gonadal secretions, both males and females experience changes in their body structures that render them capable of reproduction (see Figure 11.5).

The precise manner in which the sex hormones influence sexual motivation has remained elusive for quite some time. Recent studies, however, have begun to elucidate some of the interactions between hormones and the brain that are suggestive of possible mechanisms. McEwen (1976) has shown that there are specific receptor sites in the brain that serve as target cells for the gonadal hormones released by the testes or ovaries into the blood. In particular, the gonadal hormones seem to

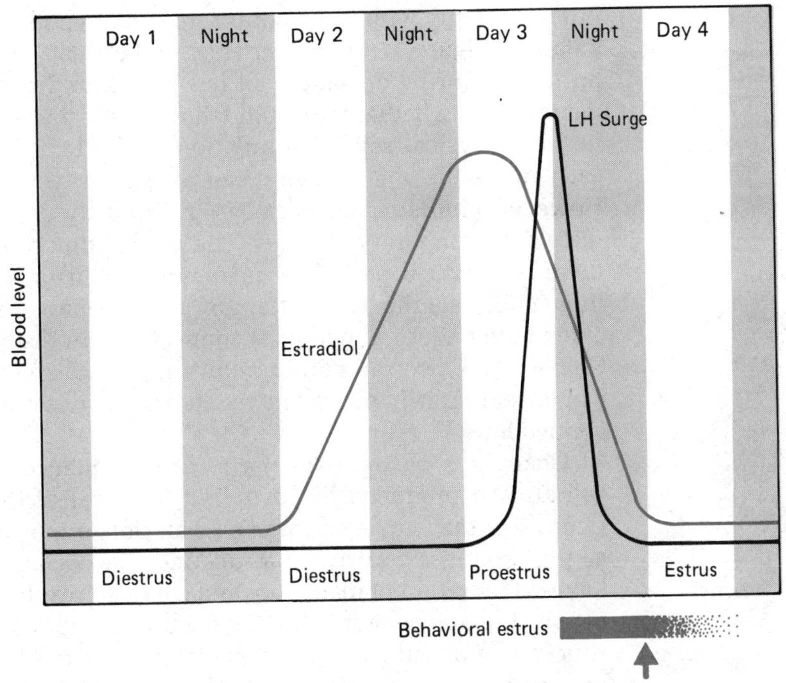

FIGURE 11.5 Sex hormones cause changes in the body that render adults capable of reproducing.

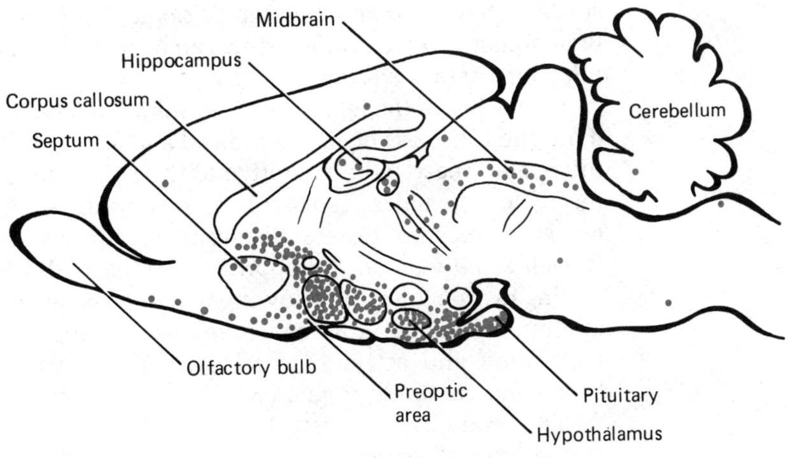

FIGURE 11.6 There are specific receptor sites in the brain that serve as target cells for the gonadal hormones released by the testes or ovaries into the blood.

interact mainly with the preoptic area, the hypothalamus, and the amygdala (see Figure 11.6). The interaction between these sites and gonadal hormones during development has been found to be a critical factor in determining whether male and female rats exhibit behavior appropriate to their physical sex. Manipulation of the brain-hormone interactions early in the life of a young rat can permanently reverse sexual behavior. However, similar manipulations in the fully developed adult rat produce only temporary changes. The implication of these findings is that there is a critical period in development during which hormone-brain interactions set the later pattern of sexual behavior in the adult by influencing the pattern of neuronal connectivity in the developing brain (see Chapter 4). Once the brain circuits are established, however, behavior can be temporarily altered by excitation or inhibition of the established connections.

Changes in sexual behavior as a consequence of hormonal changes can also be produced by castration (removal of the testes in males or removal of the female's ovaries). Castration of the adult male rat or guinea pig produces a fairly rapid decline and disappearance of sexual behavior. Castration of male dogs and cats also results in a decreasing incidence of sexual behavior, but the decline is somewhat more gradual than it is in rats or guinea pigs—especially if the dogs or cats have had the opportunity to copulate since puberty. Most male primates show little change in sexual behavior following castration, although they will not engage in sexual behavior if castrated prior to puberty. The effects of castration in the human male are tremendously affected by emotional and social factors, but it seems that the sexual urge is usually only diminished slightly, if at all. Cases have been reported, however, in which the response to castration has ranged from complete and total cessation of sexual behavior to an elevation of sexual behavior. In all species lower than humans, sexual functioning can be restored in the castrated male by injections of testosterone.

Castration in the female of all infrahuman species results in an immediate and total loss of sexual arousal and sexual behavior. Not only does the female cease to be receptive to the male; she often violently resists the male's sexual advances. Loss of hormones in the human female, however, does not necessarily result in diminished sexual activity. Although some women do report reduced sexual drive and behavior following ovariectomy or following menopause, most report no decrement at all in sexual drive. Indeed, many women report an increase in sexual motivation and activity, which is, perhaps, triggered by the freedom from concern about pregnancy.

The production of testosterone, and therefore its influence on male sexual arousal, is usually relatively constant from puberty until death, but the production of female hormone is cyclic in nature, and coincides with changes in fertility. Prior to ovulation, during the period when the egg is being prepared, the ovaries secrete estrogen. Egg preparation is, itself, under the control of other hormones secreted by the pituitary gland: follicle-stimulating hormone (FSH) and luteinizing hormone (LH). Estrogen secretion increases gradually as egg preparation continues and reaches a maximum when ovulation is actually taking place. This is the only time at which females of most infrahuman species are sexually receptive to the advances of males. Conveniently, this is the only time when fertilization is possible and likely. After ovulation, both progesterone and estrogen are produced. Progesterone helps prepare the body for maternal behavior, and if fertilization does not occur, it also acts upon the pituitary to inhibit the release of FSH and LH. In the absence of these pituitary hormones, estrogen and progesterone production drops and the uterine wall containing the unfertilized ovum is sloughed off, becoming menstrual flow and ending the cycle. At this point, estrogen production resumes and the cycle begins again. Birth control pills contain synthetic estrogens and progesterone and act to inhibit FSH and LH, thus preventing egg development and ovulation. Some of these relations are depicted in Figure 11.7.

In most mammal species below primates, female sexual arousal is a function of the level of estrogen present in the blood, resulting in cycles of sexually motivated behavior that match the animals' estrous cycle. When sexual arousability is at its peak, it is often said that the animal is "in heat." Estrous cycle length varies from species to species; in the human it is 28 days on the average; in chimpanzees, it is 36 days; in mice and rats it ranges from 4 to 6 days. Hormonal levels have less of an effect on arousability in primates, however, than they do in lower mammals. Female monkeys show some amount of sexual behavior, including copulation, throughout the entire estrous cycle. Among primates, humans are the least influenced by the estrous cycle.

There is evidence to suggest that another class of hormones—androgens—is responsible for sexual arousal in both males and females (Money and Ehrhardt, 1972). Women patients who suffer with cancer are often treated surgically by removal of their adrenal glands. Androgens are produced in the adrenals of both sexes, and associated with this decrease in androgen these women report a marked decrease in sexual desire. In males, the greatest source of androgens is the testes. Androgen replacement therapy in castrated men restores their lost sexual functioning. Since androgen levels seem to correlate well with levels of sexual arousal in both males and females, it is possible that these hormones exert a strong influence on sexual motivation.

In general, however, sexual motivation in humans is much less controlled by hormones and subcortical neural functions than it is in other animals. Not only are the ways in which humans seek gratification of

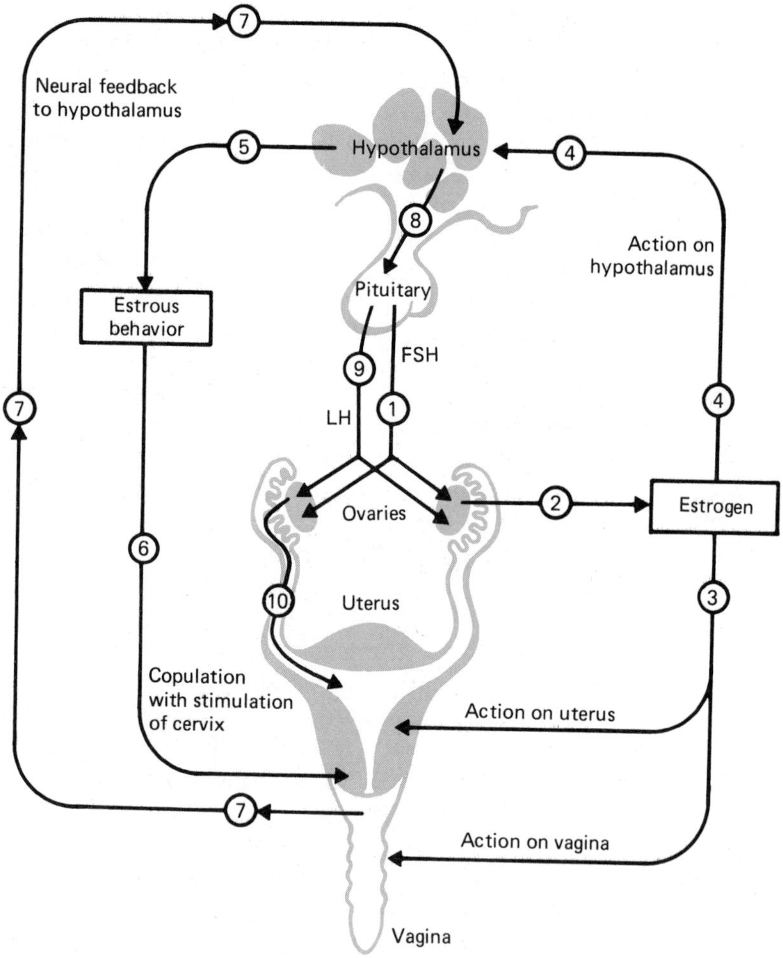

FIGURE 11.7 A schematic representation of how the hypothalamus interacts with endocrine systems.

their sexual drives extremely diverse; the stimulus situations that induce these drives vary immensely from individual to individual. Large cultural differences can be delineated, but even within a given culture, the extent and methods of sexual arousal run the gamut of possibilities. Kinsey et al. (1953) related that men report greater sexual arousal when viewing erotic stimuli than women report. However, recent work suggests that there may be few, if any, differences between the sexual arousal of men and women if physiological responses are reported. While it is true that men claim greater arousal when shown erotic stimuli, there is little difference between them and women when such responses as penile erection, vaginal lubrication, and genital sensations are reported (Buck, 1976).

Brain Stimulation, Reward, and Motivation

There are obvious connections between the psychological conceptions of reward and motivation. A reward is something that an organism will work to obtain. Thus, hungry rats will press a lever in order to obtain food. The food reinforces or rewards bar pressing. Once the animal is satiated, food is no longer reinforcing and bar pressing will stop. An alternative description of the situation is that the animal was motivated by hunger to press the bar for food. Once the need was satisfied, the rat was no longer motivated and thus bar pressing ceased. These are both acceptable accounts of the situation, and in the following, we shall examine the interaction and overlap of reward and motivational systems in the brain.

In the 1950s, Olds (1958) discovered that there were places in the brain where electrical stimulation through implanted electrodes was so rewarding that the animal would actually learn and vigorously perform a response in order to receive the current. In other words, the animals were motivated to work to reach the goal of receiving brain stimulation. This discovery came about when Olds noticed that a rat with an electrode in what he thought was the reticular formation kept returning to the spot on a table where it had been when it received stimulation. Olds followed up on this observation when he discovered that the electrode was not in the reticular formation at all, but was in the septal area. Subsequent observation confirmed that septal stimulation was in fact rewarding and in addition demonstrated that a variety of other areas, including the lateral hypothalamus (of aphagia and adipsia fame, as described earlier), were also rewarding sites.

The stimulation technique has been used extensively in situations where animals control the frequency of stimulation. That is, every time an implanted rat presses a bar or emits some other predefined response, it recieves stimulation. Thus, this approach commonly is referred to as self-stimulation (see Chapter 5, p. 113).

Brain stimulation of rewarding sites has proven to be a powerful source of motivation. Olds (1958) has shown that rats will cross an electrified grid in order to receive rewarding stimulation (see Figure 11.8). The techniques of rewarding brain stimulation have been refined to such an extent that, at an optimum site, rats prefer electrically exciting their own brain tissue to any native activity. Olds reported that one rat with

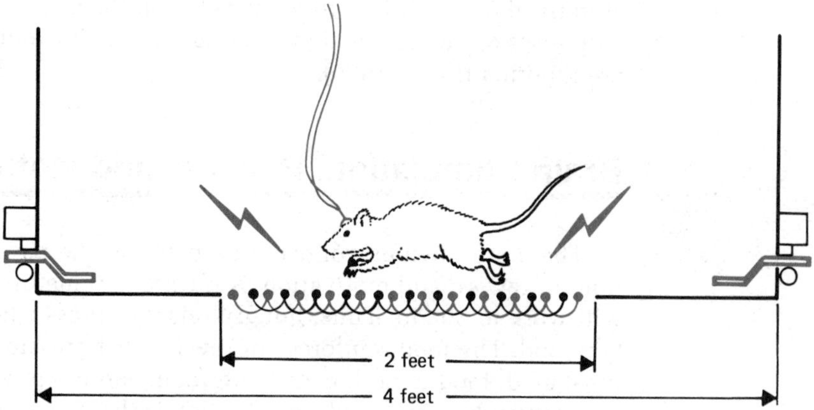

FIGURE 11.8 Rats find self-stimulation of some brain sites so reinforcing that they will cross a grid delivering a painful shock in order to stimulate themselves.

an electrode implanted in its medial forebrain bundle (MFB) pressed a lever at a rate of 2000 times per hour for a period of 26 hours before becoming exhausted (see Figure 11.9). Other rats having electrodes in the MFB have been unwilling to stop performing instrumental responses long enough to eat; they would rather starve than terminate the brain stimulation, even for an instant.

Other regions in the brain give effects opposite of those obtained from reward centers. When stimulation is administered through electrodes implanted in one of these "negative" regions, the animal stops responding as though the stimulation were aversive. Actually, this quite literally may be the case; stimulation in these areas may simply be noxious in much the same way that painful stimulation to the body's surface is

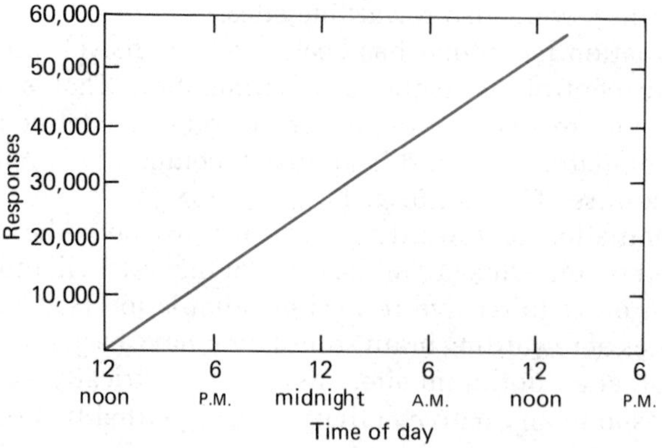

FIGURE 11.9 A cumulative response curve for self-stimulation for a 48-hour period. The animal started at noon and pressed for 26 hours at a rate of 2000 responses per hour.

aversive. It is difficult, both experimentally and conceptually, to distinguish between a brain area that may be mediating aversive motivation in general and an area that may simply be involved with transmitting information from pain receptors in some other part of the body. So, suppose you were given a rat with an electrode in one of these negative areas and each time the rat turned left, you stimulated it electrically. You soon noticed that the rat quickly ceased to make left turns. You could have been stimulating its aversive motivation center, or you could have been stimulating a relay station for painful stimulation to the left leg (you may have made his left leg hurt). Or you could have given him a headache or a stomachache, or made him nauseated. Perhaps you caused an old frightening memory to occur. The point is that there are a number of alternative explanations for the results. You need not assume that you have located the seat of punishment. Of the many theoretical interpretations given the vast amount of work on rewarding and punishing brain stimulation, one that was inevitable was that these areas are involved in the mediation of drive reduction and drive elevation. Other theorists have taken a more hedonistic view and simply referred to these areas as "pleasure centers" and "pain centers," and subsequently reduced motivation to the seeking of pleasure and avoidance of pain. Hedonism has been around for a long time as an explanation of motivated behavior, but because of the subjectivity inherent in such a theory, hedonistic notions fell from favor with the advent of modern scientific psychology. The discovery of pleasure and pain centers makes hedonism a much more objective concept: "pleasure" can be objectively defined (at least theoretically) as neural activity in a pleasure center, and "pain" as activity in a pain center.

A note of caution should be sounded to those readers who are tempted to conclude that brain stimulation holds the solution to all of the riddles of motivation. Although this may ultimately prove to be the case, just as we may eventually understand questions of behavior and learning in terms of psychological, neural, chemical, and physical formulations, science is decidedly not yet at such a point. Indeed, the work on rewarding and punishing brain stimulation has introduced many new problems. For example, rewarding brain stimulation does not seem to operate like "normal" rewards. Whereas a hungry animal is quite capable of performing many unreinforced responses on the way to a food reward, such perseverance is not apparent in animals working for brain stimulation as a reward. A rat that has just received rewarding brain stimulation will quickly run down a runway to stimulate itself again, but if it is restrained from running for five minutes and then released, there is a marked deficit in its running performance. Often the rat will not run at all. If rewarding stimulation is withheld for a short duration, then animals seem to lose interest in it. Some researchers have found that rats require a few free or "priming" stimulations in order to begin stimulating themselves—even when they have had a great deal of experience at self-stimulation.

Primarily on the basis of results such as these, it has been proposed that brain stimulation is a sort of self-perpetuating process, that one brief stimulation actually motivated responding for another stimulation. Or, in terms of drives, if brain stimulation is withheld for a period of time, the drive fades away and must be rekindled by a free stimulation (e.g., Deutsch, 1971).

A final curious discovery about rewarding brain stimulation is that one of the "best" regions for producing self-stimulation is the lateral hypothalamus. As you will remember, this area is often thought to be the hunger center of the brain. Precisely why an animal should find it so pleasant or rewarding to stimulate its hunger center—to, presumably, make itself hungry—is not at all clear.

Stimulation in Humans

What exactly is the nature of rewarding brain stimulation? To answer this question, psychologists have turned to humans who have had stimulating electrodes chronically implanted in various regions of their brains. All of the people investigated have had stimulation electrodes implanted in their brains for medical reasons (Mark and Ervin, 1970); none were merely subjects of experiments. These patients usually had an intractable disorder such as grand mal epilepsy, and had no success with conventional treatment. Some subjects suffered from severe schizophrenia, a few had terminal cancer, and at least one patient suffered from narcolepsy—a disorder distinguished by sudden, uncontrollable periods of sleep. In all cases, electrodes were implanted as a last resort, either to try to alleviate the disorder itself, or—in the case of the cancer patients—to reduce the pain and severe depression accompanying the disorder.

For the most part, results of stimulation in humans are similar to those obtained from animals, with the exception that the frantic self-stimulating behavior often observed in animals was never seen in humans. When asked what the stimulation felt like, subjects gave responses ranging from a very good feeling of well-being to a "drunk feeling" or to a feeling of repulsion or aversion, depending upon the areas stimulated. Stimulation in the septal region, and to a lesser extent in other regions, was very often accompanied by a general sexual feeling, or less frequently, by specifically sexual memories or urges. In very few instances did stimulation to the septal area produce sexual arousal. Only three male patients of 54 studied by Heath (1964) experienced penile erection following stimulation. One depressed female epileptic patient showed extremely strong sexual pleasure often accompanied by spontaneous orgasm, when acetylcholine (a neural transmitter substance—see

Chapter 5) was injected into the septal region. Stimulation to other areas of the brain also produces pleasurable sensations, but they are not as frequently of a sexual nature, although Delgado (1969) reported that stimulation in the region of the temporal lobes known as the amygdala produced flirtatious behavior in one male and two female patients.

When humans have been given control of their own brain stimulation, the results have been somewhat confusing. Perhaps one of the chief sources of confusion has been the conscious effort on the part of human subjects to please their experimenters. Subjects have reportedly continued to press a stimulation button even though the button has been disconnected, merely because they thought the experimenters wished them to do so. There are many reasons for self-stimulation in humans that have nothing to do with reinforcement or pleasure per se. For example, it has been reported that a patient's laughing response to stimulation could be explained by a stimulation-produced muscle twitch that tickled, rather than to a particularly exhilarating or happy sensation. Another patient was permitted to choose from among several sites for stimulation for a period of six hours. A very high rate of self-stimulation was obtained at one of the sites, but not because it felt good; stimulations there brought a long-forgotten memory to near-consciousness, and the patient continued to press the button in an attempt to fully recall the memory.

By and large, however, the results of self-stimulation studies in humans have yielded results that are roughly comparable to results obtained in animal studies. Stimulation sites that produce reinforcement in animals also produce reinforcement in humans. Similarly, sites that are aversive tend to be aversive for both humans and animals. If nothing else, this would tend to vindicate the use of animal subjects in the attempt to discover the intricacies and mysteries of reinforcement and motivation.

Emotion

In any discussion about motivation, especially human motivation, it rapidly becomes apparent that the concept is very closely linked with the concept of *emotion*. In the case of sexual behavior, for example, it is difficult to avoid terms such as love, desire, or pleasure. Indeed, some vague notion of "pleasure" (and "pain") is usually concealed furtively beneath the semantics of most theories of motivation. Fear and aggression are two additional forms of motivation that have unmistakable emotional overtones. When we see that someone is frightened, we know there is an urge to flee—the person is motivated—but we also understand that the person is experiencing an emotion. About the only distinction that can be drawn between motivation and emotion is that one usually thinks of motivation as arising from within the organism, often as a result of some biological need or hormonal influence. Emotion, on the other hand, is often thought to be a cognitive response initiated by an external stimulus. Hunger (a motivation), then, is a manifestation of some sort of nutritionally linked deficit, whereas fear (an emotion) usually results from experiencing some aspect of the outside world through the sensory system. We see, hear, or smell something that is fear-inducing. This is not a wholly valid distinction, however, because we can all think of counterexamples. There are times when hunger is induced not by internal needs, but by seeing or smelling a particularly enticing food. Fear, too, can certainly come from an internal stimulus. Extreme hunger can make one afraid. The point is that motivation and emotion are extremely closely related topics, though if anything, less is known about emotional behavior than motivation.

In this section several competing theories concerning the nature of emotion will be examined. We begin with the visceral theory.

The Visceral Theory

Although it is natural for us to think that the body reacts as a function of stressful situations, that is we run when we become frightened, or strike when we become angry, one of the earliest theories of emotion held the opposite view. William James, a famous American psychologist during the late nineteenth century, proposed that the information we receive from our body is the most important factor in determining our emotions; in effect, he proposed that our visceral and somatic reactions *are* our emotions. Thus, when confronted by an angry, snarling dog, our hearts speed up; we tremble, gasp, tense, and run away. Trembling, gasping, tensing, and running *are* fear. We do not run because we are afraid, "we are afraid because we run." "We are angry because we strike," instead of striking because we are angry. James felt that our perception of stressful situations would be purely cognitive without the visceral feedback received from our bodies. "We might see the bear and judge it best to run . . . but we could not actually *feel* afraid." A Danish physiologist named Carl Lange arrived independently at the same conclusion at about the same time as James; the theory is referred to as the James-Lange theory.

Walter Cannon (1927), a physiologist at the University of Chicago, was the earliest critic of the James-Lange theory. First, he argued that dogs appear to show fear and other emotional behavior even though their spinal cords have been cut, eliminating most visceral feedback signals. Second, internal organs are not well innervated and their responses are too slow to account for the great speed with which we experience an emotion such as fear. Third, different emotions seem to be accompanied by the same visceral changes. Thus, for example, the specific physical reactions that accompany fear are essentially indistinguishable from the physical responses that accompany anger, even though we have no difficulty in distinguishing fear from anger. Fourth, artificial production of the physical arousal (e.g., by injecting adrenalin) does not result in the experience of a true emotion.

Cannon's own theory hypothesized that the thalamus received sensory information from an emotion-inducing situation, then relayed the information simultaneously to the cerebral cortex and the various appropriate internal organs and muscles. For Cannon, then, visceral responses and cognitive responses occurred at the same time.

Recent research has not favored either of the competing theories. Instead, it indicates that we probably combine the information derived from our viscera with information provided by our environmental situation to determine the appropriate emotion to be felt.

In one recent study, 25 service veterans who had suffered spinal cord injuries were interviewed and asked to compare their emotional experiences before and after their injuries (Hohmann, 1962). The patients were divided into five groups, according to the level of the spinal cord at which they received their injuries. Those with the worst injuries had only the function of one branch of the parasympathetic system and no sympathetic function. Members of the least-injured group had injuries near the base of the spine and retained at least partial function of both parasympathetic and sympathetic systems. The remaining groups fell between these two extremes.

It was found that most patients *did* report reduced emotional experience. Furthermore, the degree of reduction of emotionality was directly related to the loss of autonomic function—the greater the loss of function, the greater the reduction of emotional experience. These results were found to hold for fear, anger, grief, and sexual excitement. Interestingly, some patients reported that they often *acted* emotionally, but did not really experience the emotion. For example, in describing his anger, one patient said, ". . . it's sort of a cold anger. Sometimes I act angry when I see some injustice. I yell and cuss and raise hell, because if you don't do it sometimes, I've learned people will take advantage of you, but it doesn't have the heat to it that it used to. It's mental kind of anger."

It seems, then, that the visceral feedback is not essential to the knowledge of the emotion, but it does flavor the experience. Without the feedback, patients recognize the appropriate situations for emotions, and can respond accordingly, but the emotional feeling is not actually present.

Cognitive-Physiological Interactions

Studies such as the one above relating levels of emotional arousal to spinal injury and concomitant loss of feedback from the body indicate that autonomic activity contributes a great deal to our emotions, although it probably does not determine them. However, there does not seem to be a great deal of difference in the body activity that accompanies various emotions. Thus, if one were to make two lists, one list of the physiological changes that take place as a result of a fearful experience, and another of the physiological changes that take place as a result of an anger-arousing experience, the two lists would probably be identical. How, then, do we distinguish our emotions?

Schachter (1975) proposed that the physiological mechanisms for some emotions *are* essentially identical, but we learn to label them differently in different situations. Thus, hearing noises in the attic late on a dark night while you are home alone may produce the same bodily reactions as having someone cut into a line in front of you, but you know from past experience that, in the former case, you should label your state "fear," and in the latter "anger." According to Schachter's theory, then, there are two components of emotion: a mechanism for physiological arousal and a cognitive mechanism for labeling the arousal.

Schachter reasoned that, if this theory were true, an individual experiencing physiological arousal with no or incorrect information about the appropriate label to place on the emotions would tend to mislabel the emotion. As a test of this hypothesis, Schachter made use of the fact that injections of adrenalin produce physiological reactions that are, to an external observer, indistinguishable from bona fide emotional arousal. If the theory were true, a person injected with adrenalin would tend to become angry if done an injustice, become elated if told a joke, feel afraid if threatened, or fall in love in the presence of a suitable partner. If *no* information were present upon which a decision could be based, then the emotion might be labeled according to a memory of past experience, or the person might simply decide that he or she were ill.

All subjects were told they were participating in an experiment to determine the effects of vitamin C on vision, and all were given an injection, but not of vitamin C. Instead, one group of subjects received injections of adrenalin and another group received saline solution as a placebo. The group receiving adrenalin was further divided into three groups. Subjects in one of these were correctly told what they could expect to experience as a result of their injections: pounding heart, flushed face, and tremor. Subjects in the second group were misinformed about what was to be expected: They were led to expect a headache, numbness, and itching. The third adrenalin-injected group, as well as the placebo group, were not told to expect any effects.

Each subject was then told to wait in a room occupied by another person. Although the other person was presumably also a subject, he was actually an actor (a "stooge") who was to provide a cognitive set of information about the proper label to place on their emotions. For one-half of the subjects in each group, the stooge acted as though he were angry at having to wait and angry at having to fill out a questionnaire, which he tore up before stalking out of the room. For the remaining subjects, the stooge provided a happy, boisterous, euphoric manner. He shot paper wads, threw paper airplanes, played with toys, etc.

Subjects who were informed about their physiological states of arousal were not greatly affected by the stooge's behavior. Nor were members of the placebo group, who actually were not physiologically aroused. Subjects who were misinformed or told nothing of what to expect *were* influenced by the stooge's antics. They were more euphoric in the situation designed to produce euphoria and angrier in the situation contrived to produce anger. Presumably, these subjects had no explanation for their arousal, so were more influenced by their immediate environment.

Brain Mechanisms and Emotion

It would appear that cognitive and visceral factors are thus capable of explaining emotional experience. However, it should be apparent that such theories largely ignore the brain mechanisms underlying emotion. Although Cannon suggested that the central nervous system plays an important role, the controversy over the role of visceral feedback largely overshadowed this suggestion.

As early as 1937, Papez proposed a brain theory of emotion, arguing that the critical neural structures involved a circuit interconnection between the hypothalamus, the anterior thalamus, the cingulate gyrus, the hippocampus, the septa, and the amygdala. This circuit came to be called Papez's circuit, and all of the critical structures and fiber connections are part of the limbic system.

Damage to or electrical stimulation of a limbic system has been shown to produce a variety of changes in emotional behavior. For example, Hess (1957) found that stimulation of the hypothalamus in cats could produce rage and attack behavior. Studies by Bard (1948) showed that cats with hypothalamus damage seemed resistant to rage.

A very interesting series of studies by Kluver and Bucy (1937) revealed that monkeys with amygdala lesions showed a variety of emotional changes. In general, monkeys resist being approached by humans. However, following amygdala damage, the animals would allow humans to approach close enough to be touched. In addition to this, the animals were hypersexual.

In humans brain disease involving the temporal lobes causes a wide variety of emotional disturbances. A good example of this is the story of Tavi.

Tavi edited a suburban weekly magazine that was rapidly increasing in circulation. A journalist for 20 years, he had left his newspaper job to embark on this new venture. Saddened and discouraged through the months of the magazine's inception, he now looked forward, as circulation climbed, to adding more intellectual substance in the form of political commentary, book reviews, and a space for poems.

In the last few months his wife, Maria, had noticed great changes in him. He was irritable, easily aroused to argument. He displayed far more than his usual level of energy; in fact, he was positively manic. At times he would work day and night for 72 consecutive hours, sleep little, and then start the cycle again. Recently he had been keeping a journal, a bit late in life to start a diary, his wife thought, and too early to write his memoirs. But the magazine seemed to flourish as did his personal journal. Breakfast, a routine of reading the dailies for each of them, had become crowded with Tavi's notes which were pompous admonitions and homilies added to his journal.

Maria decided a vacation in the warm Caribbean islands and a rest would cure him. It was really a pipe dream, for his effort to record every experience and each inner feeling was now a major obsession. Hoping to divert him, she brought scores of books—being an avid reader herself—and for a while he focused on one of the recent conversion stories of a former corrupt government official. Suddenly he was obsessed, not only with his journal keeping but also with God. In fact, his journal notes became a record of personal conversations with God. Maria saw the sudden personality change as a real danger signal now, and she insisted they return home.

His strange behavior was becoming uncontrollable, and although he had always been affectionate, she now found his displays of fondness excessive and was even frightened by his insatiable libidinous urges. After another 72-hour episode of manic behavior he collapsed in an exhausted state and was taken to the hospital. The triad of hypergraphia, extreme religious stances, and hypersexual behavior indicated an affective (pertaining to emotion or a mental state) disorder and a manic state. His neurologic examination, including an evaluation of his mental status, revealed flight of ideas, pressured speech, and, as he regained full wakefulness, true mania. Further diagnostic procedures revealed an abnormal right ventricle. The ventricular system within the brain is the origin of the cerebrospinal fluid; it has a very specific configuration, and abnormalities in shape or size may indicate a tumor.

Tavi was treated with antimania drugs and antipsychotic drugs. The combination made him quite lifeless, without spunk or drive. He seemed to sleep all day. After two weeks the drug doses were decreased and he improved but did not assume his former agitated state. His condition was followed very closely with monthly outpatient visits and special brain scans. That temporal lobe tumors or seizures can cause strange behavioral phenomena was known, and remained highly suspect in Tavi's case.

It has often been reported that tumors or vascular disease of sudden onset in the temporal lobes can produce a cluster of behavioral changes as described above. Deepening of religious belief, or changing of religions, hypergraphia manifested by extensive note taking, and also increased sexual desire and activity can form the symptom complex of temporal lobe dysfunction. It is further important to remember that neural structures that are thought to be critical for emotional expression are part of the temporal lobe. The hippocampus and the amygdala are deep temporal lobe structures completing Papez's circuit.

Summary

Understanding emotion and motivation remains a major problem for brain and behavioral science. Motivation, you will remember, is the tendency to behave, and to understand motivation reliable predictions about those tendencies are necessary. Attempting to understand why, when, how long, or how vigorously we behave is a monumental task.

Behavior is often motivated by a perturbed homeostatic state. These homeostatic mechanisms attempt to balance the biochemical and physical chemical reactions of the body. Even vegetative behaviors of temperature control, drinking, and eating have extraordinarily complex biochemical systems. For example, the body temperature set at 98.6°F is a closely guarded value. In case of change, a thermostatic set point controlled probably in the hypothalamus signals peripheral mechanisms for action. Too much heat leads to peripheral vasodilation and loss of water through sweating. Too much cold leads to vasoconstriction and shivering. On another order of analysis, heat or cold can act as motivating factors for the organism to seek the homeostatic set point. We seek the shade of the willow by the lake on a hot day, and a cold day prompts the wearing of a coat and sweater.

The act of drinking reflects another of the body's rigorously defended homeostatic set points. Body volume and body tonicity (the balance of water and biochemical elements) are set very specifically, and deviation of only 3 percent in either direction motivates protective metabolic mechanisms to stabilize the internal environment.

Eating is more difficult to understand. Pat's experience of voracious appetite after removal of a tumor pressing on his hypothalamus is an example of this complexity, for the specific neural control of the motivation for hunger remains unclear. Much experimental work examines hunger in animals. Lesions of different parts of the hypothalamus are associated often with extraordinary changes in behavior, some even leading to starvation and death.

Consider the preoccupation of humans with eating and body weight, even those people not so extreme as Pat. The perpetual quest for thinness because of the inevitable state of fatness has made small fortunes for a number of diet theorists, but has consistently motivated only a very few to change their eating/hunger patterns. Even fewer become thin and stay thin.

Perhaps Tavi's striking behavioral changes are more difficult to understand, for neither hypergraphia nor hypersexuality involved homeostatic mechanisms. The sexual experience, some great thinkers believe, is the central core of human existence. This is not the place to debate the importance of sex; it most certainly is an important life experience. The motivation of sexual behavior remains a mystery. Study in animals of the relation between estrogen/androgen hormones and behavior provides clues for the human models. Brain stimulation experiments, more complete descriptions of brain anatomy, and neurochemical discoveries all contribute to the rapid but small steps forward to achieve some understanding of the interrelation of brain mechanisms and motivation.

References

Anand, B. K., and J. R. Brubeck. 1951. Localization of the feeding center in the hypothalamus of the rat. *Proc. Soc. Exp. Biol. and Med.* *77*:323–324.

Bard, P., and V. B. Mountcastle. 1948. Some forebrain mechanisms involved in expression of rage with special reference to suppression of angry behavior. *Res. Publ. Ass. Nerv. Ment. Dis.* *27*:362–404.

Buck, R. 1976. *Human Motivation and Emotion.* New York: Wiley.

Cannon, W. 1927. The James-Lange theory of emotions: A critical examination and alternative theory. *Amer. J. Psychol.* *39*:106–124.

Coons, E. E., M. Levak, and N. E. Miller. 1965. Lateral hypothalamus learning of food-seeking response motivated by electrical stimulation. *Science* *150*:1320–1321.

Delgado, J. M. R. 1969. *Physical Control of the Mind.* New York: Harper & Row.

Deutsch, J. A. 1971. Appetitive motivation. In: J. L. McGaugh, ed. *Psychobiology.* New York: Academic Press.

Gallistel, C. R. 1964. Electrical self-stimulation and its theoretical implications. *Psychol. Bull.* *61*:23–24.

Gallistel, C. R. 1969. The incentive of brain stimulation reward. *J. Comp. Physiol. Psychol.* *69*:722–729.

Hardy, J. D. 1960. The physiology of temperature regulation. U.S. Navy Bureau of Medicine and Surgery. Task, MR 995.15–2002.1.

Heath, R. G., ed. 1964. *The Role of Pleasure in Behavior.* New York: Harper & Row.

Hess, W. R. 1957. *The Functional Organization of the Diencephalons.* New York: Grune & Stratton.

Hetherington, A. W., and H. W. Ranson. 1940. Hypothalamic lesions and adiposity in the rat. *Anat. Rec.* *78*:149–172.

Hohmann, G. W. 1962. The effects of dysfunctions of the autonomic nervous system on experienced feelings and emotions. Paper presented at the Conference on Emotions and Feelings at the New School for Social Research. New York, October.

James, W. 1884. What is an emotion? *Mind* 9:188–205. (Reprinted in M. Arnold. 1968. *The Nature of Emotion*. Baltimore: Penguin Books.)

Keller, A. D. 1950. Thermal regulation. *Phys. Therapy Rev.* *30*:511–519.

Kenshalo, D. R., and J. P. Nafe. 1962. A quantitative theory of feeling. *Psychol. Rev.* *69*: 17–33.

Kinsey, A. C., W. B. Pomeroy, C. E. Martin, and P. H. Gebhard. 1953. *Sexual Behavior in the Human Female*. Philadelphia: Saunders.

Kluver, H., and P. C. Bucy. 1939. Preliminary analysis of functions of the temporal lobes in monkeys. *Arch. Neurol. and Psychiat.* 54:223–229.

Manning, A. 1967. *An Introduction to Animal Behavior*. Reading, Mass.: Addison-Wesley.

Mark, V. H., and F. R. Ervin. 1970. *Violence and the Brain*. New York: Harper & Row.

McEwen, B. 1976. Interaction between hormones and nerve tissue. *Sci. Amer.* *235*:48–67.

Money, J., and A. A. Ehrhardt. 1972. *Man and Woman, Boy and Girl*. Baltimore: Johns Hopkins University Press.

Murgatroyd, D., A. D. Keller, and J. D. Hardy. 1958. Warmth discrimination in the dog after hypothalamic ablation. *Amer. J. Physiol.* *195*:276–284.

Olds, J. 1958. Self stimulation experiments and differential reward systems. In: H. Jasper et al., eds. *Reticular Formation of the Brain*. Boston: Little, Brown.

Schachter, S. 1971a. Some extraordinary facts about obese humans and cats. *Amer. Psychol.* *26*:129–144.

Schachter, S. 1971b. *Emotion, Obesity and Crime*. New York: Academic Press.

Schachter, S. 1975. Cognition and peripheralist-centralist controversies in motivation and emotion. In: M. S. Gazzaniga and C. B. Blakemore. *Handbook of Psychobiology*. New York: Academic Press.

Schachter, S., and J. Singer. 1962. Cognitive, social and physiological determinants of emotional state. *Psychol. Rev.* *69*:379–399.

Sem-Jacobsen, C. W. 1968. *Depth-Electroencephalograph Stimulation of the Human Brain and Behavior*. Springfield, Ill.: Thomas.

Sheffield, F. D., J. J. Wulf, and R. Backer. 1951. Reward value of copulation without sex-drive reduction. *J. Comp. Physiol. Psychol.* *47*:349–354.

Teitelbaum, P. 1955. Sensory control of hypothalamic hyperphagia. *J. Comp. Physiol. Psychol.* *48*:156–163.

Teitelbaum, P. 1961. Disturbances in feeding and drinking behavior after hypothalamic lesions. In: M. R. Jones. *Nebraska Symposium on Motivation*. Lincoln: University of Nebraska Press.

Teitelbaum, P., and A. M. Epstein. 1962. The lateral hypothalamus syndrome recovery of feeding and drinking. *Psychol. Rev.* *69*:74–90.

Wrywicka, W., and C. Dobrzecka. 1960. Relationship between feeding and satiation centers of the hypothalamus. *Science* *132*:805–806.

Zeigler, H. P. 1973. Trigeminal differentiation and feeding behavior in the pigeon. *Science* *182*:1155–1158.

Zeigler, H. P., and H. J. Karten, 1974. Central trigeminal structures and the lateral hypothalamic syndrome in the rat. *Science* *186*:636–637.

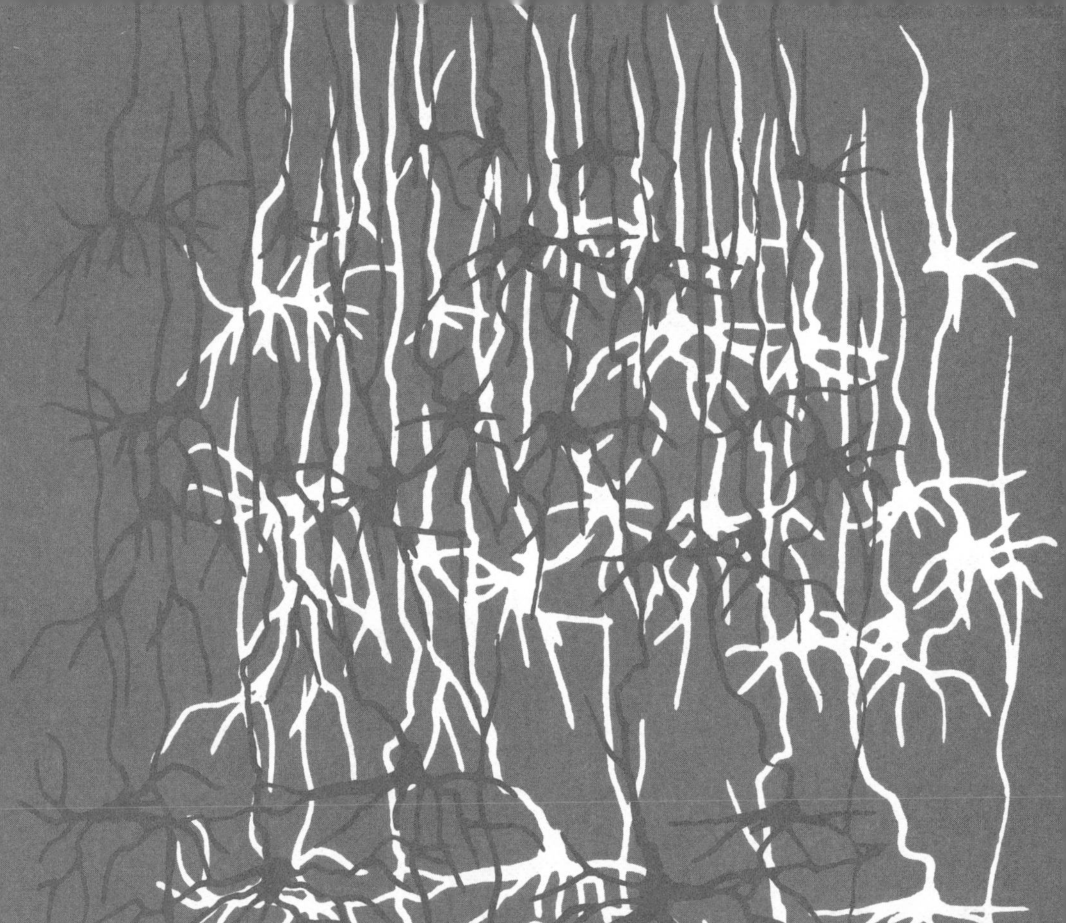

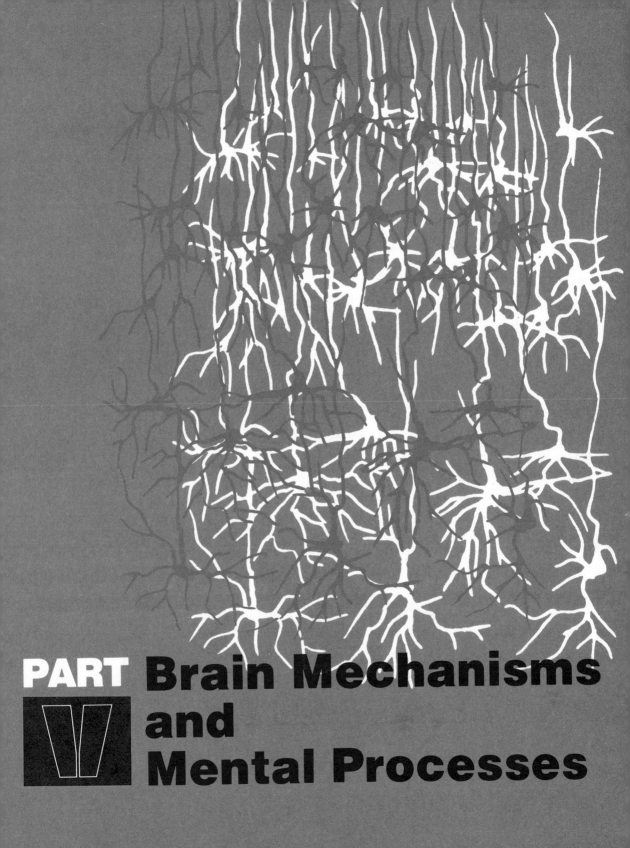

PART V Brain Mechanisms and Mental Processes

CHAPTER 12

The Biology of Learning and Memory

Another basic problem in neuroscience is the search for the physiological basis of the storage of information in the nervous system—the formation of memory, which necessarily accompanies any learning in an organism. The problem is one that has long baffled scientists. So far, neither the formation of memory in the learning process nor the storage and retrieval of memory can be explained. Consequently, disorders of memory remain something of a mystery.

A good example concerns Sandy, a 62-year-old surgeon who suffered a transitory stroke that disrupted the sight in the right halves of both eyes. He made a remarkable and complete recovery over a two-week period. Thus, within 14 days he went from normal cognitive functioning into a state that totally disrupted these processes and back again to normal functioning. The observations that are of special significance to the mechanisms of memory in this case have to do with the course of recovery commencing five days after the onset of the stroke. When a red carnation was held up in full view and the patient was asked what it was, he said, "flower." When asked what color, he said "red." But when the patient was asked what kind of flower, he was unable to say "carnation." Indeed, even when a list of names of familiar flowers was read aloud, he was still unable to make the match. This was true despite the fact that the patient's most active hobby was gardening. When the examiner finally said it was a carnation, the patient said the word aloud and accepted the assertion with equanimity. Then, spontaneously, the patient reached for the carnation, put it in his lapel, and smiled his satisfaction. On the following day, when the edema had subsided even more, thus making active more extensive brain areas, the patient was able to name all the flowers in the room (there was quite an assortment) with little or no difficulty.

At the same time in the recovery period, the patient asked about some flowers he and his daughter had planted "down by the road at the bottom of the hill." "What was that?" he asked. When the answer was given as Gazania, *a plant commonly known to him normally, he said, "Oh, Oh." Again, it seems that the category of specific names given to plants or flowers was not yet available for recall or recognition.*

These observations suggest that memory or engrams for things or events are multiply represented in the brain because the experiences themselves have multiple aspects.

Our concern here is with the questions of the neuropsychological and biochemical processes underlying the formation of memory. It is inevitable that the investigation of the neural basis for information has implications for the more macroscopic questions concerning human memory. For example, there is a continual evolution of the stored knowledge within the memory system as a human grows from childhood. This may have profound effects on the way that new information is acquired. The same new information may be encoded differently depending on whether a child or adult is involved.

There is no clear understanding of the continuum between storing a specific bit of stimuli and something like an internal representation of a fairly complex situation in the environment or the presentation of the more abstract human concepts. An integrated view of mental functioning and physiological processes will, at the least, require conceptual clarification of many of the psychologically distinct functions we attribute to the brain. These clarifications may come from the actual biochemical processes discovered in the brain.

Memory is intimately related to learning. The task of defining "learning" and "memory" precisely has been a confounding one for the psychological literature. Any study of the storage mechanisms responsible for memory is dependent upon changes in the nervous system due to the learning process during which it was instilled. We shall not attempt to make any sharp distinctions between the two, but rather will concentrate on what appear to be processes in the storage of information by vertebrate brains.

Memory as a Component System

Memory can have different durations. Remembering a phone number or a street address for a few seconds is quite different from some virtually permanent memories. A great deal of modern research essentially supports the idea that memories can be identified as having approximately three time courses and that different underlying processes may be responsible for them. These have been termed: Short-term sensory store (or iconic memory), which lasts a few seconds, short-term memory (STM), which has a duration measured in minutes, and long-term memory (LTM), which could last a lifetime. In the neuropsychological clinics iconic memory is tested by asking a subject to repeat a series of numbers. Of course, the examiner must remember the numbers too, and usually the examiner's phone number or social security number is used. Thus while the patient's iconic memory is being tested, so are the examiner's own long-term stores. Most individuals can successfully repeat seven numbers when given this test. As for short-term memory, the examiner will give the subject three familiar objects and a street address to remember. Then the subject will be asked to recall these objects and address in 5-minute intervals for the next 15 minutes. Long-term testing of memory is less formal, and conclusions are often drawn from simple interviewing.

The Consolidation Model

A very prominent theoretical framework for much of memory research is the *consolidation model of memory formation*, which states that information storage in the brain involves sequential processes (Figure 12.1). Consolidation refers to the idea that there is a short-term memory which can become permanent memory. The physiological bases for these two memories are also assumed to be two distinct processes that require a transitional neurochemical process.

It is quite clear that immediately following learning, memory is very susceptible to interference and loss, whereas older memories seem to be almost impervious to loss. Because of this shift in susceptibility, it has been postulated that the physiological basis of a given memory shifts from initial neurobiological processes with short lifetimes (e.g., electrical activity) to processes with long lifetimes (e.g., altered synaptic anato-

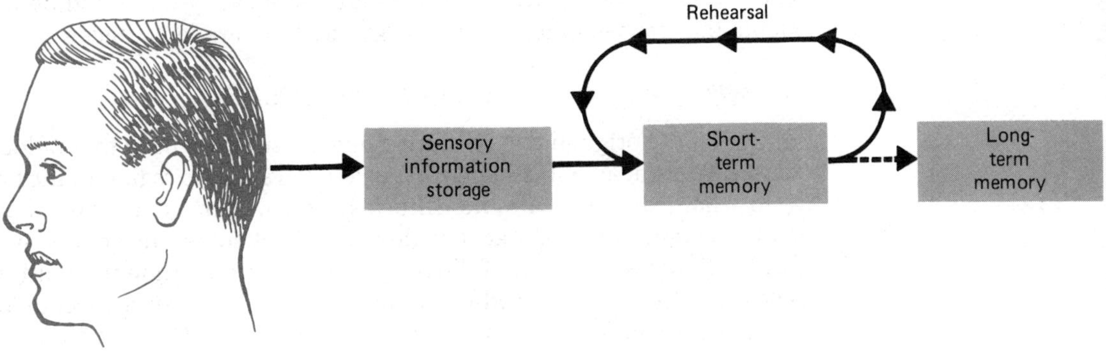

FIGURE 12.1 Information processing view of human memory. The division between the sensory systems and memory systems is not distinct; for instance, iconic memory or short-term sensory store can be viewed as part of either system. Rehearsal appears to allow material to be retained in short-term memory for an indefinite period of time and consequently to aid in its transfer to more permanent storage in long-term memory.

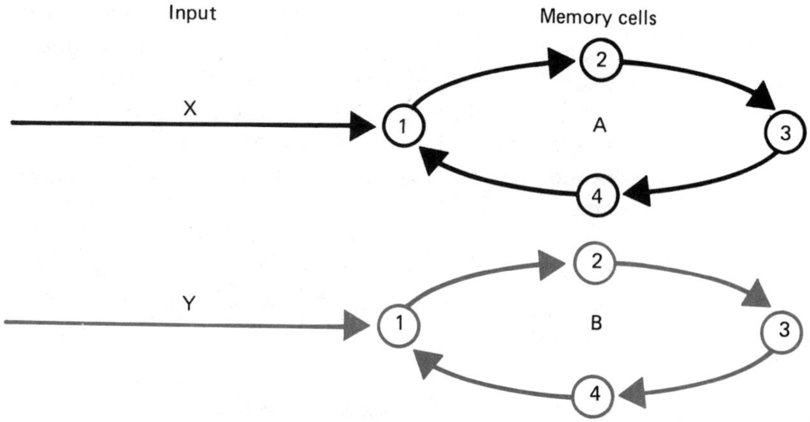

FIGURE 12.2 Model of simple reverberating circuits: A closed logo qualifies as a memory circuit in that a sensory stimulus at either X or Y initiates a sequence of electrical events around loop A or B that persists long after the original signal has stopped. Cell groups would actually be much larger and involve complex interacting patterns, which would give any specific memory a limited duration before disruption by adjacent or subsequent events.

my). Consequently, short-term memory has become associated with a reverberating neuroelectric circuit theory, easily disrupted by shocks (Figure 12.2). Long-term memory, on the other hand, is thought to entail some permanent change, involving protein synthesis and altered synaptic organization.

The evidence for successive processes comes from the fact that there are differential interference effects of drugs or electrical shock depending on when in the time course following learning they are administered. The earlier stages of these processes are more easily disrupted by treatments that cause amnesia, such as shock, than are later stages.

How Much of the Brain Is Important?

One of the original and still unresolved issues has been that of localization. To what extent is memory located in a specific region of the brain or to what extent is it a more diffuse system of storage utilizing a great deal of cerebral tissue? Karl Lashley (1950) set some precedents on the localization issue when, following extensive experiments with rats whose brains were lesioned in a systematic fashion with respect to location and size, he formulated his principles of *mass action* and *equipotentiality*. He concluded that memory was critically affected by the amount of cortex removed (principle of mass action), but did not depend on the area removed. In other words Lashley felt that all areas of the cortex were equally important for memory (principle of equipotentiality). He arrived at these conclusions because he was unable to reduce significantly a rat's performance on a learned task following small extirpation of brain tissue from any of a great many regions of the brain. However, in destroying a rather large portion anywhere he significantly affected the rat's "memory" of what it had learned.

Problems with Lashley's Principles

Lashley's conclusion that the engram – or the memory trace that must develop in the brain whenever learning occurs – cannot be localized remains generally true today. However, the principles of mass action and equipotentiality turn out to be much too simplistic. There is a great deal of modern knowledge that contradicts these principles. An example can be given from split-brain research.

A very general mass action principle is shown to be erroneous by a good deal of clinical evidence. One obvious piece of evidence is the fact that little impairment is evident in memory in either split-brain animals (Nakamura and Gazzaniga, 1974) or split-brain humans (LeDoux et al., 1977) when the subjects are tested in a manner in which only one hemisphere can perform the task (see Chapter 10). Yet two small discrete lesions within the inferior temporal lobes can alter learning quite radically. We see then a disconnection of an entire half a brain doing less harm to memory storage than, perhaps a specific 5 percent cortical lesion.

The principle of equipotentiality also makes little sense in light of the results of partially severing certain connections between the two hemispheres. In studies involving both monkeys and split-brain human patients (Gazzaniga and Freedman, 1973; Gazzaniga et. al. 1975) it was shown that rather dramatic differences were produced in the interhemispheric exchange of information, via sectioning specific sites of the interhemispheric commissures. This is not in keeping with the idea that all cortical areas are equipotential.

Memory as a More Diffuse Process

It is becoming more apparent from clinical human data (Gazzaniga, 1976) that the search for the engram should become more the search for the network that interconnects a variety of different processing systems, all contributing information to the reconstruction of past experience. The engram has been a hypothetical construct referring, in a loose way, to the physiochemical alterations that in some form must exist in the nervous system when there are changes in behavior and learning. It is very likely that the physiological basis for the notion of even the simplest type of memory involves the interaction of many systems incorporating biochemical changes in many specific areas of the nervous system. Memory, then, has aspects of a system of component parts that are widespread throughout the brain.

The Experimental Approaches

We know that all forms of learning must involve alterations somewhere between the input and the output of the central nervous system. All known forms of specific interactions between neurons occur at synapses. Therefore, it is assumed that the alterations we are searching for that are involved with memory involve some kind of changes at synapses. The obvious question is, what are the changes? Another question is, how do changes at many synapses interact to represent stored information?

The former question has become more or less the realm of the biochemical approach to memory—the search for specific changes in the chemistry of neurons and neuronal junctions. On the other hand, electrophysiological studies of electroencephalograms (EEGs), evoked potentials, and single-cell activity during behavior change attempt to uncover some of the more integrated aspects of cell activity in the formation of memory. Lastly, lesion studies in animals and clinical evaluation of brain-damaged humans also contribute a more macroscopic view of brain functions involved in memory.

All approaches obviously have to integrate and eventually present a consistent picture of what the physiological mechanisms behind learning and memory are. For example, neurochemical changes should map onto the structure of the brain in a manner consistent with the anatomical loci of memory-related electrical events.

Electrophysiological Studies: EEGs, Evoked Potentials, and Single-Unit Recordings

Investigating the relationships between electrical measures of brain activity and learning and memory has been both an active and a very disputed aspect of brain research (Figure 12.3). Most traditional studies of this type centered around EEGs and surface evoked potentials, both of which are measures of average responses of large populations of neurons.

A more recent and very promising approach involves recording, via microelectrodes, from single neurons. This is a very difficult technique, but it has the advantage of perhaps eventually being used side by side with biochemical studies, since the electrophysiological and biochemical processes are intimately related at the single-cell level, the electrical characteristics along a neuron's axon or at a synapse being determined by ionic and biochemical levels (Figure 12.4).

EEG's It has been shown (Chow, 1961) that EEG arousal occurs at the beginning of learning and diminishes as learning proceeds. Arousal is

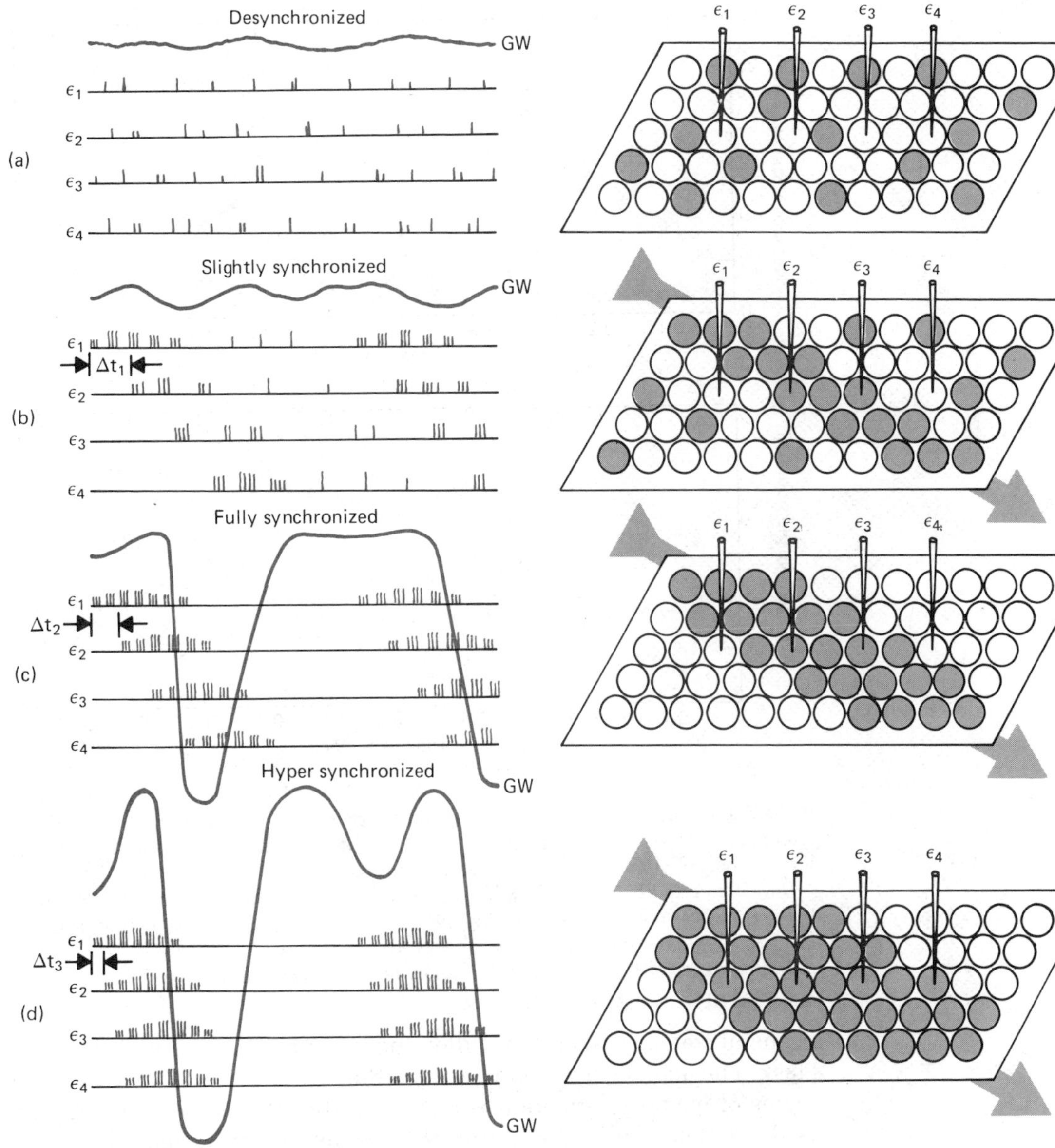

FIGURE 12.3 Some implied relationships between discharges of neurons and gross brain waves (EEGs). The left diagrams show discharges recorded from four very closely spaced microelectrodes (E_1, E_2, E_3, E_4) near the brain surface. The lines marked G.W. are oscilloscope tracings of the gross waves recorded from the scalp. On the right are hypothetical diagrammatic two-dimensional representations of the neuronal fields involved in the recording. E_1, E_2, E_3, E_4 represent the microelectrode positions and the circles represent individual neurons. The degree of darkness represents the degree of excitation of that neuron and the arrow represents the direction of neuronal activity. (From John, 1967.)

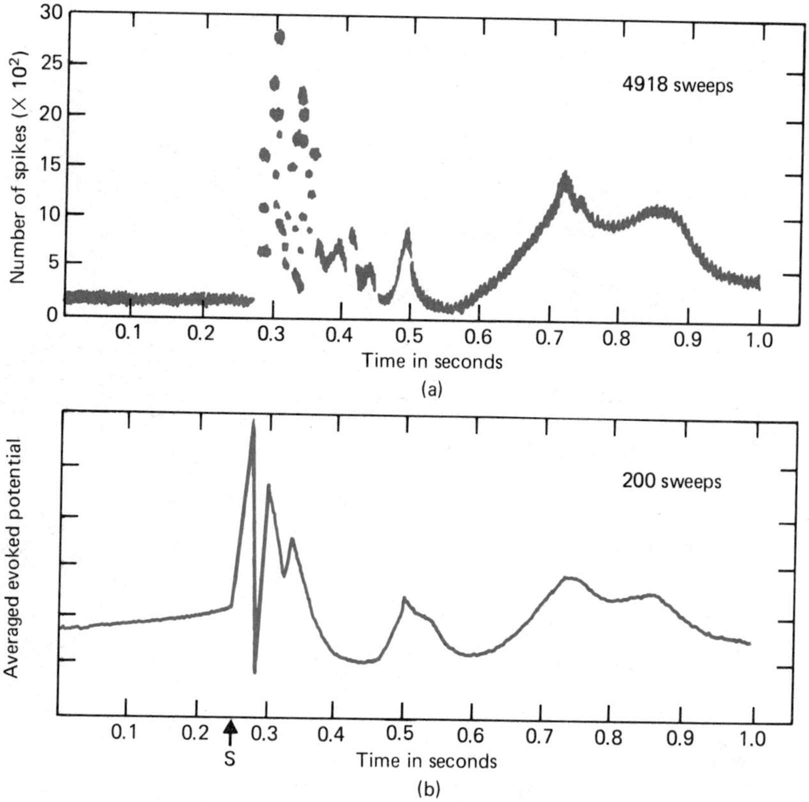

FIGURE 12.4 Implied relationship between the firing of a single neuron and an evoked potential waveform recorded from the same location. Diagram (a) shows a distribution during a period of one second recorded by a microelectrode of a neuron's action potentials in relationship to a light flash stimulation occurring at time marked S. The distribution was obtained by repeating the stimulation 4918 times. Diagram (b) shows the averaged (200 oscilloscope sweeps) evoked potential recorded from the same location with an electrode not located in any single live cell. (Data from Fox and O'Brien, 1965.)

a general state of wakefulness allowing the subject to focus attention on a task. The actual correlation between the degree of EEG arousal and the degree of memory formation is rather questionable at this time. A standard problem with interpreting the results of experiments involving memory formation is discerning between the general physiological processes ("performance variables") that occur during learning from those that actually involve changes in the memory store. At least to the extent it is understood now, EEG activity is too general an indicator of brain activity and is very likely an indicator of some of the performance variables that should be distinguished in our quest for the mechanisms of memory.

Evoked Potentials E. Roy John and associates have done a great deal of work with cortical evoked potentials and learning (Figure 12.5). John et al. (1973) carefully analyzed waveforms of evoked potentials in a series of learning experiments with cats. The cats were trained to make two different behavioral responses depending on which of two stimuli signals were presented. The cats learned to avoid a forthcoming shock by jumping a hurdle when a short-duration light flash was presented (an example of conditioned avoidance learning). They also learned to avoid a similar shock when a long-duration light was presented (conditioned lever press). Two different evoked potential waveforms were recorded from the scalp, each characteristic of the appropriate stimulus-response pair (see Figure 12.6).

What was most significant, however, was that when the animals made a wrong response, which they did at times even after they were considered well trained, the evoked potential waveform recorded was

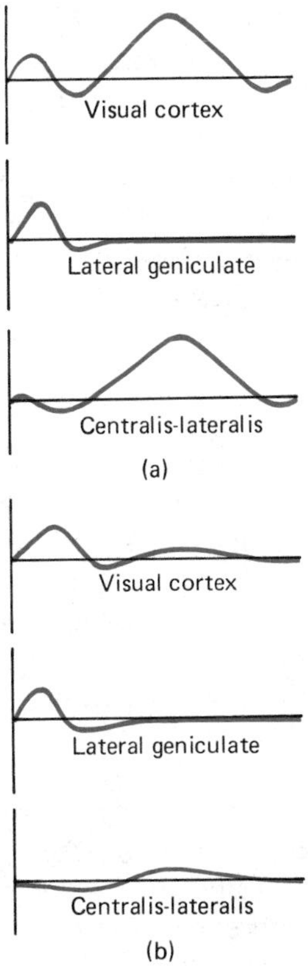

FIGURE 12.5 Some idealized examples of averaged evoked responses seen in different areas of the brain during a testing situation. Diagram (a) shows potentials during a correct response to a visual conditioned stimulus while diagram (b) shows evoked potentials in the same areas during failure of behavioral response to the signal. Note that there are two components to the waveforms in the visual cortex and nucleus centralis the second portions of which are attenuated (reduced in amplitude) during a failure-to-respond situation. The waveform of the lateral geniculate is simple and appears unaltered in the two situations. (From John, 1967.)

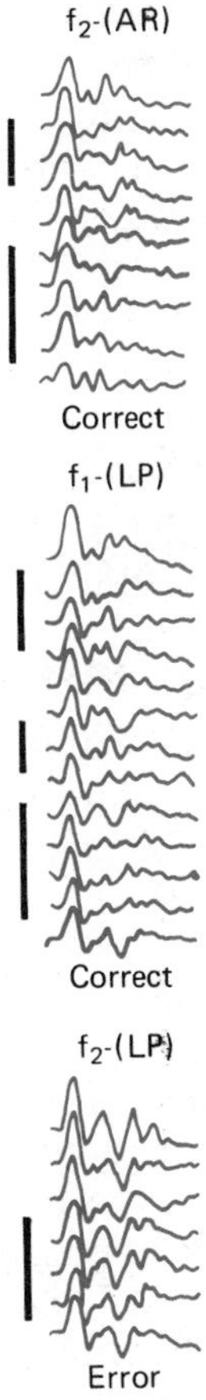

FIGURE 12.6 Waveforms of evoked potentials to light flashes of two different frequencies in cats trained to make different responses dependent on which stimulus was presented. An avoidance response (AR) was conditioned to stimulus frequency f_2, while a lever press (LP) was conditioned to a stimulus frequency f_1. Note that when they erred by responding to an f_2 stimulus with a lever press (LP), the waveform was similar to the f_1-(LP) waveform and thus characteristic of their behavior (LP) rather than the stimulus f_2 they observed. See text.

characteristic of their erroneous behavior rather than of the evoked potential waveform associated with the light stimulus they had been presented. In other words, one could determine from the evoked potential following the stimulus presentation which response the animal would make, and even predict errors. This made it clear that the evoked potential was not an indicator of the stimulus input into the organism but rather an indicator of a set of actions that had been learned by the organism.

John interprets these characteristic waveforms as "memory readout potential," which reflects a neural system of encoding learned behaviors via statistical ensembles of neurons. This is a "field theory" of learning as opposed to the more usual theories, which hold that more discrete and localizable changes are at the heart of learning. If memories are indeed sorted by statistical ensembles, then the engram will be even harder to identify or pinpoint. Not only does such a system require the most miniscule of changes at the single-neuron level, or even at the level of any particular region of the brain, but essentially it does not require any kind of structural "hard-wiring" changes to occur at all. Memories would be coded by complex interactions of diffuse groups of neurons, distinct only in terms of minute differences in firing probabilities. Such a system of memory can probably only be analyzed by examining firings of large populations of neurons over large regions of the brain. This, of course, would make the electrophysiological approaches the most fruitful in the study of memory.

There are, however, alternate explanations of the learned behavior linked waveforms that would make them less an indicator of memory processes, per se. The waveforms could, for example, reflect differences in motoric codes associated with the actual physical movements the animal prepares to make.

Synapses and Synaptic Changes

The search for the neural basis of learning involves looking for plasticity within the nervous system itself, that is, seeking out relatively enduring changes in neural function as a consequence of some experience of the organism or perhaps some manipulation of its nervous tissue. Neurons interact at synapses, and changes at synapses lead to changes in the ability of nerve cells to transmit information to one another. It is very likely, then, that learning involves the alteration of neural pathways through some type of biochemical effects at the synapses.

Hypothetical processes that might account for the modifications in activity of neuronal nets include: changes in the distance of the presynaptic and postsynaptic neurons at the synapse due to the outgrowth of axonal or dendritic processes; changes in the area of specific contacts between presynaptic and postsynaptic neurons due to expansion of the presynaptic axonal terminals or of the transmitter receptor sites on the

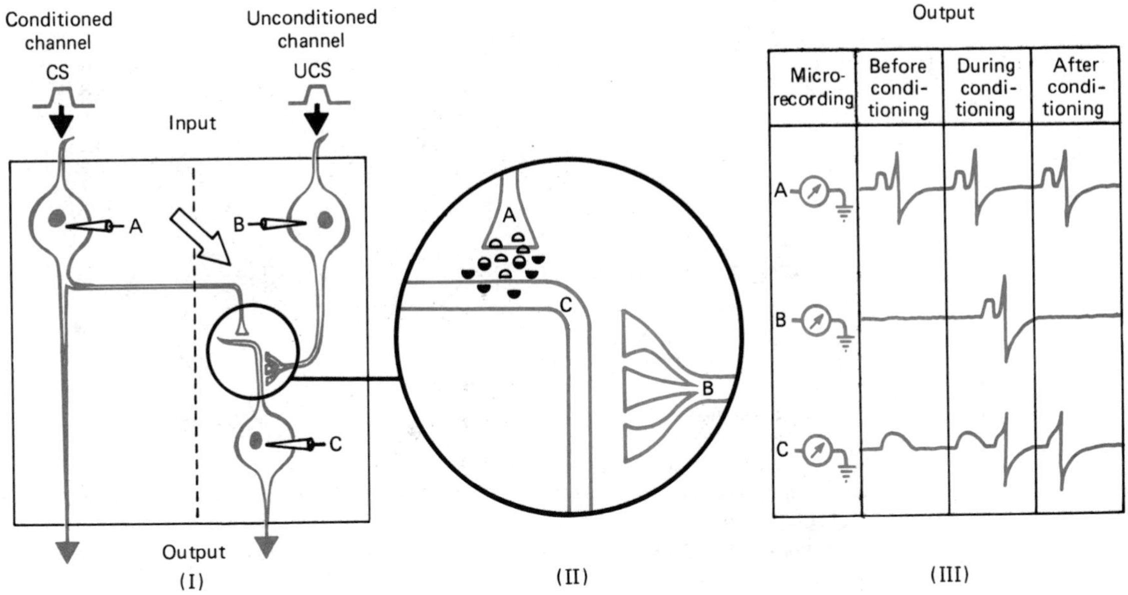

FIGURE 12.7 Classical conditioning of a single neuron and some possible synaptic changes underlying it. I is a schematic diagram of an experiment that has been performed on neurons of certain invertebrates. II is an expanded, essentially hypothetical view of the area outlined by the circle line in I. In I an electrical conditioning stimulus is applied to neuron A. The action potential produced causes a postsynaptic potential in neuron C (the recordings are shown in III) not quite sufficient to produce an action potential in C. The unconditioned stimulus is a shock applied to neuron B and the consequent action potential produced in B is sufficient to raise C to threshold and produce another action potential. If A and B are repeatedly stimulated in the above order, it turns out that after a while C becomes "conditioned" to spike in response to stimulation of neuron A above, which it did not do at first. In II it is hypothesized that the transmitter released by A (open half-circles) reacts with a substance released by the postsynaptic neuron C (dark half-circles) every time it is discharged by B. The combination of these neurochemicals is thought to induce changes in the membranes and thereby increase synaptic efficiency. (From Berlucchi and Buchtel, 1975.)

postsynaptic membrane; changes in the synthesis and release of the transmitter substance by the presynaptic neuron; changes in the transmitter binding action of the postsynaptic neuron (Figure 12.7) (Berlucchi and Buchtel, 1975).

There are many other possibilities. It is still not known how synaptic changes are brought about. Many seem to occur simply as a result of development (see Figures 12.8 and 12.9), and there is a great deal of evidence that they occur in certain learning situations. There has also been anatomical evidence of branching in cortical nerve cells and changes in synaptic spine density as a result of rather extreme environmental situations (Figure 12.10).

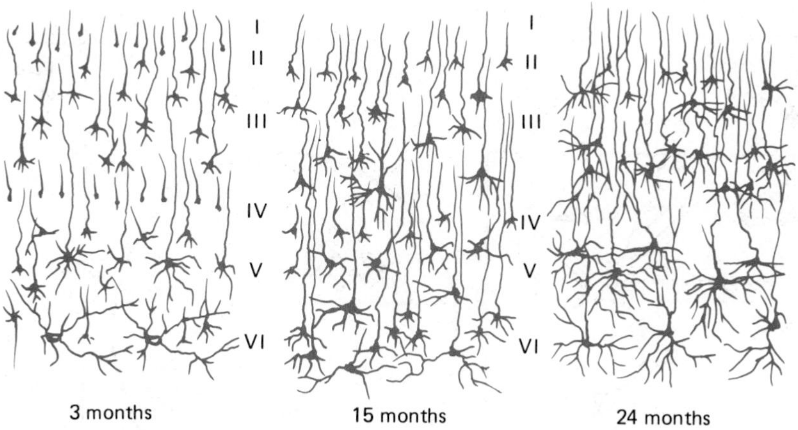

FIGURE 12.8 Tracings of pyramidal cells of human cerebral cortex. Sections were taken from human children aged 3, 15, and 24 months. The numerals I–VI mark the cortical layers. Note the branching of neurons and density of dendritic spines with increasing age. (From Hirsch and Jacobson, 1975. Based on work of Conel, 1939–1963.)

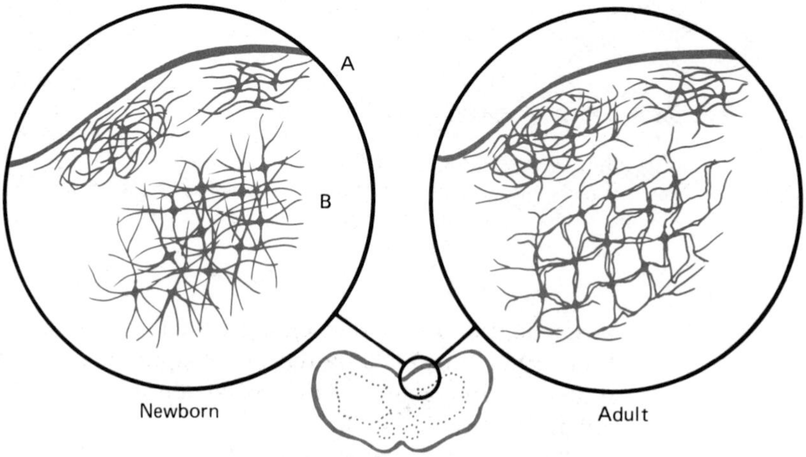

FIGURE 12.9 Dendrite arrangement in the reticular formation of the medulla of newborn and adult cat. The regions A and B of the newborn are characterized by radiating dendrites with many spinelike growths. In the adult the dendrites appear to have been rearranged; they are now grouped in tightly packed bundles around myelinated longitudinally running axons. (From Scheibel and Scheibel, 1973.)

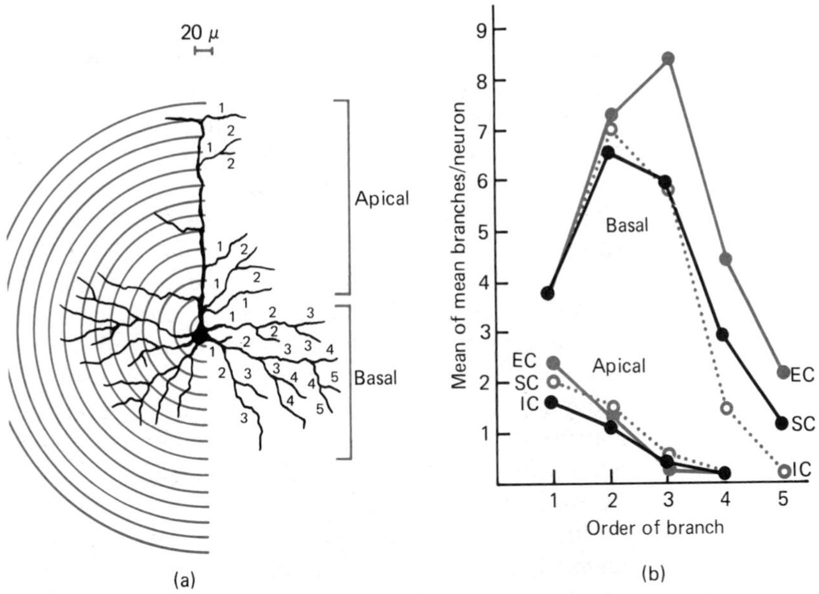

FIGURE 12.10 (a) Analysis procedures for camera drawing of stained neurons. The concentric rings on the left side of the neuron drawing are used for recording the number of intersections with dendrite per ring. The right side shows branches numbered in terms of their order away from the cell body. (From Greenough, 1976.) (b) Mean number of branches at each order away from the cell body (basal, upper diagram) and from apical dendrite (apical, lower diagram) in three sets of rats reared under different conditions: complex (EC), social (SC), isolated (IC). (From Greenough, 1976.)

A recent study (West and Kemper, 1976) reports a decrease in synaptic spine density and reduced dendritic length in rats kept on a low-protein diet from birth. Diet can also affect memory in humans. The story of Smithie illustrates one aspect of nutrition and its effect on the brain.

During his younger days Smithie played the blues. His horn was the hottest on the river, and he had been the performer who packed all the clubs after the Great War, though the culture changed rapidly, too rapidly for Smithie. Not only did the music change, but the towns expanded up and down the river, leaving few interesting places for clubs amidst planned recreational and boating facilities. He was not ready to leave the magnetic force of the river culture in which he was raised, and he stayed while others left to seek fortunes in the coastal cities. Staying meant finding a new job, for without audiences his play was only for friends and his own pleasure. Jobs for unskilled men were scarce and ordinary living expenses were often overwhelming. But that was 20 years ago, and the real problem that had recently developed was his failing memory.

In the past few months Smithie suffered a progressive behavioral change most prominently characterized by a memory defect. This defect reflected Smithie's inability to incorporate any new information into his store of old knowledge, and was expressed by his frequent fanciful response to questions whose answers he did not know. This response is called confabulation. Asked to remember three unrelated but familiar objects, such as rubber ball, turkey, and umbrella, he responded one minute later with colors of the rainbow, and further insisted that color naming was the object of the memory test. Incapable of retaining anything more than a fleeting impression of immediate circumstances, he continually sought to atone for his lacunae (memory gaps) by denying what was affirmed. Lacking all insight into his repeated errors, he showed remarkable self-assurance when his denials were challenged.

In addition to this inability to incorporate new experiences into his memory, Smithie could no longer properly sequence the order of past events. Temporal foreground and background merged into one and resulted in the juxtaposition in his stories of temporally unrelated events. On being introduced to a new person, for example, Smithie asserted he had met the man before, although that had never occurred. When this man denied such a meeting Smithie persisted by noting the alleged time and place; he even went on to describe the dress of each of them and the prevailing weather conditions. This remarkable unfolding was a jumble of past and present, and was simply not true. He was blind to the obvious contradictions.

It became clear that Smithie suffered from Korsakoff's psychosis, a syndrome named after the Russian who drew attention to it in 1890. Smithie had an inability to record accurately new events, he confabulated the details of recent experiences and mixed up time sequences for remote events, and he was quite disoriented in time and place. When he was confronted with his memory inconsistencies he was unconcerned. General apathy and indifference rounded out Smithie's behavioral picture. A severe disorder of his peripheral nerves added to his clinical syndrome. Decreased sensitivity to all sensory modalities, especially in his lower limbs, caused him great difficulties in walking. The disorder did not just affect sensation, for Smithie was weak too, especially in his legs.

Korsakoff, long ago, recorded that the cause of this strange memory disturbance and peripheral nervous disorder was due to alcohol in over 60% of the cases. The aggravating factor was not so much the consumption of alcohol, he thought, as it was the neglect of vital nutrients required by the brain. Smithie was no exception. Although other causes—

metabolic, infectious, toxic, hematologic, inflammatory—were considered, none was supported by the historical evidence. Filling in the story of the last 20 years, Smithie's landlady identified the frequent, all too frequent she was quick to add, presence of bourbon bottles in the garbage. Treatment for this sad old man was intramuscular administration of thiamine (vitamin B_1), oral B complex vitamins, and adequate diet. But symptoms of memory deficits would not respond well, and Smithie would be left with his rather significant impairment.

Proteins and Neurotransmitters: The Search for the Chemistry of Memory

The search for the engram on the molecular level has involved implicating at various times one or more of a number of biochemicals as responsible for memory storage. Theories have been put forth suggesting that activity of specific neurotransmitters, such as acetylcholine (ACh), represents memory stores. The macromolecules, such as DNA, RNA, proteins, and glycoproteins have been the object of even more investigation. Neurotransmitters have been considered due to their obvious role in trans-synaptic communication of neurons. The macromolecules have been considered as having major roles in the biological processes underlying memory storage because they are principal components of cell structure and are involved in genetic control mechanisms and cell differentiation. These biochemicals are likely candidates for the process of relating the changed structure of neurons and synapses to memory encoded events, but it is unlikely that any of these substances alone can be the basis of the engram.

It is often claimed that transmitters or proteins simply do not last long enough to be very likely candidates for a permanent memory store. Proteins are continuously formed and replaced in the metabolic processes of all cells, so any particular protein molecule usually exists for less than a month. The final chemical changes of state that store long-term memory must be stable and long lasting. However, it is not clear whether this implies that the molecules involved in a memory must themselves be stable or that the stability resides in a self-regenerative system in which the longevities of the particular molecules are unimportant.

It is perhaps more plausible to search for changes in the processes or codes that generate the proteins; these would be more permanent. In this respect, at least, RNA seems a more likely candidate for the biochemical basis of permanent memory. Actually, it is more in keeping with our original postulate that learning involves changes in the interactions among neurons at synapses, if we were to assume that certain RNA and protein changes are part of a mechanism that alters synapses. If, for example, a memory involved forming a new synapse, there could be a turnover of all the molecules involved in forming that synapse. Once formed, the biochemical events would subside leaving the structural form of the synapse.

Neurotransmitters in Memory

Acetylcholine (ACh) was originally thought to be the primary neurotransmitter involved in the memory process, and the fact that it was the only well-characterized transmitter significantly contributed impetus to such theories. Studies similar to the rich vs. poor environment used in rat experiments showed increases in brain ACh levels (Rosenzweig, 1970) as well as in the number of central nervous system dendritic synapses which is not surprising if the particular synapses use ACh as transmitter. This group of experiments showed that rats living in very rich environments, where they had much to do, had an increase in the number of dendritic spine synapses on neurons in the cortex.

There have also been many experiments using pharmacologic agents to increase or decrease the amount of centrally active ACh. In training animals for approach avoidance conditioning and appetitive tasks, this work suggests that increased ACh aids performance and decreased ACh hinders performance. These results have been applied to human concepts of memory. Recent experiments by Drachman (1977) performed on young healthy human volunteers suggest that memory can be disrupted by pharmacologic interference, specifically by blocking ACh with anticholinergic drugs. Neuropsychological memory tests, well standardized over many years of use, were administered to test and control groups of young people before and after anticholinergic drug administration. The anticholinergic treated groups revealed significant decrease in performance levels after drug treatment. Further testing included the administration of different antidotes that reversed various effects of the anticholinergic. Strikingly, memory performances improved with the antidote that specifically increased ACh levels. Memory did not improve with other, less specific antidotes.

This same group of investigators has performed extensive neuropsychological testing on aged volunteers. The pattern of the multiple test scores appears to have certain similarities to the results obtained from testing the group of young, healthy volunteers who received anticholinergic drugs (that decrease ACh levels). All of these results suggest the memory decline seen in normal human aging may be a function of ACh activity. Implications for memory research from these observations in animal and human experiments have provided great promise for the future.

Proteins in Memory

It is more or less assumed within the context of the consolidation view that long-term memory is coded by structural change at synapses. As we mentioned earlier, although protein synthesis would seem to be necessary for almost any fairly permanent change in the nervous system, it is likely that there is a structural change subsequent to protein synthesis. It is prudent to examine protein synthesis in terms of a necessary event within a larger and as yet unknown process, rather than to assume that protein synthesis is the actual storage process of memory (Figure 12.11).

DNA In light of the now well-known sequence in the metabolism of nucleic acids and of proteins, it was natural for some studies to attempt linking memory formation with brain DNA because of its genetic role in the control of metabolism and its great stability (Reinis, 1972). There is little evidence, however, that the function of brain DNA is in any way distinct from that of any other organ, and it was shown in certain studies (Casola et al., 1969) that inhibition of brain DNA synthesis apparently does not impair memory formation.

RNA Much data strongly suggest that changes in RNA metabolism are associated with general stimulation at the behavioral level (Glassman, 1974). RNA level changes have also been found in experiments involving more specific stimulation at the cellular level. Holger Hydèn has done extensive work on RNA synthesis associated with learning situations.

Hyden pioneered some refined neuroanatomical techniques for analysis of biochemical events in single cells. Most biochemical analysis requires quite large tissue samples, so consequently the data concern reactions over thousands or millions of cells. Hyden attempted to separate, for example, certain large neurons (Deiters' cells) from their companion glial cells by microdissection techniques. Using the techniques, he found that RNA was lost from neurons and later replenished from glial cells during certain animal training tasks (Hyden, 1967).

Inhibitors of RNA synthesis have been shown to affect long-term memory formation. Actinomycin D was shown by Agranoff (1968) to impair long-term memory but to have minimal effects on short-term memory. These studies have never been clearly interpreted, however, because actinomycin D is known to have complicating side effects and because it appears that blockage of RNA metabolism does not cause complete amnesia. It was recently suggested (Wetzel, 1976) that actinomycin D has no direct influence on the consolidation of memory, but rather that its intoxicant effects interfere with retrieval.

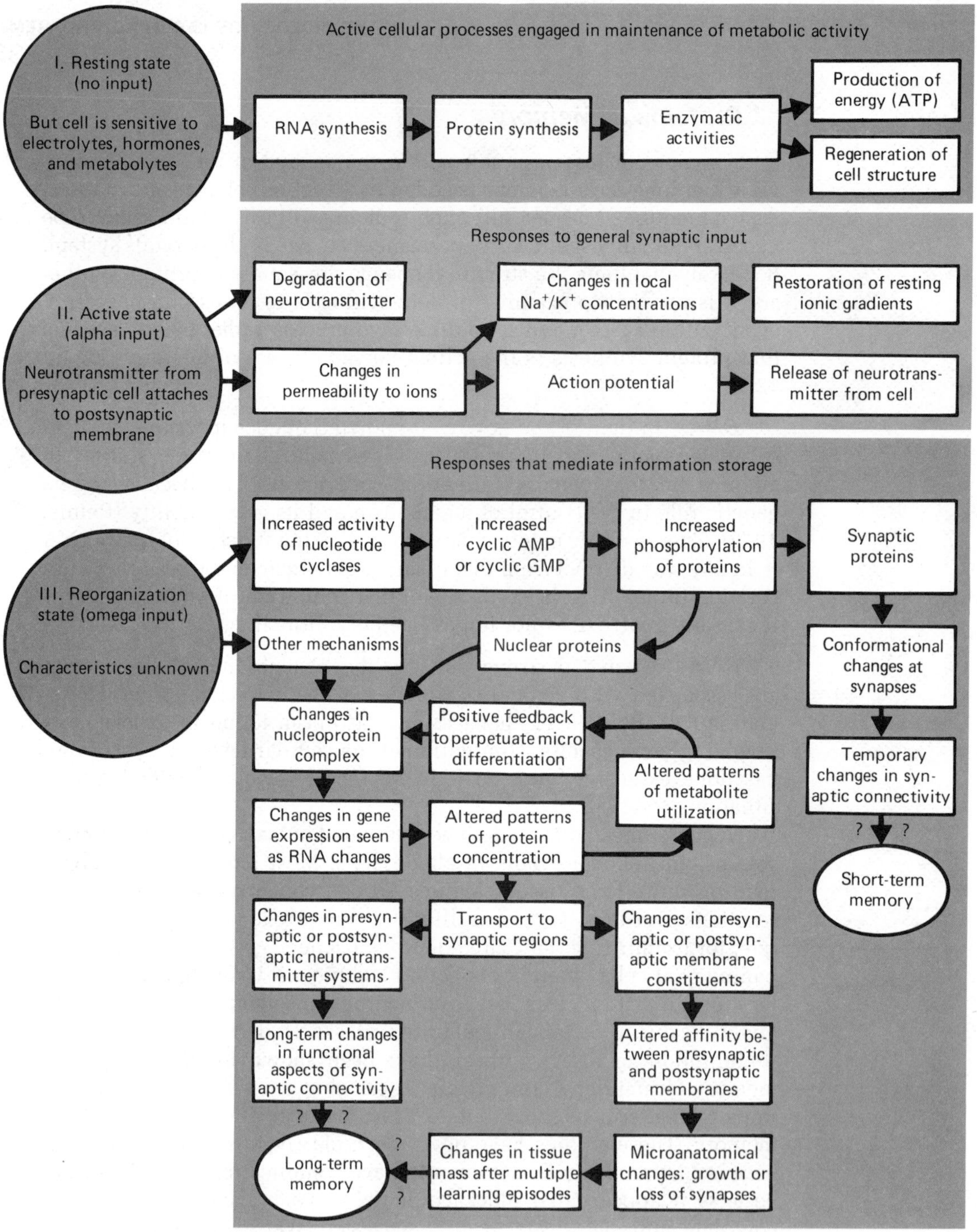

FIGURE 12.11 A perspective of some of the changes in brain metabolism that have been reported to occur after stimulation. The resting state consists of "ground state" continually occurring cellular processes. Processes associated with the active state can occur at any time. The reorganization state consists of all processes by which a neuronal cell can alter its functional relationship with its neighbors. This scheme assumes that information is stored in altered relationships between neurons and that such reorganization is accomplished at the level of individual neurons. (From Entingh et al., 1975.)

Inhibiting Protein Synthesis

Many biochemical studies of long-term memory have used drugs that interfere with protein synthesis. This is in contrast to those studies aimed at short-term memory, which test the effects of drugs that more directly affect synaptic transmission, in keeping with the postulate that short-term memory involves temporary electrical activity.

The drugs used in most protein synthesis inhibition studies have been the antibiotics puromycin, cycloheximide, and acetocycloheximide (Figure 12.12). The use of these for interfering with protein synthesis is not free from confounding side effects, though cycloheximide appears to be fairly specific and reliable. In addition, it seems that protein synthesis must be severely inhibited for the amnestic defect to appear. The brain has a high metabolic "ground state" level of protein synthesis independent of any learning situation. It would seem reasonable that severe inhibition of this synthesis would result in various and complicated impairments of function. The problem of determining relation-

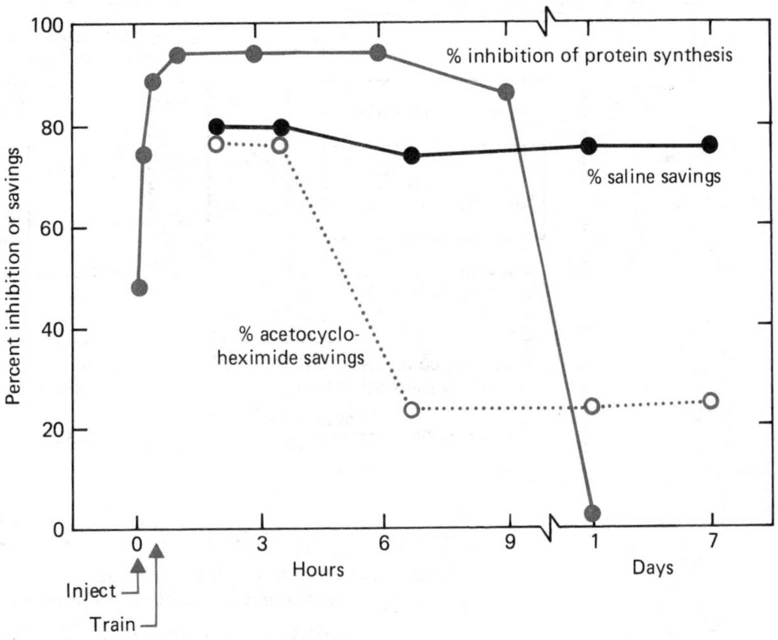

FIGURE 12.12 The effects of acetocycloheximide on protein synthesis and retention of learning in mice. The mice were injected with the inhibitor prior to being trained in a shock avoidance task. Different groups were tested for retention at the indicated times following training. The partially dotted line shows the decline in protein synthesis as the drug takes effect. The solid line shows the decline in degree of retention of the task ("memory") vs. that of saline injected controls (dotted line). (From Barondes and Cohen, 1969.)

ships between protein structure changes (and/or protein turnover) and the storage of information in the nervous system is extremely subtle.

It has been shown (Wallace, 1975) that poorly learned responses are more susceptible to inhibitory drugs than those retained after a great deal of training. The longer the training, the less effective the amnesia that is produced by subsequent drug administration. In addition, it appears that the longer the injection is postponed after training, the more areas of the brain require injection of inhibitor to produce memory deficits. This can be interpreted as suggesting the involvement of more and more neural pathways of neuroanatomical locations as a task is well learned.

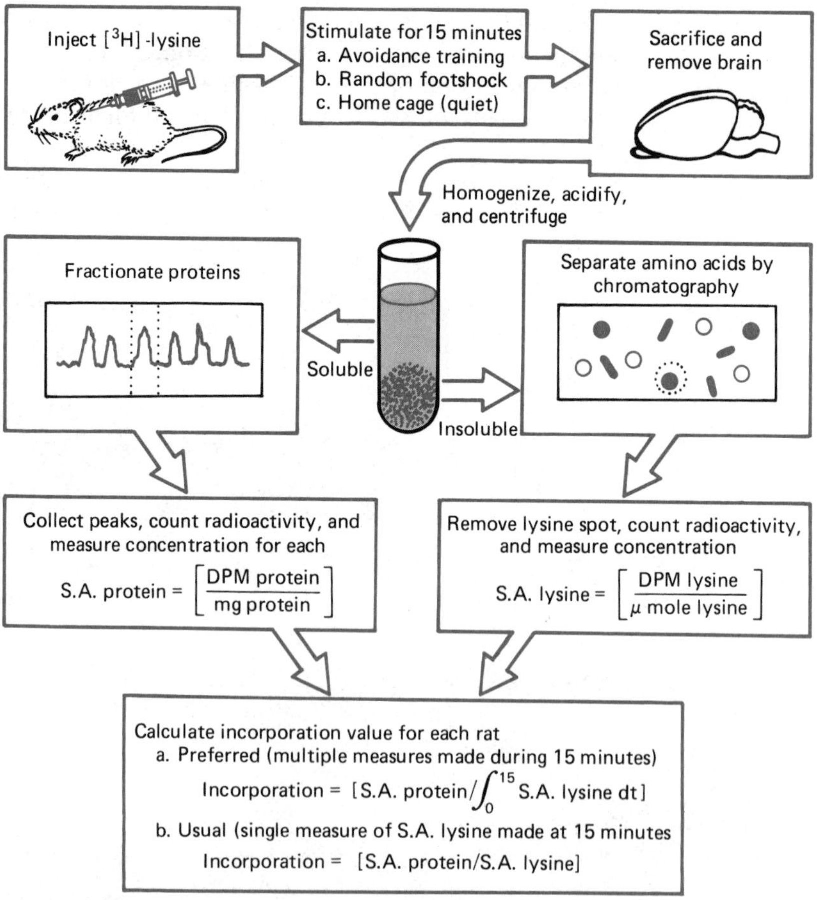

FIGURE 12.13 The general plan of an experiment studying protein synthesis through the use of autoradiography. The goal in this example is to determine if avoidance training changes the rate of incorporation of a radioactive amino acid, (^{3} H)-lysine, into specific protein groups. The "random footshock" and "home cage (quiet)" groups are controls. (From Entingh et al., 1975.)

Tracing Protein Synthesis During Learning

Reports of changes in protein metabolism induced by training have been plentiful, and there is broad agreement that cerebral protein metabolism can be altered by behavioral input (Entingh et al., 1975). The more recent studies rely on radioactively labeled proteins and amino acids as tracers in identifying specific macromolecules and structures involved in learning and memory formation (Figure 12.13).

Investigators (Popov et al., 1976) have used these microautoradiographic techniques to study the role played by constituents of glycoproteins or neuronal surfaces in regulating interneuronal synaptic relationships. They used radioactively labeled L-fucose, which is a specific carbohydrate precursor to glycoprotein synthesis, to study changes in these macromolecules during learning and memory formation. Their data showed some rather specific modifications in protein patterns in the hippocampus of trained rats, as opposed to a lack of such change in controls. This kind of evidence supports the idea that memory formation and storage involve the structure of specific macromolecules that in some way alter neuronal connectivity in distinct brain regions.

Another recent example of autoradiographic techniques is the work of Shashoua (1976), who identified specific changes in protein synthesis during a novel training situation. He isolated new template RNA molecules, used in protein synthesis, in goldfish that had been forced to learn to swim upside down by attachment of floats! Shashoua apparently determined a critical period during which macromolecular synthesis necessary for long-term memory occurs. He used two radioactive tracer versions of the amino acid leucine to isolate a protein structure formed during the learning period. Shashoua admits, however, that this is only correlational evidence of the mediation by protein synthesis of information storage in the central nervous system.

Arousal and the Transition of Short-term Memory to Long-term Memory

There is evidence that the maintenance of a level of arousal is necessary for the transition from STM to LTM to occur (Gibbs, 1976). Amphetamine and other stimulating drugs may have an influence on the consolidation of STM into LTM by increasing arousal, so the STM trace remains activated for a longer time span (Figure 12.14).

If indeed a maintenance of level of arousal is important, then the role of some endocrine system substances may be involved in consolidation. The pituitary gland manufactures neuropeptides, analogues to the adrenocorticotropic hormone (ACTH), that appear to be involved in the acquisition and maintenance of new behavior patterns. Neuropeptides have been correlated with a number of animal discrimination tasks and

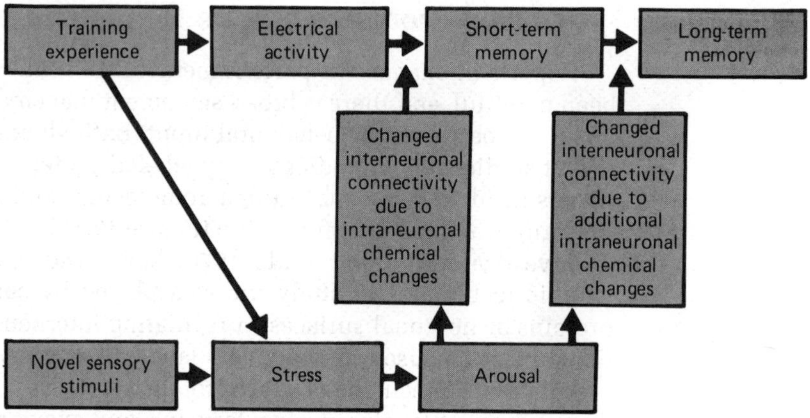

FIGURE 12.14 A schematic diagram showing some possible interrelationships between stimulation, arousal, and memory formation. (From Glassman, 1974.)

with the facilitation of memory retrieval after amnesia induced by electroconvulsive shock (ECS). The sites of activation appear to be in the limbic system, particularly the hippocampus which is normally a target for ACTH action. Electrophysiological studies suggest that neuropeptides exert an excitatory action that facilitates transmission in the limbic system. This may increase the state of arousal in these structures and also determine the motivational influences of sensory stimuli. The latter may increase the probability of generating responses to stimuli.

The transition process and neurochemical arousal have been explored by Flood and associates (1975). It was shown that a great many factors can increase the duration of memory-related protein synthesis. Variables such as training trials, amount of shock, rates of acquisition, and amount of practice seem to determine the amount of amnesia that can be subsequently caused by protein synthesis inhibitors. Flood postulates that any of these factors achieves an increase in the duration of memory-related protein synthesis due to sustaining arousal in the organisms.

Memory and Biochemical Approaches

The biochemical approach to memory may end up being integrated with other methods at a certain level of analysis. It will provide the study of the ways in which neurochemical responses within specific cells are related to the electrophysiological and anatomical organization of brain tissue networks. Biochemistry can serve as the bridge between stimulation induced changes in electrophysiological events and the much slower changes detected in anatomical structure.

Chemical findings will eventually be interpreted with respect to brain function through neuroanatomic correlations with other information about memory mechanisms. The work of tracing neurochemical responses to stimulation onto neuroanatomical structures has barely begun. There are not sufficient data really to localize memory systems in a specific set of brain loci. It is also not yet possible to distinguish between diffusely represented and highly localized storage systems.

Memory systems might very well have great duplicity at multiple neuronal networks, each participating within the same region of the brain. Memory could also be redundant in a manner that involves different neuroanatomical nuclei. We shall deal with these possibilities in the next section.

Localization of Memory: Macroscopic views from Lesion Studies and Clinical Data

We turn now to a very classic question in memory research—that of where in the brain do mnemonic processes occur? Most of the data we shall deal with concern either lesion studies of animals or human brain damage clinical data, simply because this kind of evidence has always had obvious bearing on "where" questions and because there appears to be a great deal to be learned about the "hows" of memory at this level of analysis. As we have said, tracing neurochemical responses onto neuroanatomical structures has barely begun, and much electrophysiological data could stand for more evidence of the neuroanatomical situation behind the measurements.

The Hippocampus as a Memory Site

The limbic system is thought to have a significant role in memory consolidation and storage. In particular, a number of lines of evidence have implicated the hippocampus as functionally active during learning. Some examples are as follows:

Humans with hippocampal lesions have tremendous difficulties with long-term memory—they have an apparent inability to form any but the simplest long-term memory (Penfield and Milner, 1958; Douglas, 1967).

Damage to the hippocampus in rats retards learning of active avoidance tasks (Olton and Isaacson, 1968). It has also been noted that during such learning in normal rats there are changes in hippocampal protein metabolism.

Electrophysiological measurements have shown increased theta wave (EEG) activity in the hippocampus during periods following training (Landfield et al., 1972).

It seems obvious that the hippocampus plays some role in the processes having to do with memory formation; however, it is not clear from any of these data that it is the locus of memory storage. It could, for example, play some information processing role prior to the storage of memory elsewhere in the brain (Entingh et al., 1975).

There are other reasons that make claims of evidence for storage sites such as those for the hippocampus questionable. In fact, there are reasons that perhaps make memory claims for any specific anatomical locations or even single neural processes too simplistic. We shall suggest these shortly.

One way to approach the question of localization of memory is to determine what portions of the central nervous system have the capacity to sustain the plastic changes associated with learning. It turns out that after surveying much of the literature dealing with extirpation of various portions of brains of animals, one comes to the conclusion that all sections of the nervous system can sustain forms of learning including habituation and classical conditioning, although in many test situations it is difficult to test operant conditioning for the reason that the surgery leaves only very limited sensory inputs or motor responses available.

Some Evidence from Amnesic Syndromes

A vast amount of clinical data indicates that even massive lesions to the human brain do not result in a clearly defined loss of long-term memories, as opposed to a loss of access to such memories. Most losses of past memories are impermanent. Various clinical agnosias represent memory losses in the sense of failures of recognition. Since the agnosias are limited to a particular modality such as visual agnosia, where there is an inability to recognize visually presented objects (Geschwind, 1965), it is easy to conceive of these disorders as demonstrating loss of access.

Even the harsh memory disruption of amnesia due to temporal lobe damage does not convincingly show in a true obliteration of long-term memories (Rozin, 1976) (Figure 12.15). Nor is it found, as might be expected from present knowledge of hemispheric specialization, that verbal memories are in the left or dominant side and nonverbal memories in the right. Hippocampal damage, which as we have said produces serious problems with long-term memory, still does not cause any complete obliterations (Rozin, 1976). Lastly, as we mentioned earlier, there is almost a surprising lack of any loss of old memories in either hemisphere of a split-brain human patient.

Some suggestion of localization of long-term memories comes from the literature on epilepsy cases and from reports by Penfield and associates relating to stimulation of the brain during surgery (Penfield and Roberts, 1959; Penfield and Perot, 1963) (Figure 12.16). Before removing

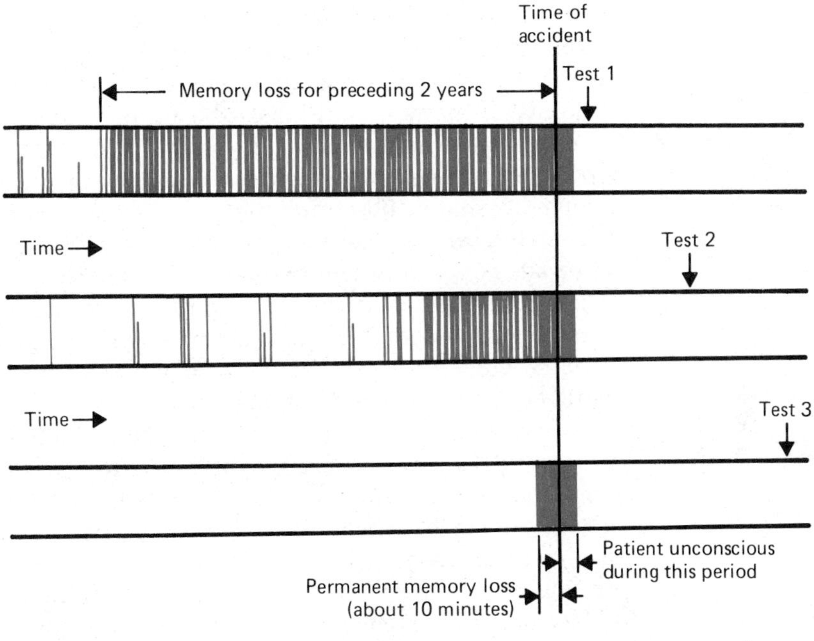

FIGURE 12.15 Typical recovery phase for amnesia victims. (From Lindsay and Norman, 1972, after data from Barbizet, 1970.)

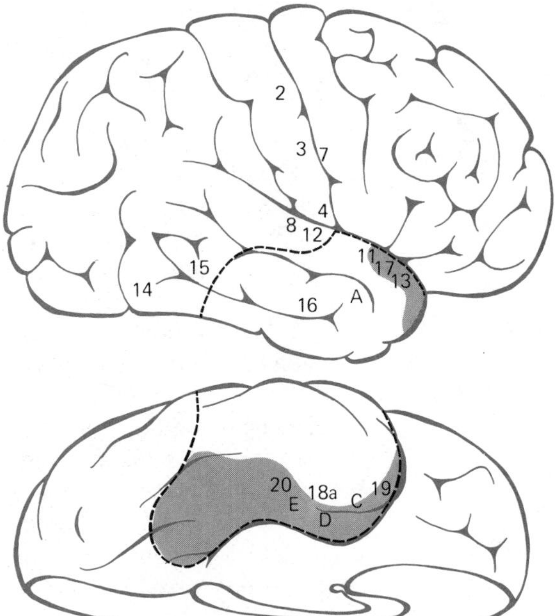

FIGURE 12.16 Diagram of stimulation sites (numbers), sites of epileptogenic discharges (letters), and extent of subsequent surgical removal of the temporal lobe of case M. M. of Penfield. Stimulation of point 17 yielded the following exclamation by the patient: "Oh, a familiar memory in an office somewhere. I could see the desks. I was there and someone was calling to me—a man leaning on a desk with a pencil in his hand." Subsequent removal of tissue (within broken line) resulted in cessation of seizures and no apparent memory loss. (From Penfield and Roberts, 1959.)

diseased tissue they electrically stimulate the patient's brain at various points in the diseased region for purposes of locating the pathology. They have reported behaviorally interesting responses from stimulation of points in the temporal lobes, the hippocampus, and the amygdala. Patients at times report visual or auditory memories and claim that these experiences are very vivid—like living them over again. They typically involve hearing or observing the action or speech of others or hearing music. However, excision of the whole area around these behaviorally active sites does not seem to erase any memories.

It has been said that most memory impairment consequent to local brain damage, in both animals and man, is not so much a removal of localizable engrams as an interference with the mechanisms that code neural events so as to allow storage and retrieval.

A somewhat different interpretation stems from the view that memory is multiply represented in the brain (Gazzaniga, 1976). Any particular experience has multiple aspects to it, and these are stored at a variety of sites in the cerebrum. Our model predicts that recalling an old experience in the presence of new brain damage may be accompanied by a breakdown in aspects of the experience. Specific lesions would "turn off" local neural processes that normally would contribute those specific aspects to a total recall.

Mitch was a talented actor/singer and worked almost all the time, an acid test for anyone in the performing arts. When he was not acting or singing he designed and constructed wigs and costumes for the opera. But he once admitted that the only reason he designed wigs was that he liked the idea of being called a perruquier *(wigmaker). That remark typified his cynical, sarcastic manner, which formed a thin but protective veneer for his true gentle nature. No matter, for the theater was his life and for 30 of his 50 years he was a constant feature of the neighborhood where all the performers lived.*

During one week last year he had a remarkable experience. He suffered total amnesia for an entire day. He had just finished a long run in the hilarious role of Nankipoo in The Mikado, *and had switched immediately the following day to finish the wigs for the opening of* La Boheme *when his troubles began. He appeared at the opera and went down to the subbasement workrooms. He worked through the entire afternoon; no one suspected that his recent memory was about to become completely disordered. As his colleagues gathered for late afternoon coffee, Mitch turned and wondered out loud, "What am I doing here?" Knowing him as they all did, they thought this statement was the beginning of a typical actor's lament. What followed, however, was more confusion, and a glazed but sincere look came over Mitch that suddenly caused fear in them all. He had no memory of any of the events of the afternoon. He did not remember working on the wigs, had no idea how he had arrived at the opera house, and did not even remember the raves of the closing performance last evening. When carefully questioned, the last events he remembered were from eight days earlier. He remembered his name, recognized familiar faces, and remembered names, but with difficulty. He easily performed dressing tasks and insisted on finishing his coffee before being taken to the hospital. He had no pains, especially no headache, and some believed this was all a hoax.*

At the hospital he was no better, and with the rush of unfamiliar surroundings and people he seemed to plunge deeper into confusion. In fact, he could not remember his doctor's face or name from one moment to the next. The examiner once walked out of the room to answer a page call from the operator. The doctor returned to find that Mitch had forgotten all the prior social interaction. Orientation to time and person had not been disturbed, but there was clearly an amnestic (related to amnesia) gap that started hours before while he was working and extended back over the last eight days of Mitch's life. Of important note was lack of seizure, headache, head trauma, or any other symptom of neurologic impairment, except for total amnesia for recent events. Otherwise, the exam was completely normal.

Mitch's electroencephalogram revealed bilateral episodic theta activity (2–5 cps), but gave no evidence of seizure activity. Theta activity represents slowing of the usual brain wave frequency and is a common finding in total global amnesia. The other possibilities of vascular insufficiency or blood vessel blockage consisting of microscopic showers of clots traveling to his brain were made untenable by other diagnostic maneuvers. Unfortunately, no one understands the pathogenesis of total global amnesia. In the many reported cases it appears benign. Mitch was no exception. By the following day the retrograde amnesia was clearing and his recent memory was improving. The EEG changes were also improving with return of normal, faster frequencies called alpha (8–13 cps) and beta (greater than 13 cps). Immediate memory and long-term memory beyond the eight-day gap had never been disordered and remained intact. Recurrences of episodes such as this are uncommon, and for that Mitch remained thankful.

The mysterious occurrence and similarly mysterious disappearance of Mitch's memory disorder are indicative of the problems facing those involved in memory research. Human memory research in general is an extensive endeavor, encompassing approaches that range from purely psychological studies of individual differences between human subjects, to the models postulated by cognitive psychologists to explain how information is processed into complex relationships, to searches for biochemical changes that occur in the brain during learning.

Summary

The recognition of the biochemical basis of memory remains a mystery for modern investigators. Biochemical approaches include the study of neurotransmitters. Here the focus on acetylcholine activity in animal and human experiments has produced some tantalizing results. Study of macromolecules, especially RNA and protein synthesis, may provide the key to permanent memory.

There are many difficulties though, including the very nature of the experimental design. Pharmacologic manipulation leads to troublesome side effects, the control of which is sometimes impossible. Presently unobtainable, ultimate proof that any specific neurochemical process is involved in memory storage requires that the actual information contained in the memory can be decoded through study of the biochemical changes in the appropriate set of neurons.

Electrophysiologic approaches, the EEG, and more recently the specific evoked potential have produced startling results. Correlations of electrophysiologic results with biochemical changes may be the integrated approach necessary for more complete descriptions of memory mechanisms. Of course, the behavioral variables must also be carefully controlled. But it is evident that more than just the reception and storage of a stimulus is involved in memory. Retention may possibly be the complete history of the experience. The events that Sandy suffered suggest that single events are multiply represented in the brain, perhaps because events themselves have multiple aspects. The dramatic example of Sandy placing the carnation in his lapel, even though he could not name the flower, vividly suggests multiple neural representation of objects. Retention does not deal with just a bit or piece of experience, but rather a whole pattern. *Memory does not have one site, nor is it a completely diffuse process spreading evenly throughout neural tissue.* It may be a complete series of impressions recorded in all the specific structures of the brain necessary to the perception of the original experience. The task of finding the engrams of even the simplest human memories seems more complex than ever in that it may involve uncovering the complete cerebral processing system with which humans deal with the environment.

References

Adair, L. B., J. E. Wilson, J. W. Zemp, and E. Glassman. 1968. Brain function and macromolecules. III. Uridine incorporation into polysomes of mouse brain during short term avoidance conditioning. *Proc. Nat. Acad. Sci.* 61:917–922.

Agranoff, B. W. 1968. Actinomycin-D blocks formation of memory of shock-avoidance in goldfish. *Science* 158:1600–1601.

Barbizet, J. 1970. *Human Memory and Its Pathology.* San Francisco: Freeman.

Barondes, S. H., and H. D. Cohen. 1968. Arousal and the conversion of "short-term" to "long-term" memory. *Proc. Nat. Acad. Sci.* 61:923–929.

Beach, G., M. Emmens, D. P. Kimble, and M. Lickey. 1969. Autoradiographic demonstration of biochemical changes in the limbic system during avoidance training. *Proc. Nat. Acad. Sci.* 62:692–696.

Berlucchi, G., and H. A. Buchtel. 1975. Some trends in the neurological study of learning. In: M. S. Gazzaniga and C. Blakemore, eds. *Handbook of Psychobiology.* New York: Academic Press.

Campbell, B. A., and X. Coulter. 1976. The ontogenesis of learning and memory. In: M. R. Rosezweig and E. L. Bennett, eds. *Neural Mechanisms of Learning and Memory.* Cambridge, Mass.: M. I. T. Press.

Casola, L., Lim, R. E. Davis, and B. W. Agranoff. 1969. Behavioral and biochemical effects of intracranial injection of cytosine arabinside in goldfish. *Proc. Nat. Acad. Sci.* 60: 1389–1395.

Chow, K. L. 1961. Anatomical and electrographical analysis of temporal neocortex in relation to visceral discrimination learning in monkey. In: J. F. Delafresnaye, eds. *Brain Mechanisms and Learning.* Oxford: Blackwell.

Conel, J. L. 1939–1960. *Postnatal Development of the Human Cerebral Cortex.* Cambridge, Mass.: Harvard University Press, Vols. 1–60.

Damstra-Entingh, T., D. J. Entingh, J. E. Witson, and E. Glassman. 1974. Environmental stimulation and fucose incorporation into brain and liver glycoproteins. *Pharmacol. Biochem. Behav.* 2:73–78.

Doty, R. W. 1969. Electrical stimulation of the brain in behavioral context. *Ann. Rev. Psychol.* 20:289–320.

Douglas, R. I. 1967. The hippocampus and behavior. *Psychol. Bull.* 67:416–442.

Drachman, D. A. 1977. Memory and cognitive function in man. Does the cholinergic system have a specific role? *Neurology* 27:783.

Dunn, A., D. Entingh, T. Entingh, W. H. Gispen, B. Machlus, R. Perumal, H. D. Rees, and L. Brogan. 1974. Biochemical correlates of brief behavioral experiences. In: F. O. Schmitt and F. G. Worden, eds. *The Neurosciences: Third Study Program.* Cambridge, Mass.: M. I. T. Press.

Entingh, D., A. Dunn, E. Glassman, J. E. Wilson, E. Hogan, and T. Damstra. 1975. Biochemical approaches to the biological basis of memory. In: M. S. Gazzaniga and C. Blakemore, eds. *Handbook of Psychobiology.* New York: Academic Press.

Flood, J. F., E. L. Bennett, A. E. Orme, and M. R. Rosenzweig. 1975. Effects of protein synthesis on memory for active avoidance training. *Physiol. and Behav.* 14:171–184.

Fox, S. S., and J. H. O'Brien. 1965. Duplication of evoked potential waveform by curve of probability of firing of a single cell. *Science* 147:888–890.

Gazzaniga, M. S. 1973. Brain theory and minimal brain dysfunction. *Ann. N. Y. Sci.* 205: 89–92.

Gazzaniga, M. S. 1976. The biology of memory. In: M. R. Rosenzweig and E. L. Bennett, eds. *Neural Mechanisms of Learning and Memory.* Cambridge, Mass.: M. I. T. Press.

Gazzaniga, M. S., and H. Freedman. 1973. Observations on visual processes after posterior callosal section. *Neurology* 23:1126–1130.

Gazzaniga, M. S., and D. H. Wilson. 1975. Neuropsychological observations following complete and partial commissurotomy. *Neurology* 25:10–15.

Geschwind, H. 1965. Disconnexion syndromes in animals and man. Parts I and II. *Brain* 88.

Gibbs, M. E. 1976. Effects of amphetamines on short term protein-independent memory of day-old chickens. *Pharmacol. Biochem. and Behav.* 4:305–309.

Glassman, E. 1974. Macromolecules and behavior: a commentary. In. F. O. Schmitt and F. G. Worden. eds. *The Neurosciences: Third Study Program.* Cambridge, Mass.: M. I. T. Press.

Greengard, P. 1976. Possible role of cyclic nucleotides and postsynaptic action of neurotransmitters. *Nature 260*:101–108.

Greenough, W. T. 1976. Enduring brain effects of differential experience and training. In: M. R. Rosenzweig and E. L. Bennett, eds. *Neural Mechanisms of Learning and Memory.* Cambridge, Mass.: M. I. T. Press.

Hebb, D. O. 1949. *The Organization of Behavior.* New York: Wiley.

Hirsch, H. V. B., and M. Jacobson. 1975. The perfectible brain: principles of neuronal development. In: M. S. Gazzaniga and C. Blakemore, eds. *Handbook of Psychobiology.* New York: Academic Press.

Huston, J. P., and A. A. Borbély. 1973. Operant conditioning in forebrain ablated rats by use of rewarding hypothalamic stimulation. *Brain Res. 50*:467–472.

Hyden, H. 1967. Biochemical changes accompanying learning. In: G. C. Quarton, T. Melnechuk, and F. O. Schmitt. *The Neurosciences: A Study Program.* New York: Rockefeller University Press.

Hydén, H., and P. W. Lange. 1968. Protein synthesis in the hippocampal pyramidal cells of rats during a behavioral test. *Science 159*:1370–1373.

John, E. R. 1967. *Mechanisms of Memory.* New York: Academic Press.

John, E. R., F. Bartlett, M. Schimokochi, and K. Kleinman. 1973. Neural readout from memory. *J. Neurophysiol. 36*:893–929.

Kelly, P. T., and M. W. Luttges. 1976. Combined electroconvulsive shock and cycloheximide inhibition of brain protein synthesis. *Behav. Biol. 17*:219–224.

Kimble, G. A. 1961. *Conditioning and Learning, 2nd edition.* Englewood Cliffs, N.J.: Prentice-Hall.

Landfield, P. W., J. L. McGaugh, and R. J. Tusa. 1972. Theta rhythm: a temporal correlate of memory storage processes in the rat. *Science 175*:87–89.

Lashley, K. S. 1950. In search of the engram. In: *Symp. Soc. Exp. Biol.*, No. 4. London: Cambridge University Press.

LeDoux, J. E., G. L. Risse, S. P. Springer, D. H. Wilson, and M. S. Gazzaniga. 1977. Cognition following commissurotomy. *Brain 100*:87–104.

Lindsay, P. H., and D. A. Norman. 1972. *Human Information Processing.* New York: Academic Press.

Machlus, B. 1971. Phosphorylation of nuclear proteins during behavior of rats. Ph.D. thesis. University of North Carolina, Chapel Hill, N.C.

Machlus, B., D. Entingh, J. E. Wilson, and E. Glassman. 1974. Brain phosphoproteins. *Behav. Biol. 10*:63–73.

Markel, E., and G. Adam. 1969. Learning phenomena in mesencephalic rats. *Acta Physiol. Acad. Sci. Hungaricae 36*:265–276.

McBride, W. J., J. W. Hingtgen, and M. H. Apreson. 1976. Neurochemical correlates of behavior: levels of amino acids in four areas of the brain of the rat during drug-induced behavioral excitation. *Pharmacol. Biochem. and Behav.* 4:53–57.

McConnell, J. V. 1962. Memory transfer through cannibalism in planarium. *J. Neuropsychiat.* 3(Suppl. 1):542–548.

Milner, P. M. 1960. Learning in neural systems. In: M. C. Yovits and S. Cameron, eds. *Self-organizing Systems.* New York: Pergamon Press.

Nakamura, R. K., and M. S. Gazzaniga. 1974. Reduced information processing capabilities following commissurotomy in the monkey. *The Physiologist 17*:294–295.

Norman, D. 1969. *Memory and Atention: An Introduction to Human Information Processing.* New York: Wiley.

Oakley, D. A. 1971. Instrumental learning in neodecorticate rabbits. *Nature 233*:185–187.

Olton, D., and R. L. Isaacson. 1968. Hippocampal lesions and active avoidance. *Physiol. and Behav.* 3:719–724.

Penfield, W., and B. Milner. 1958. Memory deficit produced by bilateral lesions in the hippocampal zone. *Amer. Med. Assoc. Arch. Neruol. and Psychi.* 79:475–497.

Penfield, W., and P. Perot. 1963. The brain's record of auditory and visual experience. A final summary and discussion. *Brain 86*:595–696.

Penfield, W., and L. Roberts. 1959. *Speech and Brain Mechanisms.* Princeton University Press.

Perumal, R. 1973. Phosphorylation of synaptosomal proteins from mammalian brain during short-term behavioral experiences. Ph.D. thesis. University of North Carolina, Chapel Hill, N. C.

Popov, N., W. Pohle, H. L. Ruthrich, S. Schulzeck, and H. Matthies. 1976. Time course and disposition of fucose radioactivity in rat hippocampus: a biochemical and microautoradiographic study. *Brain Res. 101*:283–293.

Rees, H. D., et al. 1974. Effect of sensory stimulation on the incorporation of radioactive lysine into protein of mouse brain and liver. *Brain Res. 68*:143–156.

Reinis, S. 1972. Autoradiographic study of ^{3}H-thimidine incorporation into brain DNA during learning. *Physiol. Chem. and Phys.* 4:391–397.

Roitbak, A. I. 1970. A new hypothesis concerning the mechanisms of formation of the conditioned reflex. *Acta Neurobiol. exp. 30*:81–94.

Rosenzweig, M. R. 1968. Brain functions. *Ann. Rev. Psychol.* 19:55–98.

Rosenzweig, M. R. 1970. Evidence for anatomical and chemical changes in the brain during primary learning. In: K. H. Pribram and D. E. Broadbent, eds. *Biology of Memory.* New York: Academic Press.

Rozin, P. 1976. The psychobiological approach to human memory. In: M. R. Rosenzweig and E. L. Bennett, eds. *Neural Mechanisms of Learning and Memory.* Cambridge, Mass.: M. I. T. Press.

Russell, I. W. 1971. Neurological basis of complex learning. *Brit. Med. Bull. 27*:278–285.

Scheibel, M. E., and A. B. Scheibel. 1973. Dendrite bundles in the ventral commissure of cat spinal cord. *Exp. Neurol. 39*:482–488.

Seaman, J. G., and M. S. Gazzaniga. 1973. Coding strategies and cerebral lateralization effects. *Cognitive Psychol.* 5:249–256.

Shashoua, V. E. 1976. Brain metabolism and the acquisition of new behavior: I. Evidence for specific changes in the pattern of protein synthesis. *Brain Res. 111*:347–364.

Spencer, W. A., and R. S. April. 1970. Plastic properties of monosynaptic pathways in mammals. In: G. Horn and R. A. Hinde, eds. *Short-term Changes in Neural Activity and Behavior*. London: Cambridge University Press.

Ungar, G. 1970. Role of proteins and peptides in learning and memory. In: G. Ungar, ed. *Molecular Mechanisms in Memory and Learning.* New York: Plenum Press.

Verzeano, M. 1963. Las funciones del sistema nervioso; correlaciones entre estructura bioquimica y electrofisiologica. *Acta Neurol. Latinoam* 9:297–307.

Von Baumgarten, R. J. 1970. Plasticity in the nervous system at the unitary level. In: F. O. Schmitt, ed. *The Neurosciences, Second Study Program.* New York: Rockefeller University Press.

Wall, P. D. 1970. Habituation and post-tetanic potentiation in the spinal cord. In: G. Horn and R. A. Hinde, eds. *Short-term Changes in Neural Activity and Behavior.* London: Cambridge University Press.

Wallace, P. 1975. Neurochemistry: Unraveling the mechanism of memory. *Science 190*: 1076–1078.

West, C. D., and T. L. Kemper. 1976. The effect of a low protein diet on the anatomical development of the rat brain. *Brain Res. 107*:221–237.

Wetzel, W., T. Ott, and H. Matthies. 1976. Is actinomycin D suitable for investigation of memory processes? *Pharmacol. Biochem. and Behav.* 4:515–519.

CHAPTER 13

States of Awareness

Fluctuations in levels of awareness are common. We may be groggy upon waking up, assume some semblance of alertness after a cup of coffee, perhaps function well during the morning hours, and then lapse into a postlunch slump before regaining alertness during the late afternoon. Depending on our habits, we may choose to alter our level of awareness during the evening hours, using a drug such as alcohol or marijuana. Eventually drowsiness overtakes us and we drop off to sleep, slipping into yet another level.

Defining states of awareness is not an easy task. First, one must stipulate what is meant by awareness, or consciousness (in this chapter we shall use the terms interchangeably). Briefly, consciousness implies an ability to function mentally, "the expression and awareness of an aroused mind" (Plum and Posner, 1966). Levels of consciousness, or states of awareness, include periods of decreased mental functioning, such as when a person is asleep, as well as mental activity that is outside the average realm of experience, such as meditation.

In this chapter, we shall look at physiological factors that are indicants of different levels of awareness and deal with anatomical and physiological features that are thought to be responsible for changes in levels of awareness.

In the first section, we shall look at one of the major methods for determining mental functioning: the electroencephalogram. Then we shall look at the reticular formation, the major brain area involved in gross changes in levels of awareness. Sleep and dreaming cycles will be discussed next, followed by a discussion of normal cycles of alertness. Finally, we shall briefly look at some altered states of awareness, including meditation, hypnosis, and the effects of some drugs. While in this chapter we certainly cannot cover all the levels of awareness between alert wakefulness and unconsciousness, we can at least sample some of the stages along the continuum (see Figure 13.1).

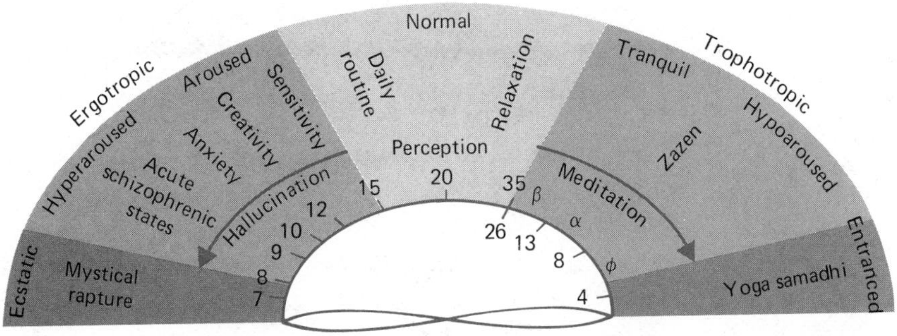

FIGURE 13.1 States of awareness range from the most highly excited and alert states to the almost semiconscious meditative state. In between these two extremes are the variations of levels of awareness we experience daily.

Brain Electrical Potentials and States of Awareness

Determining a person's state of awareness using objective criteria is not easy. A person who appears to be listening intently to a lecture may actually be quite relaxed and not thinking about the content of the lecture. The person may, in fact, not be thinking about anything at all. How, though, can the degree of mental activity be measured? One of the tools for looking at brain activity is the electroencephalogram (EEG), which measures gross brain potentials. That is, instead of recording the firing of one or a small group of neurons, as is common in research on the sensory systems discussed in previous chapters, the EEG records the patterns of bioelectrical activity generated by large areas of the brain. As described in Appendix I, electrodes are placed on the surface of the scalp of a resting subject, and the potential differences between pairs of electrodes are then measured, amplified, and recorded.

The patterns generated by the activity of the brain are complicated. Each person has a characteristic brain wave pattern, as distinct in its characteristics as individual fingerprints. Still, although no two individuals have identical EEGs, the similarities between recordings made from different people allow general EEG characteristics to be assigned to the various stages of awareness (see Figure 13.2).

The two terms significant in describing an EEG pattern are frequency and amplitude, referring, of course, to how often a particular wave occurs, generally given in cycles per second (cps), and to how large it is, usually given in terms of millivolts.

Frequencies ranging from 1 cps up to frequencies in excess of 50 cps can be measured by the EEG. The most common frequencies that are re-

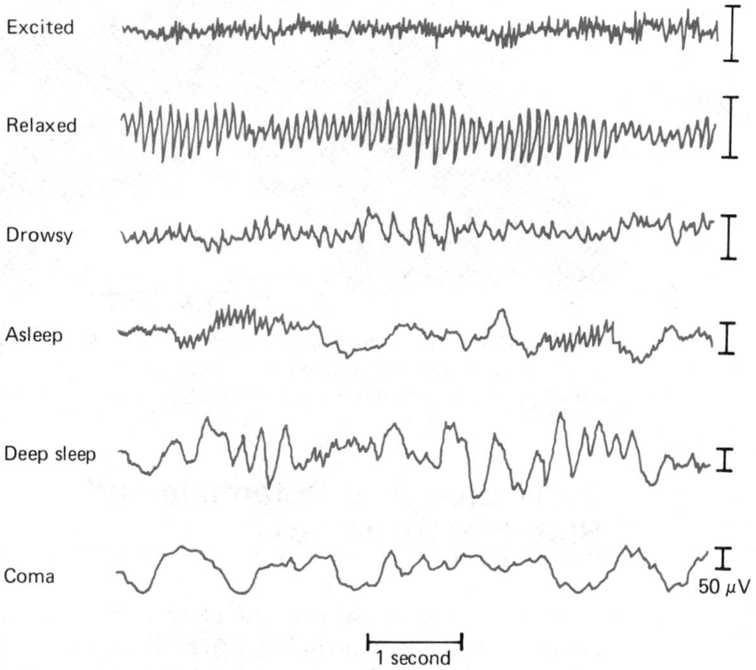

FIGURE 13.2 EEG patterns generated by various levels of awareness. The fastest waves are indicative of an excited state; the larger, slower waves indicate the less alert states.

corded are the alpha frequency of 8 to 13 cps and beta frequency of greater than 13 cps. The theta frequency of 4 to 7 cps and the delta frequency of 3 cps or less are less common in tracings of awake people.

These four wave patterns, as well as some nonpatterned electrical activity, occur during different stages of sleep and wakefulness. Also, certain wave patterns originate from different regions of the brain. During the state of alert wakefulness, for example, the EEG is marked by desynchronized activity from the entire brain. The irregular and arrhythmic waves are relatively fast (15 to 45 cps) and of small amplitude.

Alpha waves generally originate in the posterior zones of the head, in the occipital lobes, and are associated with a state of calm or relaxation. The waves are large and regular, with the amplitude being about 30 millionths of a volt. Eye opening in an awake person will generally stop the alpha waves and the desynchronized activity characteristic of the alert person returns (see Figure 13.3). However, individual differences abound: Some people produce alpha waves even with their eyes open, while others never produce alpha waves at all.

A very alert subject will exhibit a low-voltage, high-frequency wave.

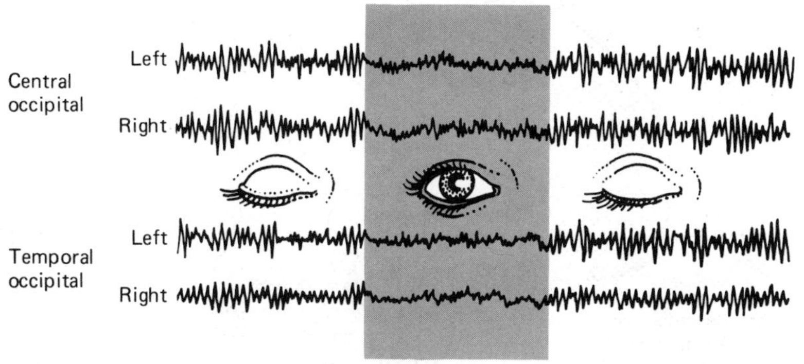

FIGURE 13.3 EEG recordings made over the occipital lobe vary according to whether the eye is open or closed. Larger, alpha rhythms occur when the eye is closed; faster activity is associated with the eye being open.

This is the beta wave, and it is generally, though not exclusively, recorded from the anterior or frontal regions of the head.

Another brain wave pattern is the relatively slow theta wave. Theta waves, which are generally largest at the sides of the head, are believed to have some relation to emotional feelings. In addition, theta waves, intermingled with alpha waves, appear as the subject becomes drowsy. During deep sleep, slow-frequency delta waves are most often recorded (Dement and Kleitman, 1957).

The EEG patterns described thus far reflect the activity of a normal, intact human brain. However, these normal brain wave patterns may vary greatly, depending on factors such as the age of the patient, the particular stage of sleep or wakefulness, whether the eyes are open or closed, and whether or not the patient is taking certain drugs (Steegman, 1970).

The Reticular Formation

The grossest classification of normal states of awareness is in terms of sleep and wakefulness. One of the primary brain structures involved in both the waking and sleeping states is the reticular formation. This central brain stem group of cells, as you will remember from Chapter 3, is a collection of cell bodies, surrounded by the sensory and motor pathways. Although its boundaries are somewhat indistinct, cells included in the reticular formation extend from the lower medulla to the thalamus. Anatomically, it consists of both small and large neurons with both short and long axons. Some of the cells are bifurcating, connecting to both sensory and motor cells in the surrounding regions. The reticular

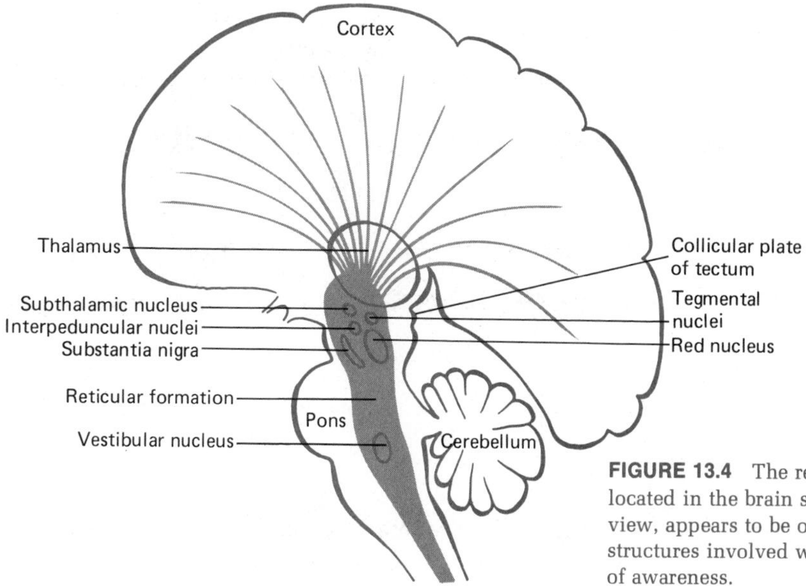

FIGURE 13.4 The reticular formation, located in the brain stem on this sagittal view, appears to be one of the major brain structures involved with maintaining states of awareness.

formation receives input from the cortex, and additionally, sends fibers to the cortex, allowing for a feedback relationship between the cortex and reticular formation (see Figure 13.4).

The first clues to the brain mechanisms involved in arousal were provided when Bremer, in the 1930s, observed that transection of the brain stem of cats at the level of the midbrain produced comatose animals. Bremer speculated that the cause of the sleep (as measured by EEG and the actual nonactivity of the animals) was the loss of sensory input from the body, as the ascending somatosensory pathways had been transected. In other words, the onset of sleep was thought to be a passive process, resulting whenever sensory stimulation failed to reach a level sufficient to maintain arousal. However, when he subsequently made transections at the point at which the brain and spinal cord fuse, the animal exhibited normal sleep-wakefulness EEG patterns, in spite of the fact that the somatosensory pathways had been transected. This proved that sleep was not simply the result of loss of sensory input, for animals without sensory input were capable of being awake. Then, in 1949, Moruzzi and Magoun found that they could produce EEG arousal in sleeping or anesthetized animals by electrical stimulation of the reticular formation. A subsequent study then demonstrated that lesions of the reticular formation produce permanent sleep (Lindsley et al., 1950). Thus, it seems that the reticular formation plays a crucial role in arousal and sleep.

The reticular formation receives collateral fibers from the various sensory projection systems en route to the cortex. These collaterals activate the reticular formation, which in turn alerts the cortex that sensory stimulation is incoming. As the lesion experiments described above suggest, without reticular formation activation, cortical arousal, which is the basis of perception, thought, and other conscious processes, is not possible. Consequently, those parts of the reticular formation concerned with cortical arousal are often referred to as the "ascending reticular activating system" (ARAS) (see Figure 13.5).

The ARAS is now believed to involve the midbrain reticular formation (especially the medial core of the midbrain) as well as parts of the diencephalon (thalamus and hypothalamus). When the reticular formation was lesioned in two stages, and the animal did not lapse into permanent sleep, it was decided that brain mechanisms beyond the reticular formation might be important in maintaining wakefulness. Gelhorn (1967) has suggested that the ARAS may extend as far as the posterior hypothalamus.

The arousal produced by ARAS excitation is general and nonspecific. That is, regardless, of which sensory system initiates ARAS excitation, the arousal is basically the same. It should thus be of no great surprise that the thalamic nuclei involved in the ARAS are the nonspecific nuclei (see Chapter 3).

Fortunately, the reticular formation can adapt to sensory stimuli, and it is the reciprocal feedback relationship between the cerebral cortex and the reticular formation that regulates the arousal initiated by a particular stimulus. While the reticular formation is capable of alerting the cortex

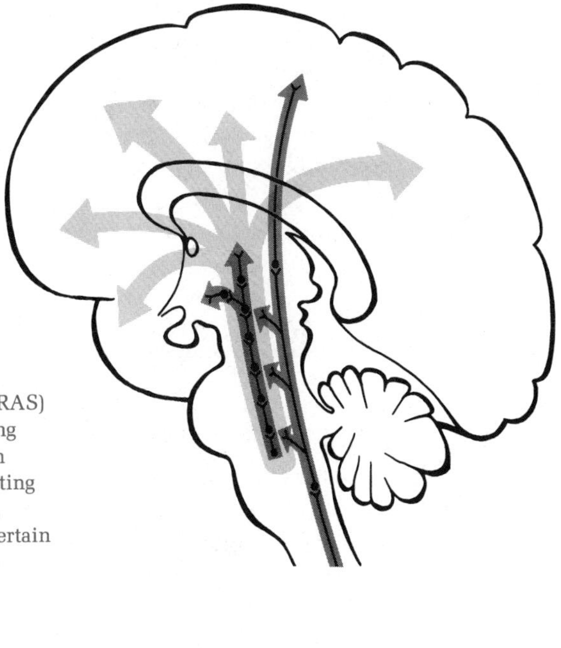

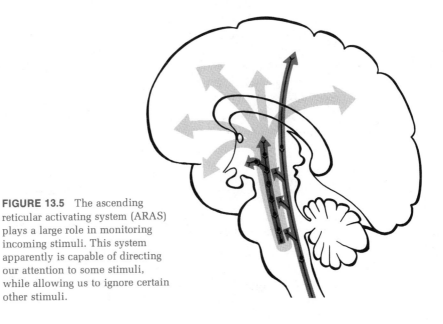

FIGURE 13.5 The ascending reticular activating system (ARAS) plays a large role in monitoring incoming stimuli. This system apparently is capable of directing our attention to some stimuli, while allowing us to ignore certain other stimuli.

to any incoming stimulus, the cortex in turn can send a message to the reticular formation, in effect notifying the reticular formation of the relative importance of each stimulus. Then, since the reticular formation is capable of producing both excitatory and inhibitory influences, it can respond in either a facilitory or inhibitory manner to a particular stimulus. Thus, a person may be able to sleep through the sounds of routine traffic or other environmental noises that may be quite loud, because the reticular formation has adapted to these stimuli. However, a novel stimulus, even a relatively quiet one such as the sound of the front door opening, may wake the person. Similarly, arousal may be influenced by the significance of the novel stimulus. A parent may be attuned to wake immediately to the sound of the baby crying, yet be able to sleep through the buzz of an alarm clock.

Sleep and Dreaming

. . . the innocent sleep
Sleep that knits up the ravell'd sleave of care
The death of each day's life, sore labor's bath.
Balm of hurt minds, a great nature's second course.
Chief nourisher in life's feast.
Macbeth
Act II, scene iii

Obviously, Shakespeare was a firm believer in the restorative power of sleep, and it is likely that a person who feels even slightly deprived of sufficient sleep will join in singing the praises of slumber. It is said that we spend approximately one-third of our lives asleep, yet sleep remains one of the most mysterious levels of consciousness. What induces sleep, how aware is a sleeping person, why do we dream? These are all questions whose answers remain somewhat speculative. It is only since the advent of widespread EEG use that sleep and dreaming have become objects of legitimate scientific inquiry.

The Anatomy of Sleep

Most people think of a "good night's sleep" as one of very deep sleep. However, in reality, normal sleep includes periods of light sleep as well as periods of deep sleep. At least four different levels of sleep have been differentiated, and each stage displays characteristic brain waves. A fifth stage of sleep, the period during which dreaming takes place, will be discussed in detail in a later section.

The stages of sleep occur in sequence several times throughout the night, with each cycle lasting about 90 minutes. The first stage of sleep is called light sleep. During this period there are small rapid changes in voltage, resembling the waking EEG pattern. Stage 2 is characterized by sudden bursts of fast wave activity from the frontal regions of the head called sleep spindles, the bursts having a frequency of about 12 to 14 cps. Stage 3 is somewhat similar to the background of stage 2, and in addition is marked by large slow changes in voltage. Stage 4, the deepest level of sleep, is characterized by the largest, slowest waves (1 to 3 cps), called delta waves.

Perhaps the most interesting aspect of sleep is dreaming, and thanks to a couple of observant researchers in the 1950s, we are beginning to solve some of the mysteries of dreaming. Kleitman and his co-workers found that periodically during the night, the eyes of a sleeping person move rapidly. These rapid movements (REM) are accompanied by a corresponding loss of muscle tone, and paradoxically, by fast cortical activity, similar to that of the waking state. Hence these periods came to be called paradoxical or REM sleep, and it is during these stages of sleep that dreaming is believed to occur. Dreaming was first discovered to occur during REM sleep when experimenters woke their subjects during the period of time in which rapid eye movements were observed. Seventy-four percent of the subjects reported detailed accounts of their dreams when awakened during REM sleep, while only seven percent were able to report their dreams when awakened during any other stage of sleep (Aserinsky and Kleitmen, 1953). This fifth stage of sleep takes place during what is normally stage 1 sleep; however, it is distinguished from normal stage 1 sleep by the presence of rapid eye movements and the "marked decrease in muscle tone." Figure 13.6 shows the patterns of sleep throughout the night, including the periods of stage 1-REM sleep.

What physical mechanisms cause the REM and the loss of muscle tone? Why do a person's eyes move during dreaming? Why the accompanying loss of muscle tone, yet the active cortical pattern? Apparently, the cortical activity corresponds to the dream sequence. It may be that the decreased muscle tone is a safety feature that prevents a person from acting out the dream. The biochemical theory of dreaming discussed later in the chapter provides a possible physiological explanation for the seeming paralysis of muscles during dreaming, since it may be that the neurotransmitter released during dreaming may act to inhibit the motor neurons from firing impulses transmitted to the motor neurons.

Locus of Dreaming

It has often been said that the right half-brain, which is assumed to be more involved in visuospatial tasks than the left half-brain, is responsible for dreaming. However, a recent study of dreaming indicates that

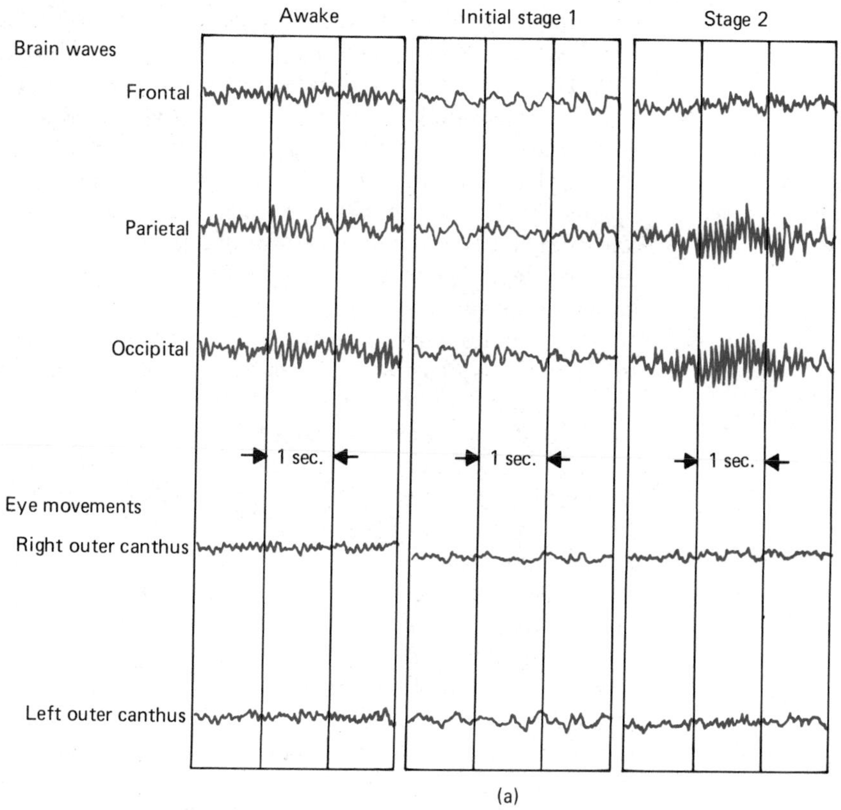

FIGURE 13.6 Brain wave patterns characteristic of the various stages of sleep. Part (a) shows the patterns of a person who is awake, in initial stage 1, and stage 2, while part (b) shows the patterns associated with the deeper stages of sleep and dreaming.

both hemispheres are involved in dreaming. The study centered on three split-brain patients, those with partial or complete section of the corpus callosum and anterior commissure (the two fiber connections between the two halves of the brain). Because the left side of the brain is known to mediate verbal processes, it was assumed that if the right brain were the only site of dreaming these patients would be unable to report their dreams, since in split-brain patients there is little or no transfer or verbal information between the two hemispheres. However, all three patients were able to report visual and verbal dreams, and EEG records indicated periods of REM sleep in both halves of the brain (Greenwood et al., 1978).

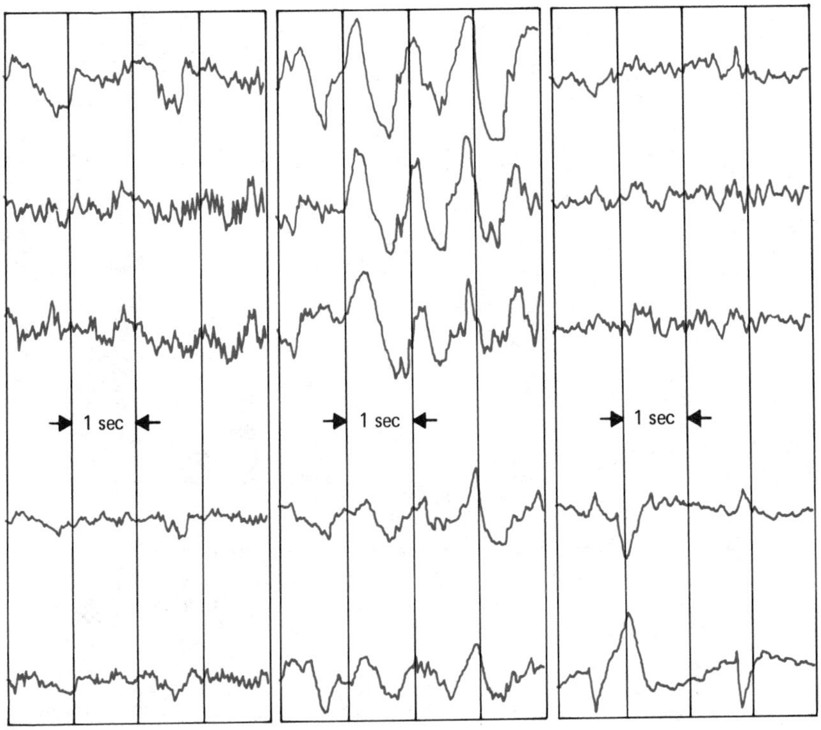

(b)

Who Dreams and How?

Dreaming is believed to occur almost exclusively in mammals, including, of course, humans (see Figure 13.7). One exception is that some birds are thought to exhibit paradoxical sleep. Some generalizations can be made, although individuals vary in their sleep and dreaming requirements. For example, cats spend about one-fourth of their sleeping time in paradoxical sleep. Likewise, average young adult humans spend about one-fourth of their sleeping time in paradoxical sleep. Stages 2 and 3 account for 60 percent of their sleep cycle, while stage 4, deep sleep, accounts for the remainder (about 15 percent) of the sleeping time. In contrast, infants spend a very high percentage of their time asleep in the

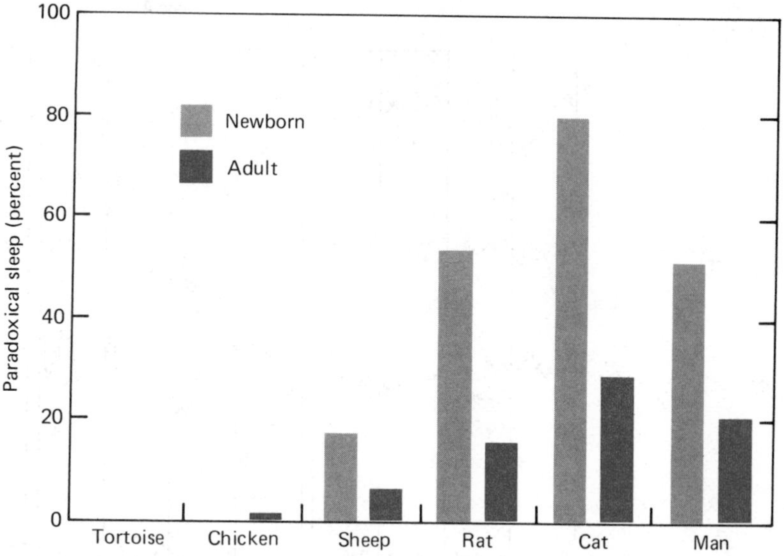

FIGURE 13.7 The amount of time spent in paradoxical sleep varies from one species of animal to another. For example, a tortoise is not believed to spend any time dreaming, while an adult cat spends about 30% of his sleep time in paradoxical sleep.

REM stage, with the percentage varying from 50 to 80 percent (See Figure 13.8). However, the percentage of time spent in paradoxical sleep decreases with age, sharply at first, and then gradually. After the age of 30, people spend progressively less time in both REM sleep and stage 4 sleep.

The full-term neonate (that is, a baby who is not born prematurely) experiences quiet sleep (QS) and active sleep (AS). Quiet sleep is grossly similar to slow-wave (deep) sleep of adults, and active sleep resembles the paradoxical sleep of adults. Still, important differences exist between newborn and adult sleep. For one thing, the active sleep of infants is accompanied by gross and localized body movements, while in adults REM sleep is marked by a loss of muscle tone (Dement, et. al., 1957, 1958).

The characteristic sleep spindles of stage 2 sleep do not appear in the EEG of infants until around 6 weeks of age. Then the sleep spindles appear immediately after the onset of QS and persist for the duration of QS, disappearing with the beginning of AS.

Having established the fact that paradoxical sleep is a regularly occurring phenomenon in the normal sleep pattern of mammals (and some birds), we now turn to ask, why? One attempt at finding an answer to this question involved an experiment wherein subjects were selectively deprived of REM sleep (Dement, 1960). Each time their EEG and eye movement indicated that they were dreaming, they were awakened. No observable aftereffects were reported. However, the deprived subjects did compensate for their loss of REM sleep on subsequent nights by spending more time in stage 1-REM sleep. Control subjects who were awakened periodically throughout the night but not during periods of REM sleep did not show the same increase in REM sleep afterwards. Some REM deprivation experiments using drugs have reported subtle disturbances of personality such as changes in aggressive patterns or in sexual behavior. However, it may be that aftereffects should be attributed to the drug administered rather than to the loss of REM sleep (Jouvet, 1974).

Similarly, cats deprived of sleep have been studied in the following manner: A cat is placed on a platform above a pool of water. The cat may doze without being awakened, but the instant it slips into paradoxical sleep and its neck muscles relax, it is abruptly awakened when its head reaches the water. The main effect from this deprivation of paradoxical sleep is that the cat develops a heart rate that is somewhat faster than

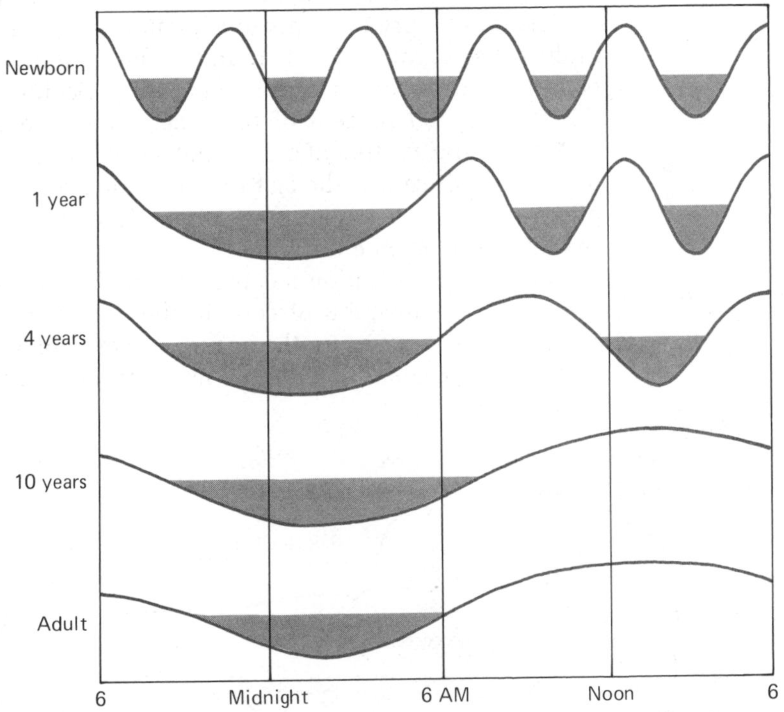

FIGURE 13.8 Sleep patterns vary with age. An infant spends a high percentage of time in paradoxical sleep, going through many short cycles of light sleep and paradoxical sleep.

normal. Like human subjects, cats seem to compensate after the experiment by spending a greater than usual percentage of time in paradoxical sleep. When the animal's sleeping pattern is back to normal, its heart rate also slows to the normal rate.

Thus it is obvious that a person needs to dream, and it is ironic that sleeping pills (barbiturates), because they suppress both stage 1-REM sleep and stage 4 sleep (deep sleep), actually leave a person in worse need of sleep than before taking sleeping pills. Too much alcohol before bedtime can have a similar effect: Stage 1-REM sleep is suppressed and the sleep cycle may be thrown off for the night.

Biochemical Basis of Sleep and Dreaming

The reticular formation has already been implicated in the control of sleep, but only in a very general way. A more specific explanation for sleep and dreaming involving a biochemical basis is being investigated by several sleep researchers. Although still in a somewhat unpolished form, the hypothesis involves two brain stem collections of cells and the neurotransmitter found in each of these collections (See Figure 13.9).

The first theory attempts to explain sleep, as an active process. The raphe cells, a group of cells found in the midline of the brain stem, are believed to be involved in producing sleep. Backward evidence points to this: Destroy 80 percent of these cells, and the animal almost never sleeps. But destruction of cells is not a sufficient explanation. What may be more significant is the fact that the raphe cells are the principal suppliers of serotonin, a neurotransmitter. Thus it may be that a decrease in serotonin brings on a decrease in sleep.

A similar explanation has been found for why we dream. The locus ceruleus is a collection of cells in the dorsal area of the pons, and it seems to be necessary for the occurrence of paradoxical sleep. The cells of the locus ceruleus contain the neurotransmitter noradrenaline, and it

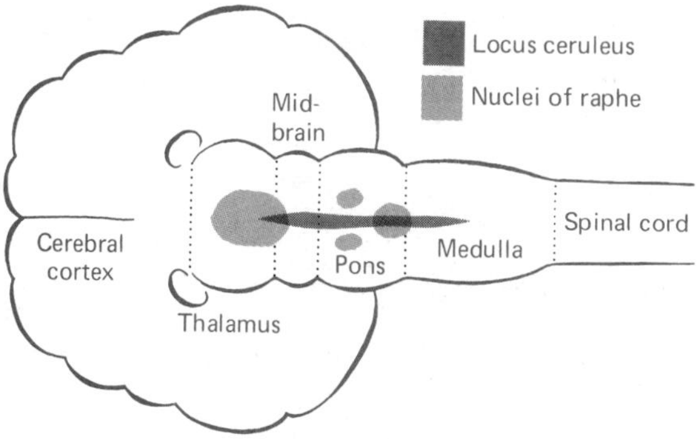

FIGURE 13.9 Two nuclei in the brain stem involved in the control of sleep and dreaming are the nuclei of raphe and the locus ceruleus. Each cell group is believed to secrete a substance that affects sleep and dreaming.

may be that this chemical substance plays a role in producing paradoxical sleep just as serotonin plays a role in producing light sleep.

An interaction between the cells of the raphe system and the cells of the locus ceruleus may account for the cycle of sleep and dreaming. When serotonin predominates, we sleep; when noradrenaline predominates, we dream. It may be that both structures within the brain stem function to counteract the effects of the ARAS. This is consistent with the idea that sleep is by an active, rather than a passive, mechanism. Jouvet has even hypothesized that our need for dreaming may have a chemical basis. It may be that a substance accumulates in the brain that is dissipated only by the chemical action that takes place during dreaming. Consequently, when we are deprived of paradoxical sleep, the subsequent increase in dreaming that is required may have a chemical physiological basis.

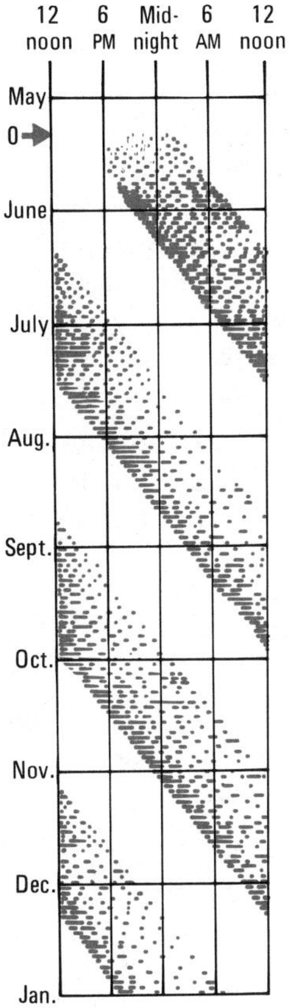

FIGURE 13.10 Even congenitally blind rats show a daily rhythmical cycle close to the normal 24-hour cycle exhibited by normal rats.

Variations in States of Awareness: The Circadian Rhythm

Variations in levels of awareness during the day tend to follow a sequence that is almost as regular as that found in the sleeping state with its five stages. This pattern is called the circadian rhythm (from the Latin *circa*, around; *diem*, day).

Richter's work with rats showed that the circadian rhythm is exhibited on an invariant schedule independently of the light/dark cycle. He had assumed that the activity pattern of normal rats was heavily influenced by the light/dark cycle, since periods of nocturnal activity and sleeping during illuminated conditions were most common among rats. To eliminate the influence of light conditions, Richter blinded the rats. Monitoring their activity periods, he found that the rats adhered very closely to the same 24-hour schedule they had been on before being blinded. The average variation was seldom more than 20 minutes either side of 24 hours. Even congenitally blind rats exhibited this 24-hour cycle (give or take about 20 minutes), so it cannot be claimed that the rats became conditioned to the normal 24-hour day/night cycle before they were blinded (see Figure 13.10). The circadian rhythm, at least in rats, is definitely an "inner clock."

On the other hand, experiments with light/dark cycles longer than the normal 24-hour period have shown that the circadian rhythm of humans can be altered. Under constant light or dark, a person's cycle may or may not change from the normal 24-hour cycle. Two male volunteers who lived in a cave where light and dark could be completely controlled showed different patterns of adaptation to a 3-week period of constant light. One man's cycle gradually changed to a 48-hour cycle: 34 hours awake, then 14 hours sleeping. The other man's adhered much more closely to a normal 24-hour cycle. However, when a 48-hour light dark cycle was imposed (as opposed to light around the clock), both men adapted to the schedule and existed well for two months (Jouvet et al., 1974).

Several physiological factors, principally within the autonomic nervous system, have been observed to follow a regular series of fluctuations, and it seems that some of the factors can at least be correlated with (if not held responsible for) variations in the level of awareness during the day. While no single one of the physical measures outside the EEG is statistically significant in affecting behavior, all of the factors together may influence performance on certain tasks at different times during the day.

Experiments monitoring these factors have found that one variable that may be indicative of the other factors affecting performance is the oral body temperature, which is one of the simplest autonomic indicants to monitor. Temperature fluctuates over the course of the day, being at its lowest at 4:00 A.M., and then gradually rising until late evening when it begins to drop (see Figure 13.11). What the temperature cycle indicates is not clear, but there is some correlation between the temperature cycle and performance on a variety of simple tasks (Blake, 1971). Except for a postlunch lag in performance, people seem to become more efficient as the day wears on. Obviously, this correlation cannot be so simple as suggesting that higher body temperature produces higher standards of performance. The fluctuation in body temperature is only one

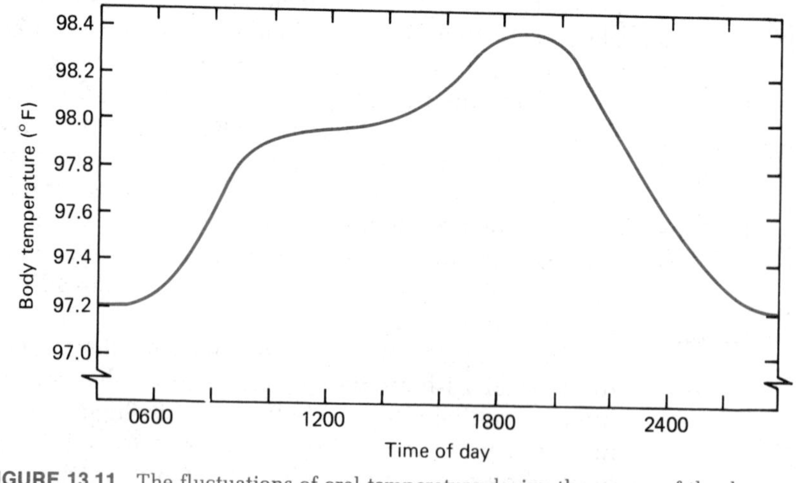

FIGURE 13.11 The fluctuations of oral temperature during the course of the day are indicative of the complex biological rhythm of the body.

of the changes going on in the body over the course of the day. Blood pressure fluctuates during the day, as do electrical resistance of the skin, heart rate, breathing, and other biological indices.

One biological index that has been linked with performance on certain types of tasks is the level of adrenal cortical steroids, that is, the hormones secreted by the covering of the adrenal gland. There seems to be a direct relationship between steroid level and the sensory detection threshold. A high level of steroids is correlated with a high sensory detection threshold, meaning that the stimulus must be fairly intense in order for the person to experience the sensation. Conversely, when the steroid level is low, the sensory threshold is low, meaning that a person is more easily stimulated (Henikin, 1970). Patients with insufficient (subnormal) levels of adrenal cortical steroids with decreased sensory threshold have a corresponding improvement in reaction times. They responded faster than normal subjects. The steroid level generally follows a fairly regular cycle, similar to that of the body temperature. The maximum level of steroids occurs about 4:00 A.M., then gradually decreases over the course of the day until late evening, when it again begins to rise.

Altered States of Awareness

The daily changes we all go through are by no means the only states of awareness known to humans. There are also the many altered states of consciousness brought on by drugs, disease, meditation, or hypnosis.

Pete, for example, represents a case of a person whose level of awareness was sometimes altered because of disease called epilepsy.

Pete wrote poetry. All of the poems were excellent, some of the poems were published, but not many of the poems were sold. So Pete worked in a factory outlet selling sport coats and suits. His work performance was sporadic, for his mind was often elsewhere. In fact, this was more literal than figurative. Pete suffered with temporal lobe epilepsy.

As a child of 8 he had been hit by a car and had sustained a fractured skull. Although he had been unconscious for a time, he had made a quick recovery, and really had not experienced any neurologic deficit. Some 10 years later he experienced the sudden onset of a rising feeling in his abdomen, accompanied by a feeling of intense anxiety. There were no visual or aural hallucinations, but he did experience the sense of smelling burning garbage; there was clearly no burning garbage around. His mother described a series of motor activities that began after his complicated feeling, technically called a visceral aura. Of course, Pete lost conscious awareness of any subsequent activity. He would smack his lips repetitively as though he were sucking a lollipop. Following this activity, his arms moved aimlessly in a hand clapping procedure, and then he would gently sit on the floor. All this would last for about three minutes, to be followed by an equal period of confusion. Waking up fully, he would then be amnestic for all activity except the aura. He remembered the anxiety, even fear, and the unpleasant smell and then nothing. Often he had a headache for a day or two.

These lapses of awareness, which characterize temporal lobe epilepsy, occurred about three or four times per year. The fear of anticipation of an attack was clearly more limiting than the attack itself. Now the seizures were part of a 10-year history, and better control was achieved with the newer antiepileptic drugs. Although he was fearful of experiencing an attack while at the clothing store, he felt that the seizure disorder helped him write.

One division that can be made in altered states of awareness is between ergotropic arousal, which includes creative, psychotic, and ecstatic experiences, and trophotropic arousal, experienced by a person meditating (Fischer, 1971). The first state is a *hyper*arousal condition; the second is a *hypo*arousal condition. Much of the measurement of both of these states is through indicants of the autonomic nervous system activity, and research has been slow since measurement of many of those factors is complicated. Still, progress is being made, and we present here some of the results of this research. The first state we shall examine here is that induced by meditation.

Meditation

With the contemporary emphasis on self-improvement and development, many persons are turning to various forms of meditation in an effort to find a spot of tranquility in an otherwise chaotic world, and, they hope, to achieve a state of enlightened self-awareness.

The meditative state introduces a variation of normal brain wave patterns. Alpha waves, normally prominent only when a person is thoroughly relaxed with eyes closed, increase in amplitude and regularity, particularly in the frontal and central regions of the brain. Subjects with a great deal of experience in meditation show other changes: The alpha waves slow from the usual frequency of 12 cps to 7 to 8 cps, and rhythmical theta waves at 6 to 7 cps appear (Wallace and Benson, 1972). As meditation progresses, the alpha waves give way to fast-wave activity at the rate of 40 to 45 cps (see Figure 13.12).

The changes in the autonomic nervous system indicate a hypo-

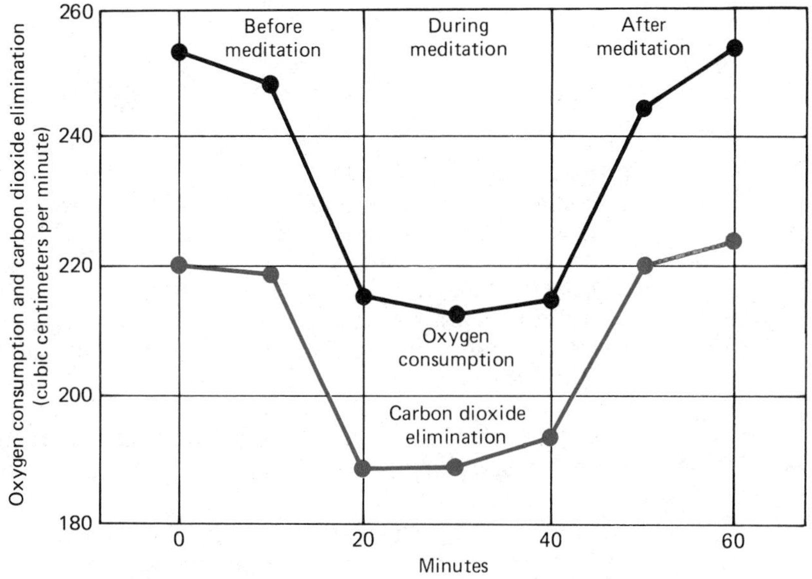

FIGURE 13.12 The physiological effects associated with meditation are a decrease in oxygen consumption and carbon dioxide elimination.

arousal state. Levels of oxygen consumption and the rate of respiration slow considerably, and the person demonstrates a very relaxed body posture.

Hypnosis

Scientific opinion diverges on the question of whether hypnosis is an altered state of awareness. There are those who firmly believe that the EEG and other physiological indicators are clear evidence that the person under the influence of hypnosis is neither sleeping nor awake. Others dispute these claims, saying that hypnosis may be easily simulated by any person so inclined. Nonetheless, some remarkable feats by hypnotized persons have been reported, and the scientific use of hypnosis as a valid means of controlling both anxiety and pain is a real possibility. It is possible that persons can unknowingly control or be oblivious to some of the functions of the autonomic nervous system. Generally, the physiological state of a hypnotized person bears similarity to the suggested mental situation. For example, if a hypnotized man were asked to recount how he felt running up a hill, his heartbeat and breathing rate would increase, while if he were told to relax, his bodily functions would slow down.

Five characteristics of the hypnotized person have been noted (Hilgard, 1965).

1. The person no longer plans activities, but becomes a passive subject, waiting for directions from the hypnotist.
2. The person is able to narrow and select attention mechanisms according to the hypnotist's directions.
3. The person will accept distortions of reality suggested by the hypnotist. In this state the person easily imagines past visual memories and seems to experience them as though they were real.
4. Distilling the three previous characteristics, the person displays an increased willingness to accept suggestions and to act out suggested roles.
5. Usually, but not always, the person is unable to remember what transpired during the hynotic state.

A person who is believed to be hypnotized may be tested according to the scale in Table 13.1 to determine the depth of the hypnotic state.

TABLE 13.1 The Stanford Hypnotic Susceptibility Scale

Suggested Behavior	Criterion of Passing
1. Postural sway	Falls without forcing
2. Eye closure	Closes eyes without forcing
3. Hand lowering (left)	Lowers at left 6 inches by end of 10 seconds
4. Immobilization (right arm)	Arm rises less than 1 inch in 10 seconds
5. Finger lock	Incomplete separation of fingers at end of 10 seconds
6. Arm rigidity (left arm)	Less than 2 inches of arm bending in 10 seconds
7. Hands moving together	Hands at least as close as 6 inches after 10 seconds
8. Verbal inhibition (name)	Name unspoken in 10 seconds
9. Hallucination (fly)	Any movement, grimacing, acknowledgment of effect
10. Eye catalepsy	Eyes remain closed at end of 10 seconds
11. Posthypnotic (change chairs)	Any partial movement response
12. Amnesia test	Three or fewer items recalled

(From Weitzenhoffer and Hilgard, 1959.)

Marijuana Euphoria

Another altered state of awareness can be induced through drugs for a number of reasons—escape, stimulant, tranquilizer, etc. Marijuana, or *Cannabis sativa*, (see Figure 13.13) is classified as a mild euphoric, and current trends toward legalizing or at least decriminalizing it are evi-

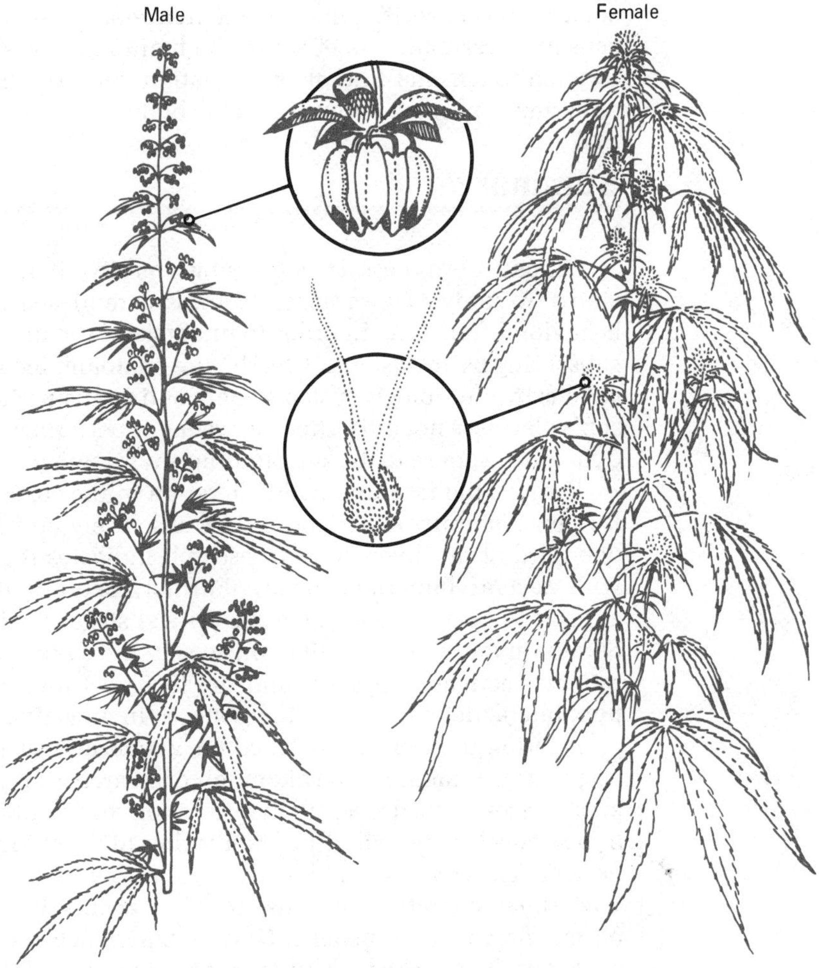

FIGURE 13.13 Marijuana produces an altered state of awareness, although its action on the brain is not fully known.

dence of its growing acceptance by a public long familiar with the pleasant effects of alcohol. Although marijuana has been used for many years, it has only recently enjoyed a surge of popularity among the general public. Most of the intoxicating effects of marijuana can be linked to various isomers of tetrahydrocannabinal (THC). A description of these effects is very often tinged with subjective reports. Physiologically, we can say that the effects of marijuana are similar to those produced when the sympathetic nervous system is mildly excited: Pupils are dilated and systolic blood pressure is raised. Additionally, certain spinal reflexes such as the knee jerk may be elicited more easily, indicating a lower sensory threshold. The effect in the brain remains something of a mystery, although one line of investigation suggests that the THC acts by adhering to post-synaptic sites in the brain.

Summary

Human awareness is not a single entity; it is a complex field of study. A study of awareness requires careful analysis of the variable behavioral functions in order to understand the interrelationship of the subserving brain systems. Clearly, the anatomic locus and neurochemical/electrophysiologic systems contributing at a particular time to a person's alertness not only affect subsequent performance but also reflect a dynamic response to the surrounding environment.

Perhaps the most dramatic alteration in the conscious awake person is sleep. Naturally experienced with absolutely no effort, sleep occupies one-third of our lives. Recent research indicates it is an active process with several important stages. Further, neurotransmitter interaction appears to be associated with the critical stages of sleep and dreaming. Serotonin and noradrenaline, present in the deep midbrain areas of the reticular activating system, and the locus ceruleus work through complex interactions to induce these stages in an active process.

Altering the delicate balance on which awareness is based occurs frequently. Sometimes the alteration of awareness is a deliberate act one experiences with drugs, or hypnosis, or medication. Hyperarousal or hypoarousal is measured by monitoring EEG activity and sympathetic nervous activity such as blood pressure, pulse rate, and respirations. Sometimes alteration of consciousness occurs because of disordered normal processes. Remember Grace's experience in Chapter 3. Driven by acute depression she took an overdose of drugs and lapsed into lethargy, then coma. Her recovery was marked by the progressive integration of the central nervous system; first regaining automatic and reflex function and finally higher cognitive functions. Pete's story is different but also represents a disease process that affects awareness. Patients with temporal lobe epilepsy are afflicted with paroxysmal loss of awareness. These moments are preceded by complicated sensory messages, clearly not apparent in the external environment. During the seizure these people often act out complicated motor schemes of which they are unaware. Medications are often available to stop seizure activity.

Whether a natural process, a voluntarily induced process, or a disease process, alterations in awareness can be commonplace daily events. Finding the biochemical mechanisms and behavioral circumstances that interact to cause the various states of mental alertness remains a key issue for neuroscience today.

References

Aserinsky, E., and N. Kleitman. 1953. Regularly occurring periods of eye motility and concomitant phenomena during sleep. *Science 118*:273.

Berger, R. J. 1963. Experimental modification of dream content by meaningful verbal stimuli. *Brit. J. Psychiat. 109*:722–740.

Blake, M. J. F. 1971. Temperature and time of day. In: W. P. Colubroun, ed. *Biological Rhythms and Human Performance.* New York: Academic Press, pp. 109–148.

Bremer, F. 1936. Nouvelles recherches sur la mécanisme du sommeil. *Comptes Rend. Soc. Biol. 122*:460–464.

Dement, W. 1960. The effect of dream deprivation. *Science 131*:1705–1707.

Dement, W. C., and N. Kleitman. 1957. Cyclic variations in EEG during sleep and their relations to eye movements, body mobility and dreaming. *Electroenceph. and Clin. Neurophysiol. 9*:673–690.

Dement, W. C., and Wolpert, H. 1958. The relation of eye movements, body mobility, and external stimuli to dream content. *J. Exp. Psychol. 55*:543–553.

Fisher, R. 1971. A cartography of the ecstatic and meditative states. *Science 174*:896–904.

Gazzaniga, M. S., and S. A. Hillyard. 1973. Attention mechanisms following brain bisection. In: S. Kormblum, ed. *Attention and Performance.* Vol. IV. New York: Academic Press.

Gelhorn, E. 1967. Principles of autonomic-somatic integrations: Physiological basis and psychological and clinical implications. Minneapolis: University of Minnesota Press.

Greenwood, P., D. Wilson, and M. Gazzaniga. 1978. *Cortex* (in press).

Henikin, R. I. 1970. The neuroendocrine control of perception. In: *Perception and Its Disorders.* Research Publication ARNMD-48:54–107.

Hilgard, E. R. 1965. *Hypnotic Susceptibility.* New York: Harcourt Brace Jovanovich.

Jouvet, M. 1974. The function of dreaming. A neurophysiological point of view. In: M. S. Gazzaniga and C. Blakemore, eds. *Handbook of Psychobiology.* New York: Academic Press, pp. 499–527.

Jouvet, M., J. Mouret, G. Chouvet, and M. Siffre. 1974. Toward a 48-hour day: Experimental bicircadian rhythm in man. In: F. O. Schmitt and F. G. Worden, eds. *The Neurosciences,* third study program. Cambridge, Mass.: M. I. T. Press.

Lindsley, D. B., L. H. Schreiner, W. B. Knowles, and H. W. Magoun. 1950. Behavioral and EEG changes following chronic brain stem lesions in the cat. *Electroencephalography and Clinical Neurophysiol. 2*:483–498.

Morruzi, G., and H. W. Magoun. 1949. Brain stem reticular formation and activation of the EEG. *Electroencephalography and Clinical Neurophysiol.* 1:455–473.

Plum, F., and J. B. Posner. 1966. *The Diagnosis of Stupor and Coma.* Philadelphia: Davis.

Richter, C. P. 1967. Sleep and activity: Their relation to the 24-hour clock. In: S. S. Kety, E. V. Evarts, and H. L. Williams, eds. *Sleep and Altered States of Consciousness.* Research Publications of the Association for Research in Nervous and Mental Disease *45*, pp. 8–29.

Steegmann, A. T. 1970. *Examination of the Nervous System: A Student's Guide.* Chicago: Year Book Medical Publishers.

Wallace, R. K., and H. Benson. 1972. The physiology of meditation. *Sci. Amer. 226*:34.

Weitzenhoffer, A. M., and E. R. Hilgard. 1959. Stanford Hypnotic Susceptibility Scales, Forms A and B. Palo Alto, California: Consulting Psychologists Press.

CHAPTER 14

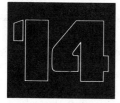

The Self, Consciousness, and the Brain

Let them perish from thy presence, Oh God, as perish vain talkers and seducers of the soul, those who observing that in deliberating there were two wills, affirm that there are two minds in us of two kinds, one good, the other evil—myself, when I was deliberating upon serving the Lord my God now—it was I who willed, I who nilled, I myself.

ST. AUGUSTINE

The idea of self is one of the fundamental dogmas of western civilization. It is the unit of the behaving organism that is ultimately held accountable for our personal actions. Our entire social structure is based on the premise that there is a unified self, and the self is considered the agent of thought and action, the force that causes a person to act.

But what of the idea that the self is *not* a unified being, that there may exist within us several realms of consciousness? It is precisely the idea of the unity of conscious awareness, of self as it is commonly understood, that comes under direct challenge from split-brain studies (Gazzaniga, 1970; Sperry et al., 1969). From these studies (see Appendix II), the new idea that emerges is that there are literally several selves in man, and they do not necessarily "converse" with each other internally. Self "one" is known to self "two" only through observing the behavior produced by self "one."

Much of the split-brain data shows that (a) it is the "verbal self" that gives us our subjective sense of self-awareness, and (b) during life it is the verbal system that is continually rationalizing our behavior and structuring our belief system by observing and reacting to actual behavior. In short, what we believe has been shown by many of the split-brain experiments is that it is the verbal system that is the essence of human consciousness. Given this information, and, through the split-brain studies, the ability to manipulate this system, we have begun to isolate and identify some of the behavioral mechanisms the verbal system uses to construct our personal sense of conscious reality.

Thinking along these lines started some years back with studies on the psychological consequences of splitting the brain in humans. These observations led to the view that the normal state of consciousness could

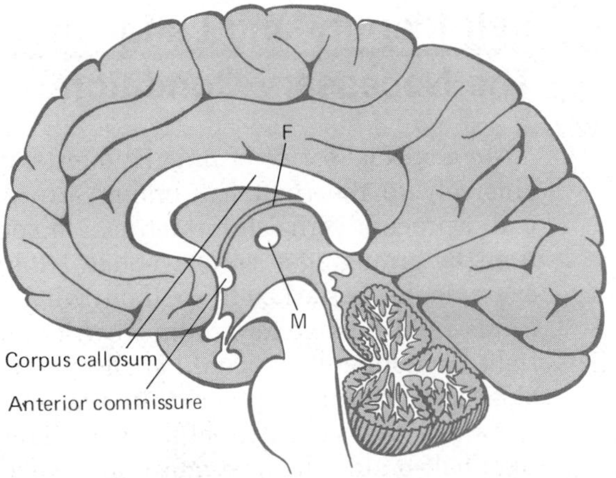

FIGURE 14.1 Midsagittal view of human brain. The major interhemispheric computation systems are the corpus callosum and anterior commissure. Some of these structures are sectioned in patients operated on for surgical control of epileptic seizures. M, massa intermedia; F, fornix.

be discretely tampered with and altered in predictable ways by dissociating the two cerebral hemispheres through surgical section of the corpus callosum (Figure 14.1).

In early split-brain reports, the claim was made that brain bisection produced two separate conscious entities. However, the two entities were never actually demonstrated; the idea of their existence was essentially just a logical extension of the fact that the brain, with seemingly identical halves, had been bisected. Thus, consciousness had been disected. However, those early split-brain studies showed the right hemisphere to be little more than an automaton. But in the last few years, new observations on split-brain patients have become available. In this chapter, we shall describe the particular observations of a truly unique individual, case P. S.

Case P. S. is unique among split-brain patients in that his right hemisphere appears to have higher than normal linguistic abilities. In most persons, language functions seem organized in the left brain, leaving the right brain without verbal processing abilities. But due to unusual early neurological development in case P. S., extensive linguistic skills seem to exist in both half-brains. In the following chapter we shall discuss the observations made possible by this special neurological circumstance. Although these observations involve P. S., a split-brain patient, this chapter is about neither P. S. nor split-brains, but instead, it is about how P. S., whose brain is split, provides a special window through which the inner workings of the human mind may be viewed.

Self-Identity and Language: The Necessary Condition

In a special series of linguistic tests, questions can be presented exclusively to the right half-brain. Surprisingly, P. S.'s right half-brain could process verbal information. He spelled out answers to the questions by arranging a set of wooden letters (Gazzaniga et al., 1977). For example, he was asked to spell out what object he saw in a slide flashed to his right hemisphere (remember, his left visual field projects to his right hemisphere). He could spell "p-e-n" or "h-a-t" or any of the other objects he saw in response to the question, "What did you see?" This test alone showed only that there was language processing ability in the right half-brain. The next question to be explored was whether the right hemisphere possessed its own self-identity.

To test this idea, subjective and personal questions were directed to P. S.'s mute right hemisphere.

Presenting questions exclusively to the right hemisphere was accomplished by verbally stating the question, except that key words in the question were replaced by the word "blank," and then the missing information was flashed in the left visual field, which effectively lateralized visual input to the right half-brain. Subsequently, P. S. was asked to spell his answer (Figure 14.2).

The first question asked was, "Who 'blank'?" The key words flashed and lateralized to the right hemisphere on this trial were "are you?" As his eyes scanned the 52 letters available, his left hand reached out and selected the "P," set it down, and then proceeded to collect the remaining letters needed to spell "Paul." Next, he was asked, "Would you spell your favorite 'blank'?" Then, "girl" appeared in the left visual field. Out came the left hand again, and this time it spelled "Liz," the name of his girlfriend at the time.

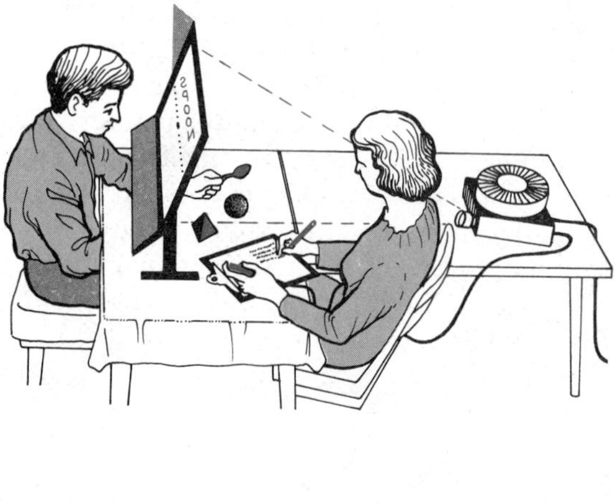

FIGURE 14.2 How a question is exclusively presented to the right hemisphere of a split-brain patient.

These observations (see Gazzaniga and LeDoux, 1978, for complete report) suggested that the right hemisphere in P. S. possesses qualities that are deserving of conscious status. It knows the name it collectively shares with the left. It has feelings, for it can describe its mood. It has a sense of who it likes, and what it likes, for it can name its favorite people and its favorite hobby. The right hemisphere in P. S. also has a sense of the future, for it knows what day tomorrow is. Furthermore, it has goals and aspirations for the future, for it can name its occupational choice.

P. S. is an active, healthy 18-year-old boy, full of spit and vinegar. His major preoccupation, other than girls, is cars and motorbikes, the latter of which he drives with daredevil skill. Circumstances were not always so pleasant for Paul, for he had intractable epilepsy.

Seizures began when he was 4 or 5, and at first these violent major motor outbursts of uncontrolled activity were managed with antiepileptic medicine. Frequent visits to the hospital for adjustment of the medical regimen were necessary. But by the time he was 14, he simply could not go to school because he was experiencing two or three epileptic attacks per week. No adjustment of medicine seemed to work.

He was admitted to the hospital and a complete evaluation revealed no clear cause for Paul's epilepsy. During Christmas, around his fifteenth birthday, he had his corpus collosum completely divided in a delicate neurosurgical operation. Postoperatively he recovered slowly, and two months later he was back to normal except for one thing—no seizures. Paul has had only one seizure in the last three years.

P. S. is the first split-brain patient to clearly possess double consciousness, and the factor that distinguishes his right hemisphere from the right hemisphere of other split-brain patients is undoubtedly the extensive linguistic representation. As we have seen, his right hemisphere can spell, and in addition, it can comprehend verbal commands and process other verbal information. While it is possible that the conscious properties observed in his right hemisphere are not solely dependent on these linguistic skills, the fact remains that other split-brain patients lack right hemisphere linguistic sophistication and so lack any evidence for consciousness.

Verbal Attribution and Multiple Mental Systems

Clearly P. S. possesses double language processing mechanisms and maybe a double self-awareness. What of the case in which mind left with its capacity for speech interprets actions explicitly produced by mind right? That is, if mind right were told to point to an object, would mind left be able to explain why the particular object was chosen?

To test this idea, each hemisphere was simultaneously presented with a different object-picture, and P. S. was required to select from a series of picture choice cards the one that best related to the flashed stimulus. Thus, if a "cherry" was one of the stimuli flashed, the correct answer was "apple" as opposed to a "toaster," "chicken," or "glass," since cherry and apple are related in that they are both fruit.

When both hemispheres were presented with stimuli, P. S. responded with both hands, his right hand pointing to the object dictated by the left hemisphere, and his left hand pointing to the object chosen by the right hemisphere. It was clear that each hemisphere could perform under the simultaneous presentation, and only rarely did the response of one side block a response from the other. In general, each hemisphere pointed to the correct answer on each trial.

What is of particular interest, however, is the way P. S. verbally explained the two responses his hands made. In the one case (right hand following the left half-brain command), P. S.'s verbal system was well aware of why the particular response had been made and thus could easily tell why he had pointed to a particular object. But in the case of the left hand's response (remember right brain command), P. S.'s robust left-sided verbal system did not have access to the information that prompted the response. However, by observing the response, P. S. quickly incorporated the left hand's response into his verbal explanation of why he had pointed as he did. For example, when a snow scene was presented to the right hemisphere and a chicken claw was presented to the left, P. S. quickly responded correctly by choosing a picture of a chicken from a series of four cards with his right hand, a picture of a shovel from a series of four cards with his left hand. The subject was then asked "What did you see?" "I saw a claw and I picked the chicken, and you have to clean out the chicken shed with a shovel." (Figure 14.3).

In trial after trial, P. S. made this kind of response. The left hemisphere could easily and accurately identify why it had picked its answer, and then subsequently, almost immediately, it would incorporate the right hemisphere's response into the framework. While any onlooker knows exactly why the right hemisphere had made its choice, the left hemisphere could merely guess. Yet, P. S.'s left hemisphere did not offer its suggestion in a guessing vein, but rather as a statement of fact as to why that card had been picked.

It is this kind of observation that suggests we are looking at a basic mental mechanism common to everyone. It may well be that the conscious verbal self does not always have access to the origin of our actions, and when it observes the person (the self) behaving for unknown reasons, it attributes cause to the action as if it knows, but in fact it does not. The verbal self looks out and sees what the person is doing, and from that knowledge, it seems to interpret a reality. Put differently, one's sense of reality, one's system of beliefs about the world, arises as a consequence of considering what one does.

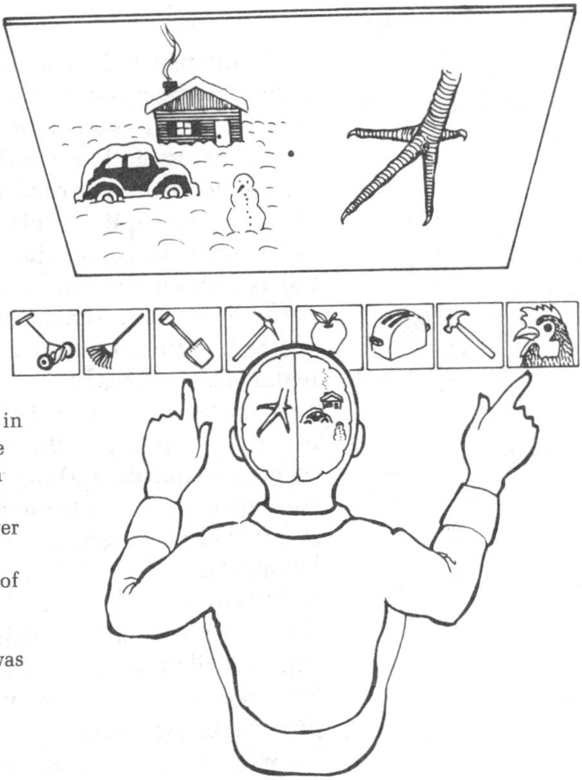

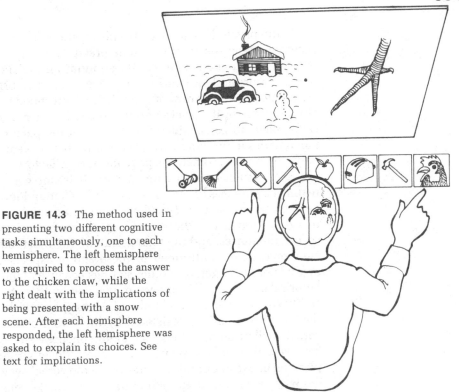

FIGURE 14.3 The method used in presenting two different cognitive tasks simultaneously, one to each hemisphere. The left hemisphere was required to process the answer to the chicken claw, while the right dealt with the implications of being presented with a snow scene. After each hemisphere responded, the left hemisphere was asked to explain its choices. See text for implications.

Verbal Identification of Mood States

Other studies show that the left hemisphere verbal system can also very accurately read changes in emotional states established by the right half-brain.

On a verbal command test, where a word was lateralized to the right hemisphere and P. S. was instructed to perform the action described by the word, his reaction to the word "kiss" proved revealing. Although the left hemisphere of this adolescent boy did not see the word, immediately after "kiss" was exposed to the mute right hemisphere, the left blurted out, "Hey, no way, no way. You've got to be kidding." When asked what it was that he was not going to do, he was unable to say. Later, "kiss" was presented to the left hemisphere and a similar response occurred: "No way. I'm not going to kiss you guys." This time, however, the speaking half-brain knew what the word was. In both instances, the command "kiss" elicited an emotional reaction that was detected by the verbal system of the left hemisphere, and the overt verbal response of left hemisphere was basically the same, regardless of whether the command was presented to the right or left half-brain. In other words, the verbal system of the left hemisphere was able to read accurately the emotional tone and direction of a word seen only by the right hemisphere. In a follow-up study this finding was reconfirmed in detail (LeDoux et al., 1977).

At the psychological level, the observation that the verbal system can accurately read the emotional tone precipitated by an external stimulus without knowing the nature of the stimulus allows speculation concerning the nature and variability of our mood states. In brief, the idea is that we are not always aware of the origin of our moods, just as we are not always aware of the origin of our actions. In other words, the conscious self appears to be capable of noticing that the person is in a particular mood without knowing why. It is as if we become subtly conditioned to particular visual, somatosensory, auditory, olfactory, and gustatory stimuli. While such conditioning can be, it is not necessarily within the realm of awareness of the conscious self. When in Florence, for example, one can be focused on *David* and feel so aroused, awed, and inspired that unbeknownst to the verbal system, the brain is also recording the scents, the noises, and the total gestalt of that most remarkable city. The emotional tone conditioned to these subtle aspects of the experience might later be triggered in other settings because of the presence of similar or related stimuli. The person, puzzled by this affective state, might ask, "Why do I feel so good today?" At this point, if the Florentine experience is not recalled (registered by the verbal system), the process of verbal attribution might take over and concoct a substitute, though perhaps very plausible, explanation. In short, the environment has ways of planting hooks in our minds, and while the verbal system may not know the why or what of it all, part of its job is to make sense out of the emotional and other mental systems, and in so doing, allow us, with our mental complexity, the illusion of a unified self.

Thus, it is evident that the verbal system's role in creating our sense of conscious reality is crucial and enormous. It is the system that is continually observing our actual behavior, as well as our cognitions and internal moods. In attributing cause to behavioral and psychological states, an attitudinal view of the world, involving beliefs and values, is constructed, and this becomes a dominant theme in our own self-image.

Toward the Normal Case

It is exactly at this point that it is necessary to ask whether multiple mental systems could be a feature of normal life. While split-brain subjects represent an explicit instance, and indeed it is the data from these studies that raise the more general questions, it must be shown that the model is useful and applicable to the normal brain.

In a study just completed, neurological patients who were not aphasic but who had left hemisphere damage of one kind or another underwent cerebral angiography (Gazzaniga, 1970; Risse and Gazzaniga, 1977). As is sometimes the case, Amytal testing was also carried out, affording a medical opportunity to study problems in memory organization. Amytal, when specifically injected into the internal carotid artery, puts the hemisphere to sleep. Prior to injection of the anesthetic, an object, for instance a pencil, is placed in the left hand and out of view. The patient is asked to identify it. When done correctly this signals that the stereognostic or touch information has coursed normally from the left hand to the right hemisphere, where it is relayed via the corpus callosum to the left hemisphere.

Then the left hemisphere is put to sleep, which means the patient is no longer conversant or capable of comprehending or producing natural language in any way. The opposite, right half of the body also becomes flaccid. At the same time, however, the left half-body and the right hemisphere are both functional because the drug affects only the injected side of the brain. Another object is placed in the left hand at this time, say a spoon. The subject feels it, and after a few seconds the spoon is removed. A few minutes later the subject awakens, the drug having now dissipated, and the left hemisphere returns to consciousness.

The patient is asked, "What was placed in your hand?," and the typical response is, "Nothing," or "I don't know." To test for a given recall ability the patient is then asked, "What was placed in your hand before?" and the common reply is, "Do you mean the pencil?"

Even with the greatest amount of encouragement or prodding, the subject cannot verbally report what object was placed in the hand during the anesthesia. But, when a card with several objects attached to it is placed in front of the patient, almost instantly the left hand points to the object, in this case, the spoon.

These data are interpreted to mean that information stored in the absence of language cannot be accessed by language when the verbal system reappears and becomes functional. The engram or memory transfer for the spoon is encoded in neural language X and speech is represented in neural language Y. The two languages are then insulated from one another and not conversant with each other inside the brain.

These data allow for the rather radical hypothesis advanced above, which is that during development, a constellation of mental systems are established within us and each has its own values and response probabilities that can remain independent of other mental systems. If this is true, then as maturation continues, the variety of behaviors that these separate systems emit are being constantly observed by the one system we come to use more and more, the verbal natural language system. Gradually a concept of self-identity (and self-control) develops such that the verbal system comes to know the other impulses for action that arise from all the other nonverbal systems, and it tries either to inhibit these or to free them as the case may be.

So far, we have indicated how studies on the split-brain patients have resisted basic behavioral mechanisms used by humans to establish our sense of conscious awareness and sense of personal unity. While it might be prudent to end on that note, we find it hard to resist pointing out some implications of these views for a variety of long-standing problems in psychology.

Implications for a Theory of Memory

The memory mechanism on which psychologists have concentrated is the verbal processing system. Yet, what if this is but one of the systems of memory, and while it is working away, simultaneous activity is going on in several other nonverbal systems, which have as their only way of responding a gesture or movement? In other words, what if the memory systems that exist, say in nonspeaking animals, are also present and working in us along with our admittedly unique language and speech systems? If humans too possess similar memory systems, then the meaning of a huge number of previous studies on human memory may be altered.

The classic distinction, for example, between recognition and recall, dissolves almost instantly. This, of course, is the well-reported and widely experienced phenomenon that a person can recall only a small part of a body of information given to him whereas he can recognize a lot more. In the present model the recall phase is only calling upon the verbal system for response. The verbal system, however, only reports a small amount of information because, just as with the other independent systems, it has a limited capacity. When the recognition phase is introduced, however, the name of the game is quite different. Now the other nonverbal systems have an opportunity to express themselves. They do this by nonverbal behaviors such as pointing to a series of objects. With that kind of response possible, all of the information the several nonverbal systems store can now be reported, making the entire system appear more resourceful.

It has long been thought that recognition tests are a more sensitive measure for information stored (memory) because they have access to information that is in some sense stored with a "weaker" value. But if there are, as these experiments suggest, several types of memory systems, then such a continuum ("stronger" vs. "weaker" memory) between recognition and recall skills becomes less viable; it is just that one memory system has a more easily accessible method of expression. Indeed, it may be that there are several equally capable storage systems, the expression of which is simply dependent on being given an equal chance for demonstration.

Implications for Cognitive Theory

It was Leon Festinger (1957) who developed the theory of cognitive dissonance, which is one of the most powerful ideas on the nature of behavioral process ever stated. The phenomenon in broad terms is this: When a person's opinion, belief, or attitudes are met with disagreement as a consequence of a freely produced behavior, a state of dissonance results. The person's cognition prior to this behavior is in conflict with the just completed behavior, and that state of dissonance is not allowed by the organism. Consonance is demanded and is usually achieved by changing the prior value or belief.

Let's take an imaginary example. George is married and full of fidelity. Then a set of circumstances develops that finds George involved in an affair with another woman. George does not believe in such behavior and does not condone extramarital affairs. So, immediately after the experience, George is very much in a state of dissonance after his recent behavior. George initially attributes it to being drunk or being seduced. That helps, but George is soon in bed again with his new friend. As this continues, his dissonance increases and something must change. What usually changes is George's attitude about his marriage. Before long he attributes his behavior to domestic tensions and comes to believe that they are much worse than he had previously thought. As a result, George shortly finds himself in divorce court. He has concluded that he must be having the affair because his marriage had deteriorated. These rationalizations and actions are the changes that resolve George's dissonance. Divorce becomes an unavoidable consequence, and George's fate was sealed after the first night.

There are millions of examples of dissonance theory at work, and hundreds have been worked out under strict experimental conditions in the laboratory. What is not understood is why the organism seeks consonance. Why can't dissonance be a viable and chronic state for the biological organism?

Let's take a step back and consider a prior question. Why did George suddenly find himself involved with the other woman in the first place? What is the mechanism for eliciting a dissonant behavior from the beginning? The behavior was clearly contrary to his existing (verbally stored) belief about such matters, and normally the verbal system can exert self-control. The reason proposed is that yet another information system with a different reference and different values existed in George, but because it was encoded in a particular way, its experience was not known to George's verbal system and, therefore, was outside of its control. That is, it wasn't known until one day it grabbed hold momentarily and took charge of his behavior and elicited a behavioral act that caused great consternation to George's verbal system. Once elicited, however, George's verbal system had no choice but to account for it and to adjust his verbal perceptions and guidelines for behavior to take this newly discovered aspect of his personality into account. In this view it is the verbal system that is the final arbiter of our many modes of consciousness, most of which we come to know only by actually behaving. Behavior elicited is the way to discover the multiple selves dwelling inside. Behavior is the way these separate information systems communicate with one another. It is probable that very little communication goes on internally. It is only after we behave in a way contrary to the usual principles of the verbal system that we may discover the multiple selves dwelling inside.

The Multiple Self and Free Will

The final implication of these explorations into the human mind is concerned with the nature of personal responsibility. If, as stated at the beginning of this chapter, most of our social institutions are built on the notion that humans are personally responsible for their actions, then implicit in that statement is a notion that humans have a unified sense of self, a single structure of consciousness. What are we now to do with that view, given the new knowledge that multiple selves exist and each self can control behavior at various moments in time?

Let's go back a step and look at the concept of free will as it has stood up in our scientific age. This is extremely important because up until now the issue of responsibility (whether it is personal or social) has been argued on the merits of a unitary self and the concept of free will. Up until recently, the scientific community has pretty much written off such concepts as free will as holdovers from the dark ages, and anyone making the case for a personal responsibility has been largely ignored. Science is reductionistic by nature, and most scientists believe, in fact, that the world is as mechanical as clockwork. Things don't just happen. There are inputs to every system and knowing the inputs will find one able to explain and predict the outputs. That's the line of thought, anyway.

At the level of human behavior, this means that when one thinks about freely choosing which person to ask to marry, one is, in fact, only acting as a result of a set of forces working already in process. That one acts freely is pure illusion. Behavior is lawful and the exacting product of past experience according to the behaviorist and reductionist, such as B. F. Skinner. Any view to the contrary is simply out of step with what is known about the physical nature of the universe.

However, D. M. MacKay (1967) deals with this problem head on and puts humans right back on top, and in personal control of their behavior. His argument goes like this.

People can be considered as mechanistic as clockwork and still be considered personally responsible for their actions and personally free in their decisions. This is true because, put simply, if you tell some people that they will eat apples for lunch because of some fantastic knowledge you possess of their past behavior, all they have to do to prove you wrong is not to eat apples. At first glance, there would seem to be an easy solution to that which would not violate the idea of reductionism. The next time, the persons whose actions are being predicted will not be told what the predictor predicts about their behavior. Instead, it will be written down and after the critical event the predictions will be examined, and with this condition the predictor will prove to be correct.

That still won't work, however, as MacKay has pointed out, because when you think carefully about it, in order for something to be true it must be valid for all people. The critical point here is that while the prediction may be true for the predictor, it is not binding on our victims and consequently not valid for both parties. A true and valid proposition must be set out for all to see, and once that is done our victims can do or not do what it says as they see fit.

It is a fascinating argument, upon which logicians and philosophers have agreed. It shows that even in a mechanistic universe there is this situation which MacKay has called a "logical indeterminancy of a free choice." While we tend to believe his point, our point is that the formulation of the problem moving from the assumptions of a unitary consciousness will not apply to the case for multiple selves. While his unique argument may well apply to a "self" system, how would it apply to a collection of "selfs"? If indeed our cranium houses many mental systems we should have to ask how his idea applies in the sociological instance as opposed to the presumed unified psychological character of the human being.

Summary

In short, what we have shown in this chapter is that the mechanisms of behavior are not fully understood. Obviously, there are biological bases for all of our actions, and we are only just beginning to discover and interpret these mechanisms.

P. S.'s story of intractable epilepsy and miraculous curative surgery serves as an important example of a special window through which the mechanisms of mind may be studied. Coordinating the extraordinary behavior of this young boy with neuroanatomic and neurophysiologic knowledge may provide greater understanding of the human condition.

So often P. S.'s robust verbal left brain does not always have access to the origin of his actions. Observing himself behaving in a particular manner, the verbal system quickly attributes cause to the action, almost as if it really knows. Does one's sense of reality, feelings, and beliefs about the world arise as a consequence of considering one's behavior?

These observations serve to stimulate ideas about memory and cognition. Study of the former system has concentrated on the verbal processing mechanism. The recall aspect of the verbal system, existing as a lone independent function separate from recognition aspects, for example, can report only a small amount of information. Its capacity is limited. Memory, or the capacity of neurons to store information, may depend on several storage systems, the expression of which depends on the chance to display action. Remember not just Paul's story, but also Sandy's story in Chapter 12; both are examples of the interdependence of verbal and nonverbal processing systems.

Is the single unitary self really a collection of "selfs"? If that is true, then which "self" of a convicted felon should receive guidance or punishment? How can the mentally ill incapacitated "self" be helped? While these questions, and other similar ones, are perhaps best left at the level of a metaphor for now, it nonetheless seems clear that brain sciences are continually, and at an ever-increasing rate, discovering facts about the psychological mechanisms active in developing and sustaining conscious experience.

It may be that the idea of self, subscribed to for so many years by those in western civilization, needs to be reexamined. The examination process will undoubtedly reveal some new fascinating philosophical and biological truths. Can there be any doubt that the brain sciences sit at the center of the primary scientific and intellectual questions of our time?

References

Eccles, J. C., ed. 1960. *Brain Mechanisms and Consciousness.* New York: Springer-Verlag.

Festinger, L. 1957. *A Theory of Cognition Dissonance.* Stanford, Calif.: Stanford University Press.

Gazzaniga, M. S. 1970. *The Bisected-Brain.* Englewood Cliffs, N.J.: Prentice-Hall.

Gazzaniga, M. S., and J. E. LeDoux. 1977. *The Integrated Mind.* New York: Plenum.

Gazzaniga, M. S., J. D. LeDoux, and D. H. Wilson. 1977. Language praxis and the right hemisphere: Clues to some mechanisms of consciousness. *Neurology* 27:1144–1147.

LeDoux, J. E., D. H. Wilson, M. D. Gazzaniga. 1977. A divided mind: Observations on the conscious properties of the separated hemispheres. *Ann. Neurol.* 2:417–421.

MacKay, D. M. 1967. *Freedom of Action in a Mechanistic Universe.* London: Cambridge University Press.

Risse, G., and M. S. Gazzaniga. 1977. Well kept secrets of the right hemisphere: A carotid amytal study. *Neurology* (in press).

Sperry, R. W., M. S. Gazzaniga, and J. E. Bogen. 1969. Interhemispheric relationships: The neocortical commissures; syndromes of hemisphere disconnection. In: P. J. Vinken and G. W. Bruyn, eds. *Handbook of Clinical Neurology.* Amsterdam: North-Holland.

Appendixes

APPENDIX

Methods of Research

In our effort to identify what is known today about the relation between psychological processes and nervous system functioning, we shall in effect be approaching psychological questions biologically. Consequently, in this section we shall review various psychobiological approaches, and their respective techniques.

In the attempt to discover the various functions and capacities of the human brain, three possible avenues of research, each with its advantages and disadvantages, come to mind. The first approach involves the use of animals as the subjects under investigation. There are several advantages to this approach. Animals are often bred for laboratory experiments, and therefore their entire environmental and sometimes genetic histories can be known to the experimenter. The scientist can also impose stringent experimental controls on these animals so that causal events may be determined with relative ease. However, the disadvantage of doing animal research is that no matter how well controlled the experiments are, it is difficult to know whether the findings in animal research are applicable to humans. Particularly when a researcher is interested in the higher cognitive functions of humans, relying on the results of animal research places the experimenter on shaky ground. For example, to our present knowledge, no other species has the speech processing and production capabilities found in humans. Many human cognitive capabilities are dependent to some extent on these linguistic capacities. It would be impossible to explore these types of functions through the vehicle of animal research.

A second possible approach is to devise experiments that can be run with normal human subjects. The advantage here is that the species of interest, to whom the results should apply, is also the species under direct investigation. The disadvantage in this case is that when everything is functioning together normally, it is difficult to tease out the specific functions of particular structures or regions in the brain. Also, for ethical reasons, many of the appropriate experimental manipulations cannot be employed.

The third approach is to study individuals with localized or known neurological damage. Using normal subjects as a base of comparison, the functions that seem deficient in the brain-damaged patient can often be attributed to the lesioned or damaged area. Again, the scientists are already dealing with the species to which they wish to generalize. This approach, however, also has a disadvantage that should be kept in mind. The brain that is being studied is a damaged brain, and not the normal one whose functions researchers are searching to discover. It is possible that the damaged brain undergoes other changes besides those involving the primary lesion that may be localized. The other changes that are not precisely known may cause some problems in the generalizability of these findings to the workings of the normal brain. However, even with this drawback, studies of neurologically impaired patients have yielded some extremely interesting findings, most of which have been validated with both animal and normal human subjects.

Obviously, it is helpful if you know the structure of something before you try to figure out how it works. Thus, the first techniques to be discussed are those of the neuroanatomical approach.

Neuroanatomical Approaches

Neuroanatomy is the study of the structure of the nervous system. Early scientists were limited to exploring dissected brain tissue with the naked eye. This approach provided the basic understanding of nervous system organization. However, it was the invention of the microscope in 1830 and the subsequent development of techniques for preparing brain tissue for microscopic examination that led to real progress in neuroanatomy.

Two early neuroanatomists who had an important impact on modern approaches were Golgi and Cajal. Golgi's studies led him to believe that the nervous system was a vast and continuous network of interconnected cells and fibers. This was called the reticular (network) theory. Cajal, on the other hand, felt that the nervous system was composed of discrete cells and their fibers. In other words, the cells and fibers of one neuron, according to Cajal, were distinct units. The separations between the neurons were called synapses. This theory is generally accepted today and goes by the name of the neuron doctrine.

Histology is the study of tissue, and histological techniques for preparing brain tissue are essential tools of the neuroanatomist. The basic approach involves the perfusion of the brain (replacing the blood with formaldehyde), removal of the brain from the skull, and sectioning or slicing of the brain. Formaldehyde (commonly known as embalming

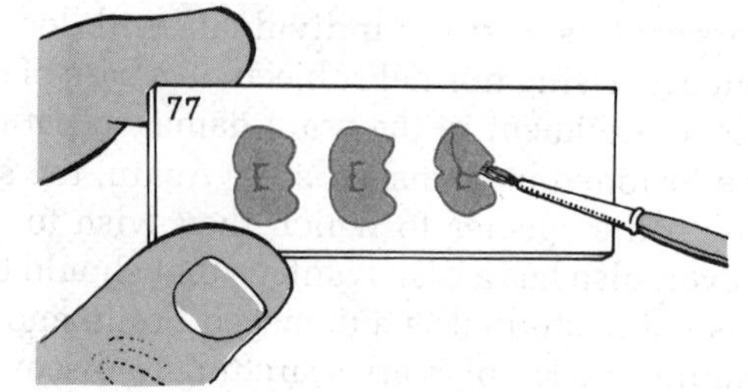

FIGURE I.1 A slicing microtome is used to section the frozen brain. The brain is sliced in very thin sections and placed in a solution. Subsequently, the sections are typically placed on slides for staining.

fluid) preserves the tissue. Prior to sectioning of the perfused brain, the tissue is generally frozen (though other approaches, such as embedding the tissue in paraffin, are sometimes used). The frozen brain is then sectioned using a slicing microtome (see Figure I.1).

Once the brain has been sectioned, the final histological step involves staining the tissue. Various stains are available, each with a unique purpose. Some stains allow the microscopic examination of neural fiber, while others highlight the nerve cells themselves.

Thus far, we have described the histological preparation of normal tissue. Most often, however, the anatomist is interested in manipulating the normal tissue in some way so as to trace the fiber connections from one area to another. In essence, experimental neuroanatomy is concerned with mapping the circuitry of the brain.

One way of tracing fiber connections is to destroy (lesion) the cell

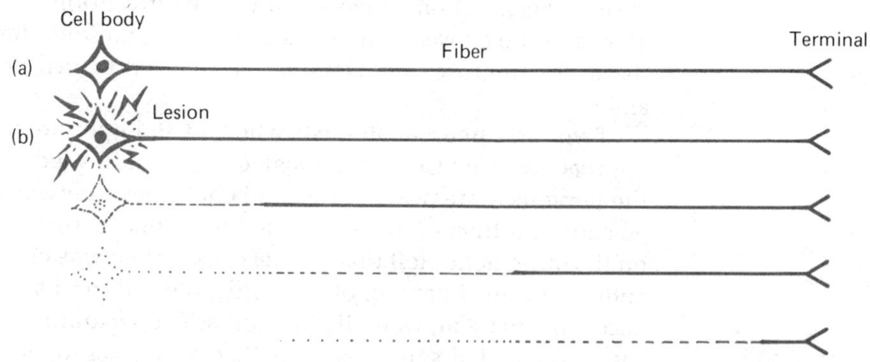

FIGURE I.2 Silver degeneration technique. Part (a) shows a highly schematized view of a normal fiber projection system. When the cell bodies are destroyed by a lesion, as in part (b), the fibers degenerate. Part (b) also depicts various stages of degeneration of fibers. The fibers degenerate near the cell body first and then progressively degenerate towards the terminal, and finally the terminal degenerates. Some silver stains allow the visualization of the degenerating fiber itself, while other stains selectively highlight the terminal degeneration.

bodies in one area of the brain of a live animal. The fibers arising from the destroyed cell bodies can then be traced in the histologically prepared brain because the fibers degenerate when their cell bodies are destroyed (see Figure I.2). Using a certain class of tissue stains called silver stains (so named because the stain is based on a silver nitrate solution), it is possible to trace the degenerating fibers. So, the anatomist can determine that lesions of area A produce silver degeneration products in areas X, Y, and Z. This suggests that fibers from area A project to these other areas. By making systematic lesions and tracing the connections, the anatomist can thus uncover the wiring scheme of the brain.

Another way of tracing fibers makes use of metabolic manipulations. Instead of destroying a group of cell bodies, researchers can inject chemicals into the area containing the cell bodies of interest. One approach, called the autoradiographic technique, makes use of radioactively labeled (or "tagged") amino acids. The amino acids are taken up by the cell bodies, are converted into proteins, and are transported to the fiber terminal (see Figure I.3). Techniques that allow the visualization of the labeled proteins make it possible to determine the areas of projection of the injected cell bodies.

In contrast to the autoradiographic technique is the horseradish peroxidase (HRP) technique, in which a chemical is injected at the terminal region rather than the cell body region. When the HRP enzyme is injected it is selectively taken up by the axon terminal and is transported to the cell bodies projecting to the injected region (see Figure I.4). Using procedures that selectively stain the HRP enzyme enables the tracing of

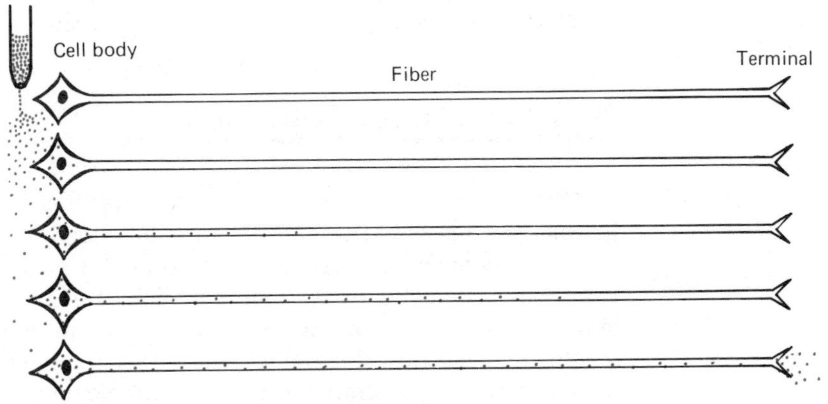

FIGURE I.3 An autoradiograph of a terminal zone. Radioactively labeled amino acids are injected into the brain and are taken up by the cell bodies in the region of injection. The amino acid is synthesized into protein by the cell body through normal metabolic processes. The tagged protein is then transported to the terminals where it is deposited.

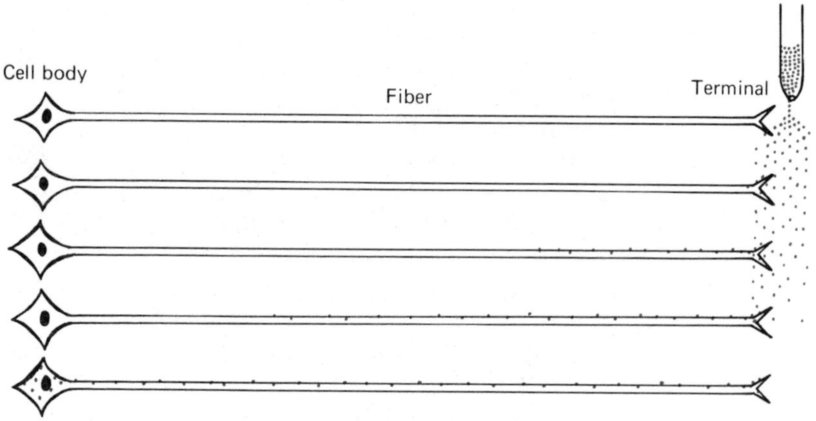

FIGURE I.4 Cell bodies infested with HRP molecules. With HRP, an enzyme is injected into the terminal zone, is taken up at the terminal, and is transported through normal metabolic processes to the cell bodies that send fibers to the injected region.

connections by starting at the terminal. So, while autoradiography gives information about all of the areas receiving fibers from the cell bodies of the injected area, HRP tells about the cell bodies projecting to the injected terminal zone.

Before leaving our overview of anatomical techniques, we must point out that the use of the electron microscope makes possible the visualization of very small structures. In fact, with the electron microscope, it is now possible to see a synapse, the junction between nerve cells hypothesized by Ramon y Cajal (see earlier discussion). In addition to confirming the neuron doctrine, Cajal's theory that nerve cells are discrete units separated by synapses, the electron microscope has made it possible for the anatomist to study the brain at levels undreamed of in Cajal's day.

Neurochemical Approaches

Perhaps the most recent set of techniques that have emerged as aids in understanding brain function are biochemical techniques. While biochemists have been grinding up brains for years and carrying out a variety of systematic assays that have determined concentrations of the brain regional levels of various amino acids, proteins, and other basic biochemical entities, it is the relatively recent developments in the neurochemistry of neurotransmitters, the chemicals that underlie the communication between most neural cells, that has caused so much recent excitement. Identification of particular brain cells and neural systems that specifically secrete certain neurotransmitters has led to some major theoretical as well as practical advances in brain science. For example, discovering the biochemical pathways of dopamine, a primary neurotransmitter, has led to the discovery that in some kinds of neurological disease (Parkinson's disease) there is a specific biochemical deficiency that can be remedied by the taking of a drug L-dopa.

There are a variety of other brain chemicals such as the endorphins and enkephalins, which are small proteins (peptides) that hold great promise as the chemicals that underlie many of our mood states. Clearly, until there is more basic understanding of the chemistry of the brain, there will be but a cursory understanding of brain mechanism. It does truly represent an exciting new area.

Neurophysiological Approaches

Neurophysiology is the study of the electrical activity of the nervous system. This discipline naturally owes its origin to the early studies that demonstrated the electrophysiological nature of nervous system functioning. Contemporary neurophysiological approaches include techniques for recording the electrical activity of the nervous system, as well as stimulation techniques.

Electrical Stimulation

Following Fritsch's and Hitsig's success in eliciting overt bodily movements, Sir Charles Sherrington adopted the electrical stimulation technique. His pioneering studies of spinal cord reflexes elucidated principles of nervous system function and organization that have held up for nearly a century and have earned him a place in history as the "father" of neurophysiology.

The stimulation technique involves the permanent or temporary implantation of small electrodes (microelectrodes) into a particular part of the brain or other area of the nervous system. The electrode is made of small-diameter metal wire that is insulated its entire length, except for an exposed tip. The other end of the electrode is connected to an electronic stimulator that produces highly controlled electric impulses. When the electrode is inserted into the brain, only the tissue in contact with the uninsulated tip receives the electrical stimulation. An increase in the current flowing through the electrode, however, can increase the radius of stimulation.

Brain stimulation was originally used in producing movement, as described earlier. Researchers systematically stimulated successive points in a surgically exposed area of the nervous system and noted all areas that produced movements. This sort of work was carried out mainly on the cerebral cortex and spinal cord. Later studies implanted stimulating electrodes below the cortical surface in subcortical regions (see Figure I.5). Using such an approach, Hess (1954) discovered that cats,

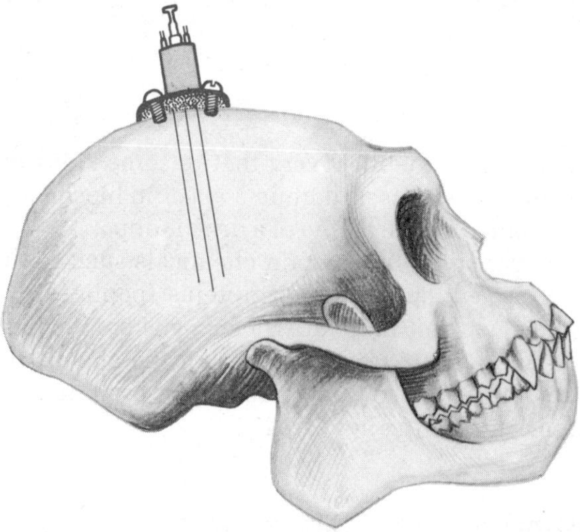

FIGURE I.5 How electrodes can be implanted deep in the brain and can be used to stimulate various brain structures.

when stimulated in certain regions, would exhibit ragelike attacks. More recently, Olds and Milner (1954) have shown that stimulation of some areas produces "rewarding" effects (i.e., animals will work to receive the stimulation) and stimulation of other areas produces aversive effects (i.e., animals will work to avoid the stimulation). These studies, which suggest that through electrical stimulation one can tap into motivational and emotional brain systems, have been described in Chapter 11.

Before leaving the stimulation approach, the brain atlas and stereotaxic instrument should be described. An atlas is a map of the brain in

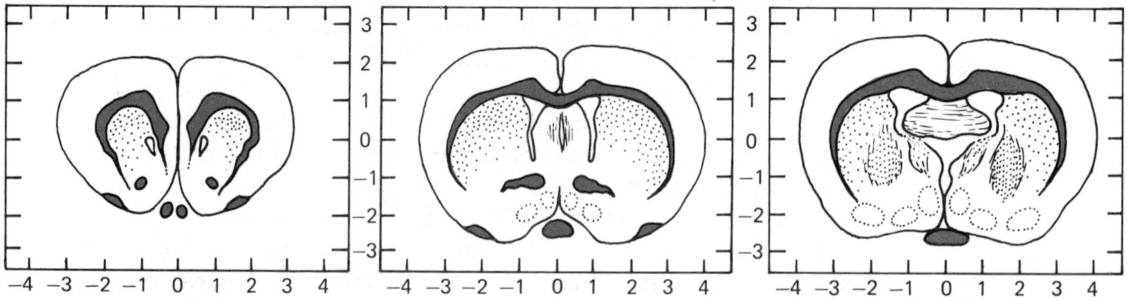

FIGURE I.6 A schematic view of a whole brain with sections etched in, showing how the brain sections appear in an atlas. Imagine the brain being sliced like a loaf of bread and then imagine looking at the slice of bread head on. The brain atlas is a collection of such slices. The slices or sections are arranged sequentially. Because the brain is smaller at the front and back than in the middle, the sections from the two ends are smaller than those for the middle. The number of each section provides the experimenter with the front-to-back location of the brain areas contained in that particular section. The grid marks around the section tell the experimenter how far from the midline of the brain and how deep in the brain each region in the section is. Thus, by looking up a particular brain area in the atlas index and then finding the appropriate brain slice, the experimenter can obtain the location of that area in three-dimensional coordinates. These coordinates are used in conjunction with a stereotaxic instrument (see Figure I.7).

three-dimensional coordinates (see Figure I.6). To stimulate a particular area, one looks that area up, and then, using the coordinates provided by the atlas, implants the electrode in the approximate area. This approach is called stereotaxic surgery (stereotaxic describes an arrangement that uses contact, especially with a solid body, as a directional factor). The stereotaxic instrument used in brain surgery holds the animal's head in a predetermined way (see Figure I.7). After the animal is securely and properly placed in the instrument, its skull is exposed and marks on the

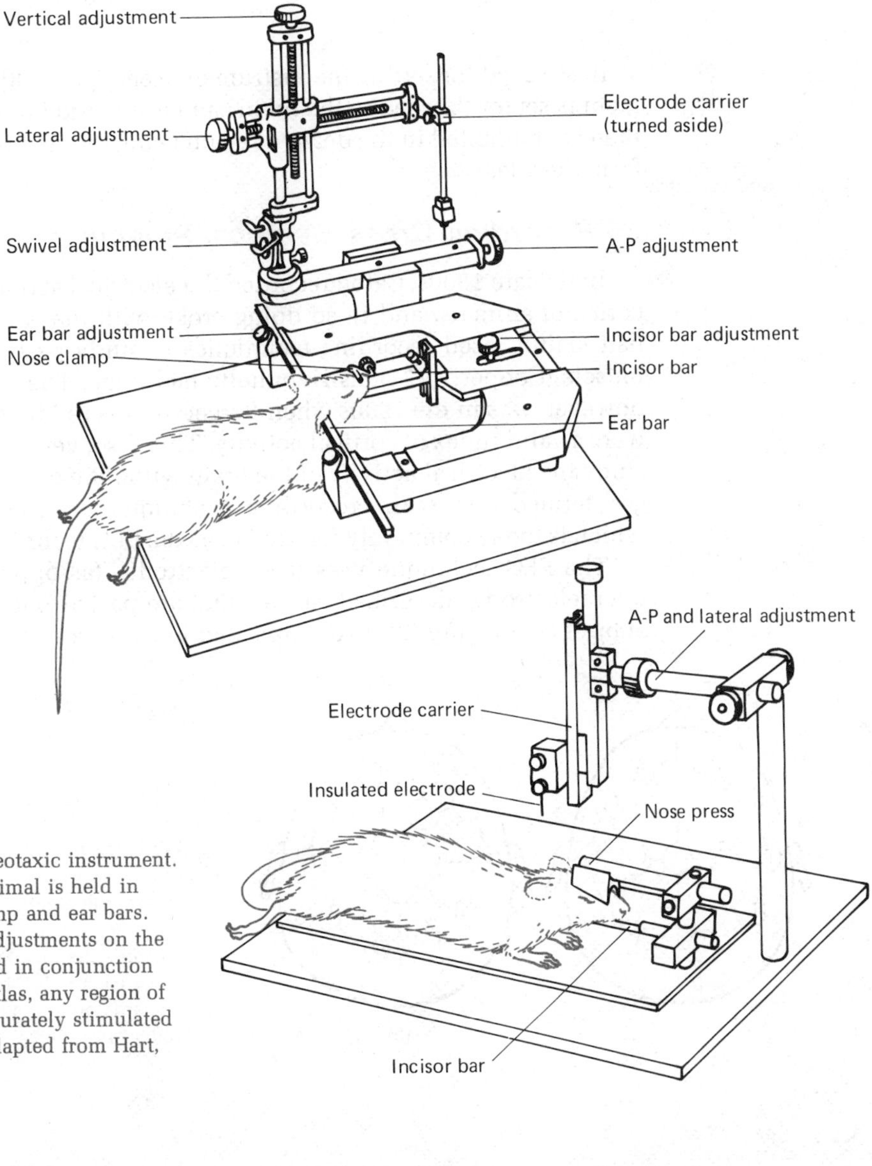

FIGURE I.7 A stereotaxic instrument. The anesthetized animal is held in place by a nose clamp and ear bars. When the various adjustments on the instruments are used in conjunction with a stereotaxic atlas, any region of the brain can be accurately stimulated with electrodes. (Adapted from Hart, 1969.)

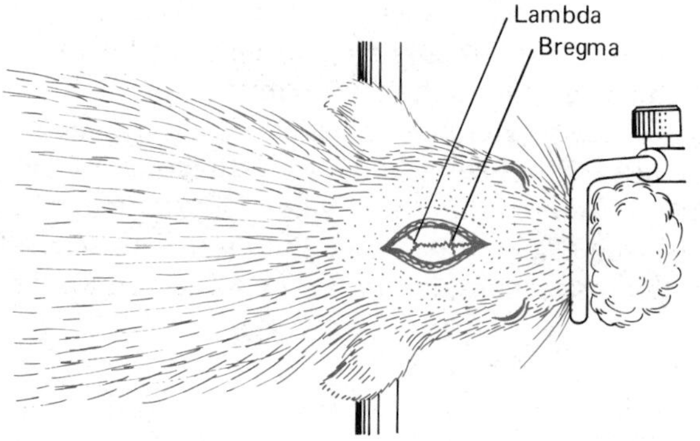

FIGURE I.8 An incision through the skin exposes the skull, and the sutures (places where bone comes together) are readily identifiable. Bregma is the one closest to the animal's eyes, while lambda is further back. These are used in setting the stereotaxic instrument for the individual animal. (Adapted from Skinner, 1971.)

skull are used for setting the instrument (see Figure I.8). Once the instrument is set (or "zeroed"), the brain can be exposed and the electrode can then be implanted in the desired region using the stereotaxic coordinates from the atlas.

Recording Gross Electrical Potentials

In the late 1800s, Caton recorded the electrical activity of the exposed cortex of animals, and in so doing broke with the earlier tradition that had mainly used recording techniques to study peripheral nerves and muscle (Cooper, 1971), as Helmholtz had done. The real breakthrough, however, was in the 1930s when Berger discovered that scalp recordings were a valid index of cortical activity. This discovery made it possible to study the electrical activity of the brain without exposing the brain. Berger termed his scalp recording technique electroencephalography, which is today commonly referred to as the EEG technique.

The EEG technique uses macroelectrodes (as opposed to the small microelectrodes described earlier) that are pasted onto the scalp of the subject (see Figure I.9) and connected to a recorder. What the electrode

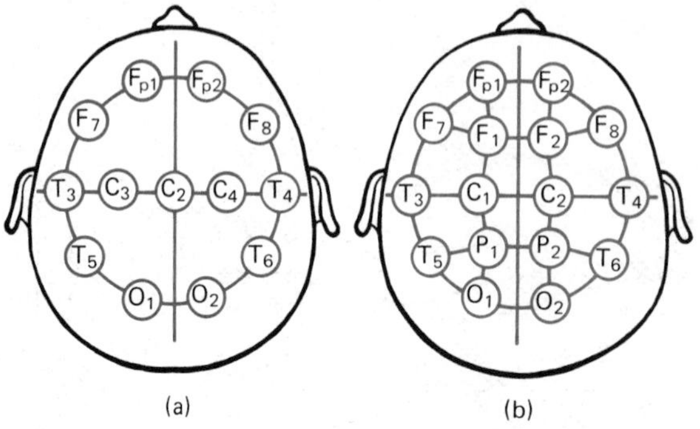

FIGURE I.9 Electrode placement for scalp recording of EEG. (Adapted from Cooper et al., 1974.) In (a) the vertex (C_2) acts as ground and the tracing records the local unipolar activity near each point. In (b) the tracing records bipolar activity between two adjacent points.

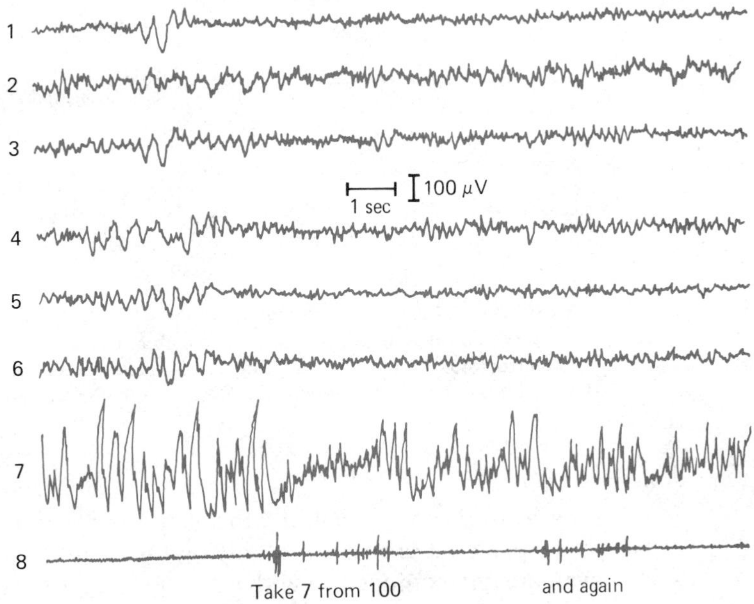

FIGURE I.10 A typical record of an EEG recording.

picks up is the average of the activity of all the central nerve cells directly below the electrode (Cooper et al., 1974). The EEG machine amplifies this activity, measures the voltage differences between pairs of electrodes, and generates a chart that depicts the activity in terms of waves of varying cycles per second (see Figure I.10). In general, the EEG has been found to measure four types of waveforms (differing in their range of cycles per second), each associated with a different state of alertness, as described in Chapter 12.

In addition to being useful in measuring various psychological states, the EEG is one of the clinical tools used to help determine if an abnormality in brain functions is present. Changes in both the amplitude and frequency of the expected electrical activity may signal the presence of a possible blood clot, tumor, or other lesion in the brain. When a patient is in a coma, the EEG pattern is exceptionally slow. The EEG is most often employed in the evaluation of convulsive disorders such as epilepsy (Figure I.11). A state of electrical hyperexcitability present in epilepsy produces a focal spike and slow wave pattern that is recorded in the EEG. However, the EEG is not always reliable or consistent. Often, lesions of different origins may produce similar electrical abnormalities. Occasionally, abnormalities in the EEG do not show up, while in fact, gross lesions of the brain are present (Steegmann, 1970). For these rea-

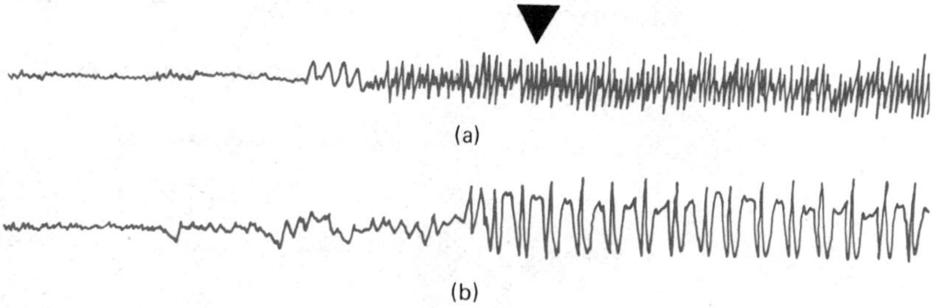

FIGURE I.11 (a) An EEG representing a tonic-clonic seizure, in a 9-year-old boy. The point at which the epileptic seizure became apparent on a behavioral level is indicated by the arrow. (b) An EEG representing a petit mal seizure, which is associated with staring, blinking, and brief losses of consciousness. (From Gardner, 1975.)

sons, as well as the variability that can occur in the EEG due to age, states of sleep, etc., it is best not to rely on the results of the EEG alone, but to evaluate it in conjunction with other neurological tests.

A special and currently popular use of EEG technology involves the evoked potentials technique. This technique is so called because an external stimulus is used to "evoke" a reaction in the brain. Scalp macroelectrodes or implanted macroelectrodes can be used to measure evoked responses. Because the amplitude (size) of the evoked response on the scalp is so small, the presence of unrelated background brain activity makes recording difficult (Cooper et al., 1974). One way of overcoming this problem is to present the response-evoking stimulus repeatedly and record many evoked responses. Then the average evoked response is computed. One especially useful application of the evoked potentials technique is in clinically diagnosing whether there is damage along the pathway from the sensory receptor to the cortex.

Microelectrode Recording

Microelectrode recording is a refined outgrowth of gross recording techniques and involves the use of small electrodes that are implanted either permanently or temporarily in nervous tissue. These electrodes, like the electrodes used in stimulation studies, are insulated, except for an exposed tip.

The use of micro recording electrodes is generally called the "single-unit" technique. Because these electrodes are so small, they are able to register the activity of a single unit (single nerve fiber or cell body). This technique has been used extensively in brain science and has made possible many of the important discoveries discussed throughout this book.

Experimental Lesions

The lesions (or tissue destruction) approach dates back to Flourens, whose carefully executed studies played an important role in the experimental verification of the brain as the organ of the mind. Flourens's lesion studies of brain function led him to speculate that the nervous system has a unity because in addition to the "action propre" of each part of the system there is also an "action commune," and removal of any one part reduces the efficiency of the entire system (Boring, 1950). The cerebral cortex, according to Flourens, functions as a whole, with its "action propre" being the maintenance of higher mental functions. Thus, while it was possible to localize motor and sensory areas in the cortex, Flourens felt that volition, learning, memory, and the like defied localization. His position was largely supported by Lashley's studies in the 1920s.

Lashley's experiments on rats led him to the conclusion that cognitive capacity depends upon the amount of cortical tissue available for processing and is independent of what tissue is available. Thus, Lashley believed that lesion size, not lesion locus, was the critical variable. Lashley identified two principles of brain function: mass action (brain capacity depends on the mass of cortical tissue available) and equipotentiality (all cortical areas are equally capable of mediating higher cognitive functions). Recent lesion studies have led to a rejection of Lashley's major points.

The surgical approach used by Lashley and those before him was the ablation approach. The animal's brain is exposed and the desired amount of tissue is either aspirated (suctioned) or dissected out. While this approach is still used today in studies of cortical function, experiments involving subcortical structures generally employ stereotaxic surgery. An atlas is used to identify the coordinates of the desired area, and the electrode is stereotaxically lowered to the proper position. The current is then turned on for a specified amount of time and the lesion is made (see Figure I.12). Because of the source of the current, such lesions are called electrolytic.

Another lesion approach is the leukotomy. A leukotomy involves the

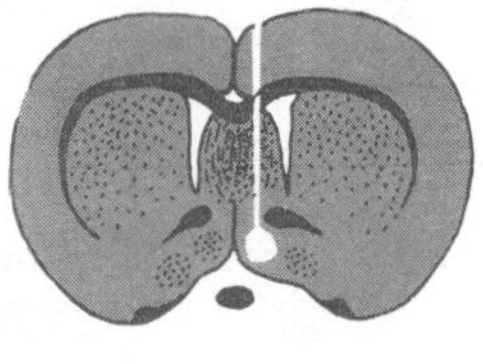

FIGURE I.12 An electrolytic lesion actually burns out an area of the brain. The hole in this section through a rat brain is of course the lesion site.

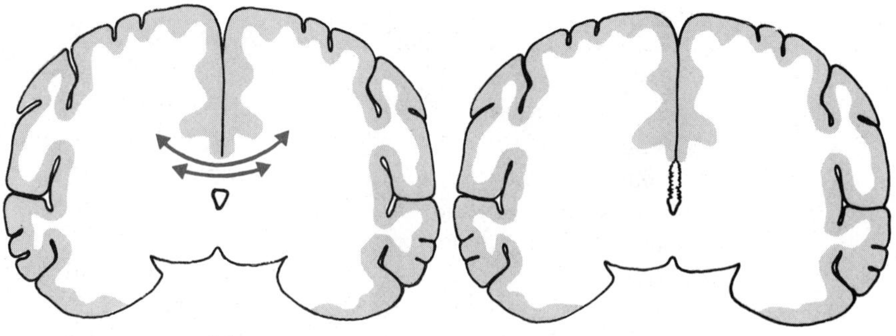

FIGURE I.13 Split-brain surgery. In part (a), the major interhemispheric pathways of the corpus callosum are intact. In (b), however, these pathways have been severed.

cutting of fiber connections (white matter), as opposed to lesioning or aspirating the nerve cells (gray matter). A special type of leukotomy that has received much attention in recent years involves sectioning of the fiber connections between the two halves of the brain. An organism having undergone such an operation is said to have a "split brain" (see Figure I.13). The behavioral consequences of split-brain surgery in both animals and man are examined in several of the last chapters.

The Clinical Approach

The clinical approach is in many respects the human lesion approach. Patients with lesions due to more or less natural causes (stroke, tumor, and the like) are the typical subjects of clinical studies. However, patients undergoing brain surgery are also frequently examined.

The clinical approach originated with the observations of Broca, a nineteenth-century neurologist. Broca observed a patient who had lost the capacity to speak, but who had no apparent damage to the vocal cords or the related musculature. Broca had the opportunity to examine the patient's brain at autopsy, and he observed an infarct (lesion due to a vascular dysfunction) at the base of the frontal lobe of the left hemisphere. This region is now called Broca's area and is believed to be the cortical representation of speech production. Subsequent investigations of brain-damaged patients by Hughlings Jackson, Carl Wernicke, Hugo Leipmann, Kurt Golstein, and other neurologists in the late 1800s and the early twentieth century led to a basic understanding of cortical organization in man. Today, the clinical approach is beginning to be recognized as one of the most powerful ways of coming to grips with the relation between brain mechanisms and psychological processes, and we shall examine some of the contributions of the early neurologists, as well as the wealth of data that have surfaced in the past few years.

The effectiveness of the clinical approach as a source of information about brain function is of course limited by the preciseness with which the locus of the damage can be identified. Fortunately, clinicians today do not have to wait around for an autopsy in order to have some indication of the lesion locus. As described earlier, the EEG technique is useful in pinpointing lesions by signifying areas of abnormal electrical activity. Another diagnostic technique involves radioisotope brain scans.

Radioisotope Brain Scans

This technique is often used to aid in the localization of brain tumors. This procedure has a relatively high degree of accuracy while posing little hazard to the patient.

A radioisotope tracer substance is injected intravenously, and after a certain amount of time has passed, a scintillation scanning procedure is carried out. X-ray films are used to show which structures in the brain take up large concentrations of the radioactive substance. Areas of the brain that are free from damage or normal possess an intact blood-brain barrier that prevents the uptake of the trace element. Tumors or lesions of the brain often cause damage to the blood-brain barrier, which then allows the radioisotope to pass through to the damaged tissue (Figure I.14).

The blood-brain barrier is comprised of capillary walls in conjunction with membranous material and processes from astrocyte cells (Figure I.15). These structures form a protective layer around the various parts of the central nervous system. An intact blood-brain barrier regulates the

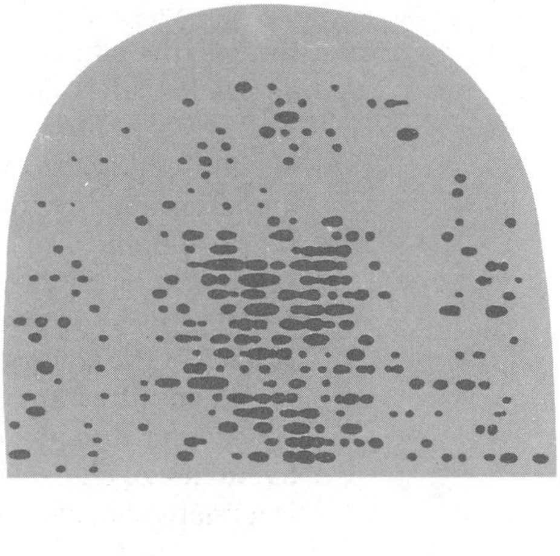

FIGURE I.14 Brain scan indicating the presence of a tumor of the corpus callosum and nearby areas of the hemispheres. The heavy concentration of the radioactive isotope reveals the location of the tumor. (From Elliott, 1964.)

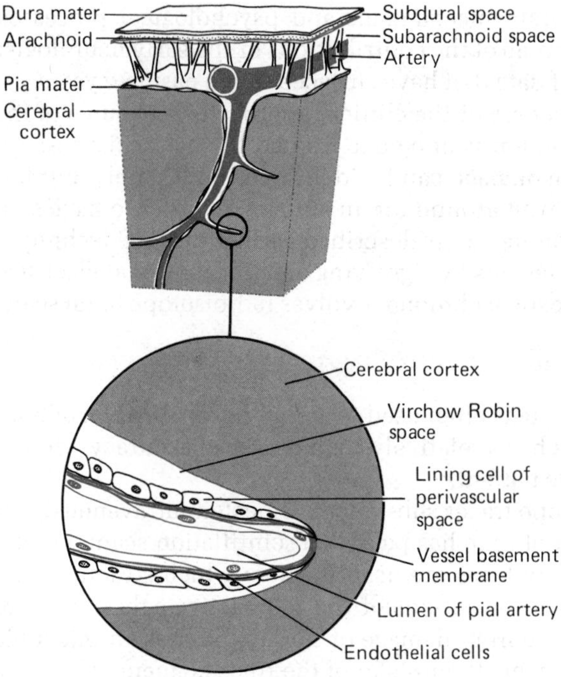

FIGURE I.15 A visual representation of the blood-brain barrier. As the vessel enters the substance of the cerebral cortex, now at the level observed by the electron microscope, the blood vessel wall is lined. (From Truex and Carpenter, 1969.)

passage of chemicals between arterial blood and the brain cells. Normally, the blood-brain barrier allows substances necessary for the health of the neurons to pass through, while it prevents the passage of toxic substances, as well as certain dyes and radioactive isotopes (Truex and Carpenter, 1969).

Pneumoencephalography and Ventriculography

The ventricular system is a system of cavities or canals running through the brain. Normally filled with cerebral spinal fluid, the cerebral ventricles can be injected with air, either through burr holes made in the skull (ventriculography) or through lumbar puncture (pneumoencephalography). When the ventricles are filled with air, x-rays of the skull are taken and ventricles appear as dark outlined areas on the film. If a tumor, hemorrhage, or other lesion is present in the ventricular system, the ventricles will appear displaced in the region of damage. Also, if cerebral atrophy is present, large collections of air can be observed in the sulci over the convex regions of the hemispheres.

When intracranial pressure is normal and either cerebral atrophy or ventricular tumors are suspected, pneumoencephalography may be the technique of choice. Under conditions of normal intracranial pressure, it is a relatively safe procedure although it is somewhat painful to the patient. Ventriculography might be a slightly more dangerous procedure because it can produce a rapid increase in intracranial pressure. However, in patients whose intracranial pressure is already raised, ventriculography is safer than pneumoencephalography and it also results in better pictures of the ventricular system (Steegmann, 1970).

Angiography

The last of the diagnostic neurological procedures to be mentioned is angiography. This test helps determine whether or not damage to the blood vessels in the brain has occurred. An appropriate contrast medium is injected into either the carotid, vertebral, subclavian, brachial, or femoral artery. This causes the blood vessels of the brain and spinal cord to appear radiopaque on x-ray films. A picture of the brain's entire vascular system results, and occluded blood vessels (caused by a stroke) or blood vessels that are displaced by tumors are revealed. Although angiography is a useful diagnostic tool, it is a dangerous procedure that poses the risk of possible neurological damage and, in some cases, even death.

The diagnostic procedures outlined above can be utilized to determine the type of neurological damage present in a particular patient. Each procedure is useful in providing information about specific types or regions of damage and each procedure also has some associated disadvantages. The advantages and disadvantages of each technique should be evaluated by trained neurologists who can decide on the best diagnostic procedures for each individual patient.

References

Boring, E. G. 1950. *A History of Experimental Psychology.* Englewood Cliffs, N.J.: Prentice-Hall.

Cooper, R. 1971. Recording changes in electrical properties in the brain: The EEG. In: R. D. Myers, ed. *Methods in Psychobiology.* Vol. 1. New York: Academic Press, pp. 156–206.

Cooper, R., J. W. Osselton, and J. C. Shaw. 1974. *EEG Technology.* London: Butterworth.

Elliott, F. A. *Clinical Neurology.* Philadelphia: Saunders.

Gardner, E. 1975. *Fundamentals of Neurology: A Psychophysiological Approach.* Philadelphia: Saunders.

Hart, B. 1969. *Experimental Neuropsychology: A Laboratory Manual.* San Francisco: Freeman.

Hess, W. R. 1954. *Diencephalon: Autonomic and Extrapyramidal Functions.* Monograph in Biology and Medicine, Vol. III. New York: Grune & Stratton.

Olds, J., and P. Milner. 1954. Positive reinforcement produced by electrical stimulation of septal area and other regions of rat brain. *J. Comp. Physiol. Psychol.* 47:419–427.

Skinner, J. E. 1971. *Neuroscience: A Laboratory Manual.* Philadelphia: Saunders.

Steegmann, A. T. 1970. *Examination of the Nervous System: A Student's Guide.* Chicago: Year Book Medical Publishers.

Truex, R. C., and M. B. Carpenter. 1969. *Human Neuroanatomy.* Baltimore: Williams & Wilkins.

APPENDIX II

Behavior Disorders and Neurological Disease

Disturbances of Motor Behavior

An apraxic disturbance is characterized by the patient's inability to perform familiar motor tasks in the absence of sensory loss, rigidity, involuntary movement, intellectual impairment, or weakness and uncoordination. In learning a particular sequence of motor behavior, it is necessary that visual, proprioceptive, and tactile memories be intact and that these various memories come together to control the specific movements necessary for the task at hand. Through observations of patients with localized brain damage, it has been suggested that these memories are stored in the parietal lobe of the dominant hemisphere, which seems to play the most important part in apraxia (Critchley, 1953; McFie and Zangwill, 1960; Brain, 1941). The dominant parietal lobe maintains a certain amount of control over the contralateral motor cortex through pathways in the corpus callosum.

Several specific types of apraxia have been observed in different patients. When a patient is unable to carry out a desired task and is not even capable of determining how to go about carrying out the task, the patient is said to exhibit ideational apraxia. This type of apraxia may occur when damage to both parietal lobes is present. In cases where the parietal lobe connections to motor and premotor cortex are not intact, ideokinetic apraxia results. In this case, the patient also is aware of making mistakes but cannot seem to prevent them. Ideokinetic apraxia is often characterized by the patient's ability to perform certain movements spontaneously while being unable to perform these same movements on command.

We mentioned in Chapter 7 that what has been labeled expressive aphasia may be a special case of apraxia. Patients with expressive aphasia know what they want to say and can understand what is being said to them, but they cannot carry out the appropriate expressive motor response. Here again, the patients recognize their mistakes.

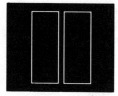

Another language disorder, which is a motor disorder as well, is dysgraphia. Dysgraphia is an inability to write even though the patient knows what to do and can recognize mistakes. It may be caused by a lesion in the premotor area of the dominant hemisphere. Dysgraphia may also be present as a result of lesions further back in the parietal lobe. In this case the patient cannot recognize letters (a form of agnosia) and this causes the difficulty in writing and the lack of recognition for mistakes.

Two other specific varieties of apraxia are often mentioned: dressing apraxia and constructional apraxia. Both of these seem to occur when the parietal lobe of the nondominant hemisphere is damaged. In dressing apraxia, patients can name their garments properly but put them on backwards or on the wrong parts of their bodies. Constructional apraxia signifies an inability in copying patterns with building blocks or match sticks, as well as an inability in copying drawings. Sometimes defects in writing such as lines intersecting each other, or being placed on top of one another, occur in patients with constructional apraxia. These patients often do not realize their mistakes (McFie and Zangwill, 1960).

The various types of apraxia mentioned in this section are associated with damage to the parietal lobes or the premotor, or the prefrontal zones of the frontal lobes.

At least partially responsible for several disturbances of both language and motor behavior are deficits related to memory. One of these memory disorders, auditory agnosia, was already described earlier in Chapter 7 under the label of receptive aphasia. We turn now to a description of additional forms of agnosia, as well as other types of memory disorders.

Disturbances of Memory

In general, agnosia refers to a failure to recognize familiar sensory patterns. The disruption seems to be related to the memory process while the primary sensory capabilities remain intact.

Tactile agnosia is described as a failure to recognize familiar objects through touch and can result from lesions of the postcentral gyrus. Damage to this cortical area interferes with the tactile memories that have been acquired and stored over the years.

In the visual realm, an area neighboring the primary visual cortex is involved in the ability to recognize (through memory) objects visually. If this area is destroyed, our visual memories of objects are also destroyed, and this results in the clinical disorder known as visual agnosia. The patient is capable of physically seeing an object, but can no longer recognize it visually when called upon to do so.

In a similar fashion, the storage site for auditory memories is adjacent to the primary auditory area (Heschl's gyrus), which is the center for hearing in the brain. In turn, olfactory, kinesthetic, and tactile memories are stored in regions of the brain that neighbor the respective primary sensory areas. To summarize, the cortical areas adjacent to the primary cortical centers for touch, vision, audition, and olfaction act as storage areas for memories acquired in each respective modality.

Regions concerned with sensory memories occur in both halves of the brain. For example, there is a storage region for visual memories in the same area of both the right and left hemispheres. Since these sensory memories are stored bilaterally, if damage is only unilateral, only slight impairment of these memory capacities will occur. On the other hand, if damage to a particular sensory region occurs bilaterally, a severe impairment in the functioning of memories within that specific sensory modality will result.

An exception to this bilaterality of sensory memories seems to be those memories associated with the written or spoken symbols of speech. These memories are often unilaterally represented in the dominant hemisphere. Unilateral lesions of the dominant hemisphere can, in this case, cause severe language deficits.

Intoxications and diseases that produce more diffuse rather than localized damage also may cause disturbances of recognition. These difficulties in recognition of familiar faces and objects contribute to the mental and behavioral confusions that many patients exhibit in the presence of diffuse cerebral damage or intoxications.

Korsakoff's syndrome is associated with these types of memory defects. It may occur in alcoholic patients and is considered a nutritional disorder of alcoholism, since it is associated with a thiamine deficiency. Less frequently, Korsakoff's syndrome may result from a subarachnoid hemorrhage, meningitis, or head injury. Autopsies of alcoholic patients with Korsakoff's syndrome usually reveal lesions in the mammillary bodies and the fornix, both in the hypothalamus, and the medial nucleus of the thalamus. It is believed that the memory defect is most closely associated with the thalamic lesions.

Patients with Korsakoff's syndrome exhibit difficulties or defects of memory for recent events. Often such patients are unable to remember things that happened only a few minutes before. They also have difficulty recognizing familiar faces and environments. As one might suspect, this results in a great deal of confusion for the patients, and they will often make up detailed stories to fill the memory gaps. These fictitious accounts of past events are termed confabulation and sometimes can be very convincing to the listener. Some of the confabulations are not entirely untrue, but simply describe events that occurred at a different time from the time of the story being recounted. It is interesting to note that confabulation usually occurs in patients with Korsakoff's syndrome, while it usually does not occur in patients with other types of amnesic disorders. Other amnesic patients will generally state that they do not remember certain events and they do not try to fill the gaps in their memory with fictitious accounts of past events. The basis for the occurrence of confabulation in Korsakoff's patients is still unknown.

Aside from the disturbances in the formation and retention of memories, impairments of perception and concept formation are also present. In the more severe cases, a combination of these symptoms can cause severe disturbances of mood and behavior. Complete recovery occurs in only a small portion of patients. Since this disorder is usually associated with a severe thiamine deficiency, treatment usually consists of the administration of thiamine, nicotinamide, and other components of the vitamin B complex.

Another type of memory disturbance can result from bilateral damage to the hippocampus (Rose and Symonds, 1960; Victor et al., 1961). In these cases, patients are not capable of remembering events in their personal lives that occurred months or sometimes years before their illness. These patients may not remember what kind of work they did, whether or not they are married, or even where they live. This type of amnesic disorder is distinctly different from the agnosias. Unlike the agnosics, patients with bilateral hippocampal damage are capable of recognizing various sensory stimuli; they can recognize familiar objects they see or hear; they can recognize what they feel or smell. The memory loss seems to be specific to personal events in the patient's life and understandably causes the patient to lack a sense of personal identity.

A disturbance that is more accurately described as a disorder of attention rather than a disturbance of memory is what is known as the "parietal lobe syndrome."

Disturbances of Attention

Patients with right parietal lobe damage who are presented with stimuli to their right and left sides simultaneously will not attend to the stimuli impinging on their left side. Often the patients will even ignore the left side of their own bodies. This may result in some rather bizarre behavior. For example, a male patient might shave only the right half of his face; he might not use his left leg or arm (which sometimes gives the false impression of paralysis); he might even try to dress only the right side of his body. However, if the patient's attention is brought to the specific stimuli appearing on his left, he is capable of recognizing them. In this way, this disorder differs from agnosia.

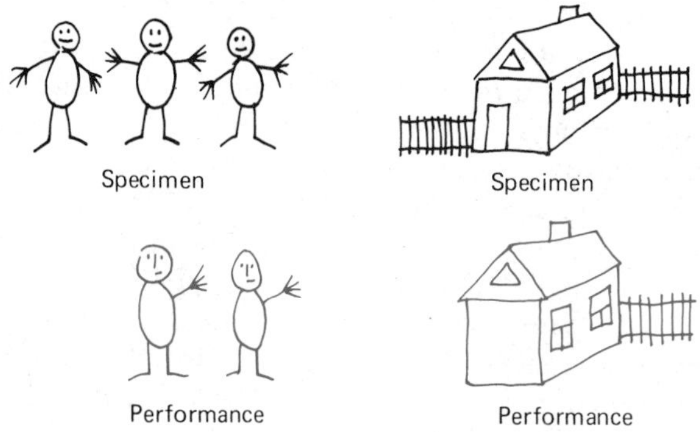

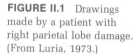

FIGURE II.1 Drawings made by a patient with right parietal lobe damage. (From Luria, 1973.)

The patient exhibits an inattention to almost anything that takes place in the left half of external space, and will ignore objects and even people who appear left of the midline. These patients often exhibit difficulties in reading, which stem from their lack of attention to the printed material on the left half of the page. When the patient is asked to draw an object, the right half will be well drawn, while the left half will be poorly represented or left out entirely (Figure II.1). Often the patient will write only on the right half of the paper. This "inattention" to stimuli in the left half of external space is thought to result from a form of perceptual rivalry between the hemispheres (Hecaen, 1969).

Having thus far described some of the disturbances of language, motor behavior, and memory and attention, we feel it is important to mention some of the research pertaining to a childhood disorder that may contain elements of each.

Minimal Brain Dysfunction

A childhood disorder that seems to be receiving an increasing amount of research attention is the syndrome known as minimal brain dysfunction (MBD). The term MBD is not clearly defined and is often used interchangeably with the term "hyperkinetic syndrome." For purposes of this appendix, the two terms will be used in reference to the same symptom cluster.

Hyperkinesis is a label used by professionals who are most interested in observable behavior without reference to the etiology of the disorder. On the other hand, MBD is the term used by professionals who believe the disorder has a biological or organic etiology because of the soft neurological signs that are often observed in these children.

For a child who is 7 or 8 years old, examples of a few "soft signs" would be clumsiness in fine motor coordination tasks (tying shoelaces or buttoning clothes), finger agnosia, pupillary inequalities, mixed laterality, and disturbances of right-left discrimination. The problem with weighing these "soft signs" too heavily in diagnosis is that the normal acquisition of skills such as finger recognition and tying shoelaces occurs over a wide range of time, making it difficult to decide when an abnormality is truly present.

Lacking a precise definition, the hyperkinetic syndrome has been described as consisting of the symptom cluster of motor restlessness, impulsivity, short attention span, learning difficulties (particularly involving learning to read), and emotional instability. The syndrome may occur alone or in conjunction with other psychiatric or neurological diseases. The prevalence of this disorder (occurring alone—not with other neurological diseases) has been reported between 4 and 20 percent for children in the general school-age population. Most researchers report an incidence of MBD in 5 to 10 percent of all school-age children.

This disorder is not selective in that children from both rural and urban areas, from different economic backgrounds, living in the United States or in Europe seem to be afflicted equally. Some sex differences, however, have been observed. The number of boys with MBD or hyperkinesis has been reported as much higher than the number of girls with the disorder. Figures range from four times as many boys as girls to nine times as many boys as girls affected with MBD (O'Malley, 1976).

The problem with determining whether or not a child has MBD stems from the vagueness of the so-called defining characteristics. When a child scores within the normal range on various psychological tests, and there is no known neurological damage, but the child exhibits several learning disabilities, is highly distractible, and in general seems to be performing on a much lower level than his age peers, the term MBD is often applied. At the present time, MBD seems to be a "catch-all" category. Further research will probably reveal that what is presently called MBD, or the hyperkinetic syndrome, is in fact a cluster of several different, although perhaps related, disorders.

A few of the more promising areas of research in this field are those studies seeking to delineate some of the electrophysiological, genetic, and biochemical correlates of MBD.

The most common clinical EEG abnormality found in children with MBD is an excessive amount of slow wave (generally theta) activity. This slow wave activity is commonly found in younger normal children. This evidence is, therefore, consistent with the hypothesis of a delayed CNS maturation in these children.

In a blindly rated study of the EEGs of 106 MBD children and their normal controls, Capute et al. (1968) found that 43 percent of the MBD children had mild to moderate EEG abnormalities. Again, the abnormality most often found was the presence of more slow waves than expected for that age. Only 17 percent of the control children exhibited any mild or moderate EEG abnormalities, thus lending even more support for Satterfield et al.'s (1973) hypothesis.

Recently there has been growing interest in a possible genetic basis for MBD or hyperactivity. Cantwell (1972) evaluated the parents of 50 hyperactive children and 50 matched controls on a psychiatric exam. Most of the control group parents were free from any psychiatric illness, whereas almost half of the parents of the hyperactive children had received some psychiatric diagnosis. Fathers rather than mothers tended to be ill more often. A greater prevalence of alcoholism, sociopathy, and hysteria was found in the parents of the hyperactive children. Eight out of the 50 fathers of the hyperactive children were thought to have been hyperactive themselves as children, while only one of the fathers of the normal children was thought to be hyperactive as a child. Two of the 50 mothers of the hyperactive children were hyperactive as children, whereas none of the control mothers were. On the basis of the above study, however, it is impossible to determine whether the hyperkinetic syndrome is genetically or environmentally transmitted.

Morrison and Stewart (1973) conducted an adoption study where they found that the hyperactive child syndrome was prevalent to a much larger degree in the biological (first and second degree) relatives of hyperactive children than in relatives of the adopted children. The incidence of the syndrome in adopting relatives was not significantly different from that found in relatives of the control group. Both the adoptive and biological parents would have an effect in passing on the disorder if it were environmentally transmitted, but only the biological parents could pass it on if it were genetically determined. Therefore, the results of Morrison and Stewart's (1973) study lend support to the genetic transmission hypothesis.

Further support for the genetic hypothesis comes from the work of Safer (1973). Safer studied the full and half siblings of 17 MBD index cases. The results showed that 10 out of 19 full siblings were thought to exhibit symptoms of MBD while only 2 out of 22 half siblings exhibited the symptoms.

Another line of research that may prove fruitful in solving the puzzle of MBD is the research seeking to determine whether biochemical differences exist between MBD and normal children. Paul Wender (1971), in his book *MBD in Children*, suggests that children with MBD show an abnormality in metabolism of the monoamines: serotonin, noradrenaline, or dopamine. Wender believes the syndrome may be at least partly due to a decreased reactivity of the monoamines in children with MBD. He points to some inferential evidence from animal studies that show that brain levels of serotonin and noradrenaline increase with age. In humans some of the symptoms of MBD, such as hyperactivity, generally decrease with age. Therefore, if a similar pattern of results is found for humans as for animals, that is to say, if monoamine levels are observed to increase with age, this would lend support tn Wender's hypothesis. Wender also cites a study in which the androgen testosterone was administered to rats and an increase in their monoamine activity occurred. To generalize these results to the human sphere, it is known that at puberty there is an increase in androgenic activity. If this human androgenic activity in turn causes an increase in monoamine activity, as it does in rats, this would help explain the decrease in some MBD symptoms that is often observed at puberty.

Looking at levels of serotonin in the blood, Coleman (1971) found a low blood concentration of serotonin in 88 percent of the 25 hyperactive children she studied (aged 4 to 12), who had no known organic or EEG abnormalities. It is still unclear whether Coleman's finding supports Wender's hypothesis, since the relationship of blood serotonin levels to brain serotonin levels is not well understood.

The final sections of this appendix contain a brief discussion of epilepsy and introduce some of the intriguing research on "split-brain" phenomena. What has come to be called "split-brain" research in humans resulted from the study of patients with intractable epilepsy who underwent neurosurgery to control their seizure activity.

Epilepsy

Epileptic seizures result from uncontrolled electrical discharges produced from scar tissue in the brain. The scar tissue may have resulted from disease or trauma and may be present at birth or occur later in life (Milner, 1970). Whether or not seizures occur depends to a large extent on the site of the disease or trauma. Certain regions of the brain have lower seizure thresholds than others. The temporal lobe, especially in the area of the hippocampus, has a lower seizure threshold than the frontal or parieto-occipital regions. Also, lesions in the gray matter are more prone to producing epileptic activity than are lesions in the white matter.

A genetic component to epilepsy has been noted by several researchers (Lennox, 1947; Metrakos and Metrakos, 1961; Lilienfeld and Pasamanick, 1954; Bray and Weiser, 1964). Lennox (1947) found a history of epilepsy in 2.7 percent of 12,119 blood relatives of 2130 epileptic patients. Although this percentage does not seem very large, it was in fact five times as large as the amount of epilepsy found in the general population during that year. Studying patients with centrencephalic (petit mal) epilepsy, Metrakos and Metrakos (1961) found that 13 percent of the patients' parents as well as 13 percent of the siblings were affected with the disorder.

Bray and Weiser (1964), in studying patients with focal or temporal lobe epilepsy, found results similar to those of Metrakos and Metrakos (1961) for patients with centrencephalic epilepsy. Bray and Weiser (1964) found diffuse EEG abnormalities in almost half of the close relatives of epileptic patients. Both groups of investigators found that the closer the relative, the higher the incidence of seizures or abnormal EEGs. To put this hereditary component of epilepsy in perspective, if one parent has epilepsy, there is a 29 out of 30 chance that the child will be normal, and if no seizures have occurred by the time the child is 4, the chances increase to 39 out of 40 for remaining seizure-free. If two epileptics have a child, the chances of the child's being epileptic are increased.

Lilienfeld and Pasamanick (1954) were interested in determining

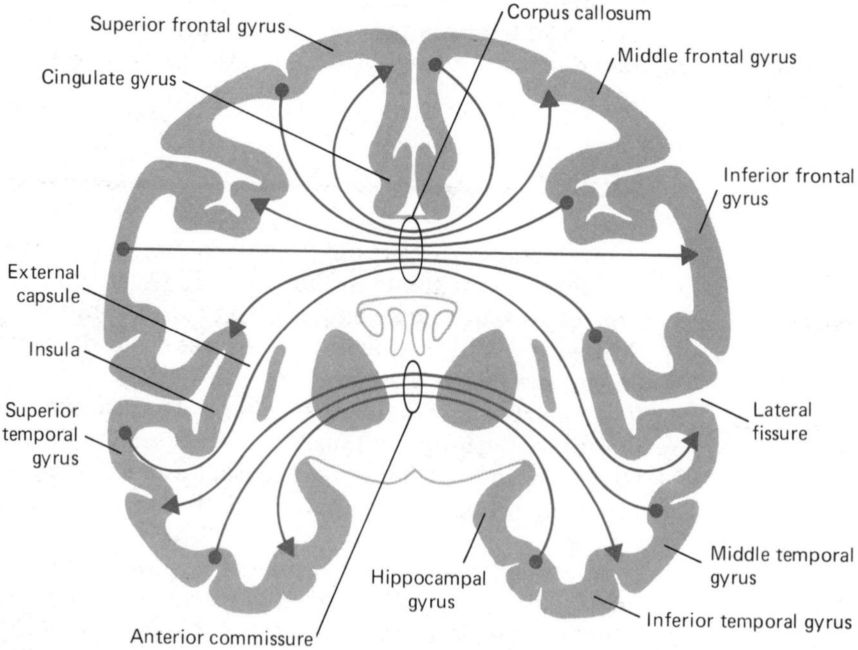

FIGURE II.2 A coronal section of the brain at the level of the anterior commissure. This drawing indicates possible anatomical pathways by which an epileptic seizure may spread from one hemisphere to the other. (From Crosby et al., 1962.)

what role acquired brain damage played for an individual who was genetically predisposed for epilepsy. By reviewing perinatal records of epileptic children and their siblings, they found an increased number of pregnancy and birth complications, as well as problems in the neonatal development of the epileptic children compared to their nonaffected siblings.

For cases of extremely severe epilepsy, where medication does not seem to relieve the seizure activity, a surgical technique has been developed that helps to control the epilepsy. This technique involves the sectioning of the corpus callosum, the major fiber tract connecting the two halves of the brain, and sometimes sectioning the anterior and hippocampal commissures, as well as the massa intermedia (see Figure II.2). This type of surgery was performed for the first time in the late 1930s on a few patients in order to prevent the spread of epileptic seizures from one hemisphere to the other.

While the effectiveness of the surgery was questioned by some, others believed that split-brain surgery should work to control epilepsy. So, in the 1960s, another series of patients was started (Bogen and Vogel, 1963). Although the medical value of the surgery is still debated today, these patients have provided the opportunity for psychological studies of a type never before possible. In the following, we shall examine some of the results and ideas that emerged out of these studies.

The Split Brain

Basic Observations

Following brain bisection, split-brain patients seem normal in most aspects of daily life. Their temperament, personality, and general intelligence are largely unaffected by the surgery. However, by using tests especially designed for the purpose, it is possible to elicit some striking and dramatic phenomena (Gazzaniga, 1970). For example, as described in Chapter 7, if a person's gaze is fixed on a central point on a screen, all information appearing to the right of the fixation point is directed to the left hemisphere and all information to the left of fixation goes to the right hemisphere (see Figure II.3).

In the normal person, the forebrain commissures (corpus callosum, anterior commissure) allow sensory input lateralized to one hemisphere to reach the other half-brain as well. In the split-brain patient, however, the commissures are no longer available, so information lateralized to one hemisphere remains there. Thus, if a picture of a spoon is presented to the left hemisphere, the patient can, using the right hand, find the ob-

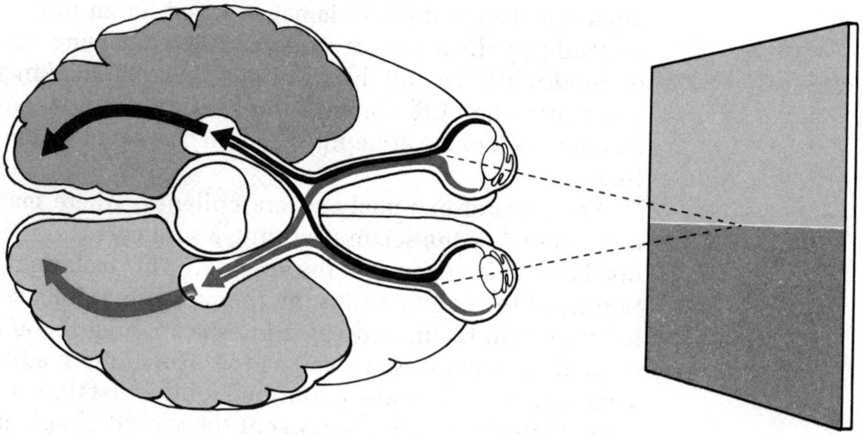

FIGURE II.3 The projection of the visual fields. Because the optic chiasm has been split, visual input can be lateralized. If the person's gaze is fixed on a center point, then information presented in the left visual field goes only to the right hemisphere, and vice versa.

ject in a group of several objects. However, the patient will have difficulty if required to find the object with the left hand after left hemisphere exposure.

Hemisphere Specialization

The right hemisphere, while lacking verbal sophistication, has proved to be superior on certain tasks, such as drawing and copying figures, arranging blocks to form geometric designs, and performing discriminations involving complex tactual patterns (Bogen and Gazzaniga, 1965; LeDoux et al., 1978; Milner and Taylor, 1972). In general, what is more striking is the fact that following the lateralized presentation of a visual or tactile stimulus to the left hemisphere, the patient is usually able to describe the information verbally. This is so because the speech and language mechanisms are usually in the left hemisphere. So, if a stimulus is presented to the left visual field or placed in the left hand, the right hemisphere gets the critical information, which is not available to the left half-brain for verbal identification. The right hemisphere excels on tasks requiring spatial skills. This observation led some to suggest that while the left hemisphere of humans is evolutionarily specialized for verbal processing, the right is specialized for spatial processing (Levy, 1974). This implies that in the course of human evolution, something new happened in each half-brain. It has recently been argued that the hemisphere differences can all be explained by evolutionary changes in the left hemisphere (LeDoux et al., 1977). If, in acquiring language, the left hemisphere sacrificed some of its spatial abilities, then there would be no need to suggest right hemisphere specialization. In other words, according to this theory, the right hemisphere advantage in spatial tasks is attributable to left hemisphere inefficiency rather than right hemisphere superiority. While this point is unimportant from the point of view of identifying hemisphere differences in humans, it is important in understanding brain evolution. As it turns out, the spatial processing region in both hemispheres of nonhuman primates and in the right hemisphere of humans is a region important in language processing in the human left hemisphere. This observation supports the idea that the superior spatial skills of the right hemisphere arose as a by-product of the fact that the left hemisphere lost its spatial skills in acquiring language in the course of human brain evolution.

References

Bogen, J. E., and M. S. Gazzaniga. 1965. Cerebral commissurotomy in man: Minor hemisphere dominance for certain visuo-spatial functions. *J. Neurol.* 23:394–99.

Bogen, J. E., and P. J. Vogel. 1963. Treatment of generalized seizures by cerebral commissurotomy. *Surgical Form* 14:431.

Brain, R. 1941. Visual disorientation with special reference to the lesions of the right cerebral hemisphere. *Brain* 64:244–272.

Bray, P. F., and W. C. Weiser. 1964. Evidence for a genetic etiology of temporal central abnormalities in focal epilepsy. *New Eng. J. Med.* 271:926.

Cantwell, D. P. 1972. Psychiatric illness in the families of hyperactive children. *Arch. Gen. Psychiat.* 27:414–417.

Capute, A. J., E. F. L. Neidermayer, and F. Richardson. 1968. The electroencephalogram in children with minimal cerebral dysfunction. *Pediatrics* 41:1104.

Coleman, M. 1971. Serotonin concentrations in whole blood of hyperactive children. *J. Pediatrics* 78:985–990.

Critchley, M. 1953. *The Parietal Lobe.* London: Edward Arnold.

Crosby, E. C., T. Humphrey, and E. W. Lauer. 1962. *Correlative Anatomy of the Nervous System.* New York: Macmillan.

Gazzaniga, M. S. 1970. *The Bisected Brain.* Englewood Cliffs, N.J.: Prentice-Hall.

Hecaen, H. 1969. Aphasic, apraxic, and agnostic syndromes in right and left hemisphere lesions. In: P. J. Vinken and G. W. Bruyn, eds. *Handbook of Clinical Neurology.* Amsterdam: North Holland Vol. 4.

LeDoux, J. E., D. H. Wilson, and M. S. Gazzaniga. 1978. Manipulo-spatial aspects of cerebral lateralization. *Neuropsychologia* 15:743–758.

Lennox, W. G. 1947. The genetics of epilepsy. *Amer. J. Psychiat.* 103:459.

Levy, J. 1974. Psychobiological implications of bilateral asymmetry. In: S. J. Dimond and J. G. Beaumont, eds. *Hemisphere Function in the Human Brain.* New York: Halsted Press.

Lilienfeld, A. M., and B. Pasamanick. 1954. Associations of maternal and fetal factors with the development of epilepsy. *J. Amer. Med. Assoc.* 155:719.

Luria, A. R. 1973. *The Working Brain.* New York: Basic Books.

McFie, J., and O. L. Zangwill. 1960. Constructional praxia. *Brain* 83:243.

Metrakos, K., and J. D. Metrakos. 1961. Genetics of convulsive disorders II. Genetic and encephalographic studies in centrencaphalic epilepsy. *Neurology* 11:474.
Milner, B., and L. Taylor. 1972. Right hemisphere superiority in tactile pattern recognition after cerebral commissurotomy: Evidence for nonverbal memory. *Neuropsychologia 1972*:10.
Milner, P. M. 1970. *Physiological Psychology*. New York: Holt, Rinehart and Winston.
Morrison, J., and M. Stewart. 1973. Evidence for polygenetic inheritance in the hyperactive child syndrome. *Amer. J. Psychiat.* 130:791–792.
O'Malley, J. E. 1976. The hyperkinetic syndrome revisited: Myths and mayhem. In: D. V. Sivasankar, ed. *Mental Health in Children.* Vol. II. pp. 303–317.
Rose, S. P., and C. P. Symonds. 1960. Persistent memory defect following encephalitis. *Brain* 83:195.
Safer, D. A. 1973. A familial factor in minimal brain dysfunction. *Behav. Genetics* 3: 175–187.
Satterfield, J. H., L. I. Lesser, R. E. Saul, and D. P. Cantwell. 1973. EEG aspects in the diagnosis and treatment of minimal brain dysfunction. *Ann. N. Y. Acad. Sci.* 205:274–282.
Victor, M., J. B. Angevine, E. L. Mancall, and C. M. Fischer. 1961. Memory loss with lesions of the hippocampal formation. *Arch. Neurol.* 5:244.
Wender, P. 1971. *Minimal Brain Dysfunction in Children.* New York: Wiley.

Index

T

79 80 81 82 9 8 7 6 5 4 3 2 1